AF832576

# TOPICS IN RENAL BIOPSY AND PATHOLOGY

Edited by **Muhammed Mubarak** and **Javed I. Kazi**

**Topics in Renal Biopsy and Pathology**
Edited by Muhammed Mubarak and Javed I. Kazi

**Published by InTech**
Janeza Trdine 9, 51000 Rijeka, Croatia

**Copyright © 2012 InTech**
All chapters are distributed under the Creative Commons Attribution 3.0 license, which allows users to download, copy and build upon published articles even for commercial purposes, as long as the author and publisher are properly credited, which ensures maximum dissemination and a wider impact of our publications. After this work has been published by InTech, authors have the right to republish it, in whole or part, in any publication of which they are the author, and to make other personal use of the work. Any republication, referencing or personal use of the work must explicitly identify the original source.

As for readers, this license allows users to download, copy and build upon published chapters even for commercial purposes, as long as the author and publisher are properly credited, which ensures maximum dissemination and a wider impact of our publications.

**Notice**
Statements and opinions expressed in the chapters are these of the individual contributors and not necessarily those of the editors or publisher. No responsibility is accepted for the accuracy of information contained in the published chapters. The publisher assumes no responsibility for any damage or injury to persons or property arising out of the use of any materials, instructions, methods or ideas contained in the book.

**Publishing Process Manager** Adriana Pecar

**Technical Editor** Teodora Smiljanic

**Cover Designe**r InTech Design Team

Additional hard copies can be obtained from orders@intechopen.com

Topics in Renal Biopsy and Pathology, Edited by Muhammed Mubarak and Javed I. Kazi
p. cm.
ISBN 978-953-51-0477-3

# We are IntechOpen, the world's leading publisher of Open Access books

## Built by scientists, for scientists

**4,000+**
Open access books available

**116,000+**
International authors and editors

**120M+**
Downloads

**151**
Countries delivered to

Our authors are among the
**Top 1%**
most cited scientists

**12.2%**
Contributors from top 500 universities

WEB OF SCIENCE™

Selection of our books indexed in the Book Citation Index in Web of Science™ Core Collection (BKCI)

Interested in publishing with us?
Contact book.department@intechopen.com

Numbers displayed above are based on latest data collected.
For more information visit www.intechopen.com

For EU product safety concerns:
IN TECH d.o.o., Prolaz Marije Krucifikse Kozulić 3, 51000 Rijeka, Croatia,
info@intechopen.com or visit our website at intechopen.com.

# Meet the editors

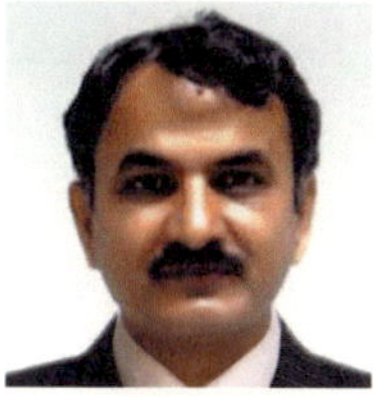

Dr Muhammed Mubarak is currently working as Associate Professor and Consultant Histopathologist at Sindh Institute of Urology and Transplantation (SIUT), Karachi, Pakistan. He graduated from Liaquat Medical College, Pakistan, and later completed his postgraduate training in clinical pathology and histopathology at Hammersmith Hospital, London, SIUT, and PNS Shifa Hospital, Karachi. He has authored, together with Prof. Kazi, more than 65 papers in local and international peer-reviewed journals, including those describing the pattern of renal biopsy pathology in Pakistan for the first time. He is a member of the editorial board and reviewer of many local and international medical journals. He is a member of many professional organizations such as Transplant Society of Pakistan, Renal Pathology Society, and Country Representative of European Nephropathology Working Group. He has participated in many national and international conferences on pathology, renal pathology, and transplantation. His areas of special interest include renal and transplant pathology, uropathology, and gastrointestinal pathology.

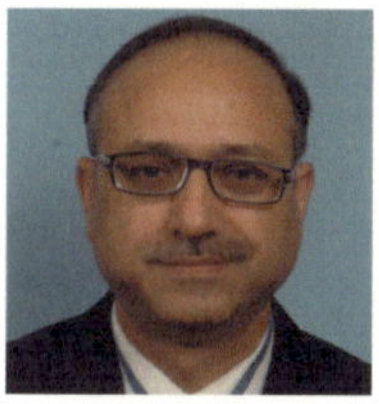

Dr Javed I. Kazi is Professor and Chairman of Pathology at the Karachi Medical and Dental College and Abbasi Shaheed Hospital, Karachi, and Consultant Histopathologist, Sindh Institute of Urology and Transplantation (SIUT). He is a Dow graduate and has trained extensively both in Pakistan and abroad, including the National University of Singapore, Addenbrook's Hospital, Cambridge, and Leicester General Hospital, where he, in collaboration with Professor Peter Furness, developed an artificial neural network for the diagnosis of early graft rejection. Professor Kazi established the department of Histopathology, including the Electron Microscopy Unit at the SIUT in 1995. Since then, he has been involved in promoting renal and transplant pathology in Pakistan.

# Contents

# Preface

We the editors, Drs. M. Mubarak and Javed I. Kazi, dedicate this book to our mentor, Professor Adeeb Rizvi, for his untiring efforts in creating a state of the art treatment facility in nephrology, urology, and transplantation, completely free for the poorest of the poor people of the third world, and having faith in us for establishing and running the renal and transplant pathology services at the SIUT.

Richard Glassock has written so vividly in his foreword to a related book in nephrology by the InTech open access publishers entitled "An update on glomerulopathies-Clinical and treatment aspects" that "The study of the fundamental and clinical aspects of glomerular disease has expanded exponentially over the last several decades." Undoubtedly, the major contribution to this exponential expansion of the knowledge of the kidney diseases has come from the systematic study of the renal biopsies. Renal biopsy is an important diagnostic and prognostic procedure that is widely used in the nephrology practice throughout the world these days. Percutaneous renal biopsy is the method of choice for the tissue diagnosis of the medical disorders of kidney, but a number of other approaches are also used in selected cases. Its indications are well established, but in practice vary considerably from center to center. In fact, as alluded to in the beginning of this preface, the systematic study of renal biopsy has revolutionized the understanding of renal pathology during the early phases of the disease evolution. Prior to the widespread use of percutaneous renal biopsy, the study of renal diseases was limited to the autopsy material, which revealed the advanced changes of end-stage renal disease with often no clue about the primary pathologic process. Moreover, renal biopsy also provided a useful raw material for the widespread application of two new techniques of pathological study, i.e., the Immunohistochemistry and the electron microscopic study in the 1960s and early 1970s. At the same time, the procedure is invasive and not entirely without risks. The later, however, have been dramatically reduced with the modern techniques available to the renal physician during the performance of renal biopsy. After procurement of renal tissue, its proper handling and processing require the highest standard of laboratory practice for an accurate pathological evaluation of the obtained material. The pathologic evaluation of renal biopsy is an integrated process, which requires not only an experienced pathologist but also input from the immunology, serology, immunoflourescene, and electron microscopy studies, and the nephrologists to arrive at a correct diagnosis.

There is no dearth of high-quality books on renal biopsy and pathology in the market. These are either single author or multi-author books, written by world authorities in their respective areas, mostly from the developed world. The vast scholarly potential of authors in the developing countries remains underutilized. Most of the books share the classical monotony of the topics or subjects covered in the book. The current book is a unique adventure in that it bears a truly international outlook and incorporates a variety of topics, which make the book a very interesting project. The authors of the present book hail not only from the developed world, but also many developing countries. The authors belong not only to US but also to Europe as well as to Pakistan and Japan. The scientific content of the book is equally varied, spanning the spectrum of technical issues of biopsy procurement, to pathological examination, to individual disease entities, renal graft pathology, pathophysiology of renal disorders, to practice guidelines.

The book has fourteen chapters that have conveniently been divided into five sections to encompass the variety of topics.

Section one of the book has three chapters which describe the historical background and the methodology of renal biopsy procedure, its indications, procurement, complications, and handling of the tissue after biopsy procurement in detail. Renal biopsy in children is also being increasingly used throughout the world and there is a full chapter devoted to renal biopsy procedure in the pediatric population. A report describing an interesting alternative to the renal biopsy for the diagnosis of kidney disease, i.e., skin biopsy, has also been included in section one of the book.

Section two has two chapters, one of which describes the post-biopsy handling and processing of the procured renal biopsy tissue for an optimal pathological evaluation. It also describes the normal microstructure of the kidney parenchyma to serve as a foundation for subsequent chapter on the pathological interpretation of the renal biopsy material. The later chapter describes an elegant algorithmic approach to the systematic study of renal biopsy tissue by the pathologists.

Section three has four chapters; one chapter each devoted to recent updates on different aspects of some common medical disorders of the kidney which are at the forefront of renal research at present. These include; collapsing focal segmental glomerulosclerosis, IgA nephropathy, IgM nephropathy, and thin glomerular basement membrane disease.

Section four contains one chapter, which describes in detail the pathological approach to the systematic evaluation of renal allograft pathology. The chapter is also supported by high quality images, which will facilitate a clear understanding of the increasingly complicated topic of transplant pathology.

The final section describes the pathophysiology of renal diseases. It includes; acute kidney injury complicating neoplasms, acute renal cortical necrosis, an update on chronic kidney disease, and an approach to the diagnosis of acid-base disorders. All these chapters are exhaustive reviews of the relevant topics and may be viewed as reference sources.

Despite the diverse origin of the authors, nearly all chapters are written in a coherent style and many are well illustrated with both schematic and original photomicrographs to help the readers comprehend the complex kidney topics covered in this book.

The book will prove useful for postgraduate students and consultants in nephrology, transplantation, and renal pathology.

**Dr. Muhammed Mubarak**
Associate Professor & Consultant Histopathologist
Sindh Institute of Urology and Transplantation
Dow Medical University Karachi
Pakistan

Co-editor
**Dr Javed I. Kazi**
Professor of Pathology, Karachi Medical and Dental College, Karachi
Consultant Histopathologist
Sindh Institute of Urology and Transplantation
Dow Medical University Karachi
Pakistan

# Part 1

## Biopsy Methods

# 1

# Percutaneous Renal Biopsy

Louis-Philippe Laurin, Alain Bonnardeaux,
Michel Dubé and Martine Leblanc
*University of Montreal*
*Canada*

## 1. Introduction

Renal biopsy is an essential tool for the diagnosis of several renal diseases. The first renal biopsies were performed in 1923 as open surgical procedures (Gwyn, 1923). The percutaneous approach has been part of the clinical practice since 1951 (Iversen & Brun, 1951). A few years later, a description of the procedure with the patient placed in a prone position was published (Kark & Muehrcke, 1954). The new technique had a success rate of more than 90% and was not associated with major complications. Percutaneous ultrasound-guided renal biopsy is now considered as the standard method. It is a routine procedure that can be done with minimal discomfort to the patient. Here we review major topics related to this frequent and useful procedure in the field of nephrology.

## 2. Indications

Although indications for renal biopsy can sometimes be a matter of debate among nephrologists, common indications include: isolated hematuria, mild to moderate proteinuria, nephrotic syndrome, glomerulonephritis, acute renal failure, renal manifestations of systemic diseases and chronic renal failure (Table 1). There is also an important role for percutaneous kidney biopsy in kidney transplantation. Percutaneous kidney biopsy is not only reserved for the diagnosis of renal parenchymal diseases, but it may also have a role in the diagnosis of renal tumor as described below in this chapter.
Impacts of diagnosis made by kidney biopsy have to take into account considerations beyond therapeutic implications. A kidney disease diagnosis within the patient's records could have psychological and financial consequences (e.g. insurances), and can modify family planning decisions (e.g. hereditary renal diseases) (Korbet, 2002). Performing a percutaneous kidney biopsy therefore implies a good communication between the attending physician and his patient.

## 3. Contraindications

In 1988, the Health and Public Policy Committee of American College of Physicians (ACP) elaborated a list of contraindications to kidney biopsy (ACP, 1988). As described below, the relevance of this policy may be actually questioned upon recent technological developments resulting in a virtual absence of catastrophic complications in recent series (Waldo et al., 2009).

### 3.1 Absolute contraindications

Several contraindications to renal biopsy have been described (Madaio, 1990). Absolute contraindications are generally recognized as uncontrolled bleeding diathesis, anatomic abnormalities, uncooperative behaviour and pregnancy (Table 1). Chronic renal disease associated with two small kidneys with cortical atrophy remains a contraindication to renal biopsy, since the bleeding risk is high, but can be considered relative if performed by a well-experienced operator. Absence of an appropriate pathologic support makes no sense to perform a biopsy and should therefore be considered as a contraindication (Korbet, 2002). Single functioning kidney is not considered as an absolute contraindication anymore because of technical and real-time imaging improvements over the last decades. As stated in a report of nine cases of normal size solitary kidney biopsy, it can be performed with good outcomes in terms of bleeding and renal function (Mendelssohn & Cole, 1995). In this series, the only complication reported was post-procedure gross hematuria in one patient. Histopathological diagnosis was made in eight of nine cases.

One can argue that an uncooperative patient is no longer an absolute contraindication in particular circumstances. Intensive care unit patients on mechanical ventilation appear to tolerate well bedside biopsy with appropriate administration of sedative agents (Conlon et al., 1995). The procedure is performed off ventilator with ventilation controlled with an ambu bag, permitting a perfect synchronization between respiratory movements and needle insertion, thereby minimizing risks of complications.

### 3.2 Relative contraindications

Relative contraindications consist in conditions that may be reversed, sometimes relatively easily; these include uncontrolled hypertension or hypotension, renal abscesses, pyelonephritis, hydronephrosis, marked obesity, severe anemia, previous technical failure, uremia, anatomic abnormalities of kidney such as large renal tumors, arterial aneurysm and cysts (Table 1) (Madaio, 1990). Correction of these medical conditions with antihypertensive medication, antibiotics or blood transfusions makes possible the biopsy to be carried out safely.

## 4. Preparation

First, the patient's past medical history information should be reviewed before the biopsy. Personal and family history of bleeding diathesis, and allergy to substances used during the procedure such as povidone-iodine should be evaluated. Second, a thorough physical examination should be undertaken to look for skin infection as well as anatomic anomalies (e.g. obesity) that could interfere with the procedure. An assessment of blood pressure control is also essential.

A pre-biopsy laboratory evaluation is also made routinely and includes complete biochemical profile, complete blood count and urinalysis. Baseline coagulation parameters, including platelet count, prothrombin time, partial thromboplastin time and fibrinogen, are usually documented before biopsy procedure. Bleeding time is also commonly analyzed prior to the biopsy, but its role to predict post-biopsy bleeding remains controversial; it will be discussed in detail later in this chapter. Stopping all the medications that could disrupt normal coagulation should normally prevent post-procedural bleeding. Antiplatelet agents and non-steroidal anti-inflammatory drugs have to be withdrawn prior to the procedure for at least seven days. Performing a renal biopsy in patients on anticoagulation therapy is

always a medical challenge. Decision to stop the anticoagulants before the biopsy should be based on the patient's thromboembolism risks. If the decision is made to do the biopsy, an anticoagulation bridge with intravenous anticoagulation (e.g. heparin) is needed in most cases.
A good preparation is an essential step to minimize the risk of bleeding complications as well as to intervene promptly in case of an adverse event.

| Indications | Contraindications |
|---|---|
| Isolated hematuria | **Relative** |
| Mild to moderate proteinuria | Uncontrolled hypertension |
| Nephrotic syndrome | Hypotension |
| Nephritic syndrome | Renal abscesses |
| Glomerulonephritis suspicion | Pyelonephritis |
| Renal manifestations of systemic diseases | Hydronephrosis |
| | Marked obesity |
| Acute renal failure | Severe anemia |
| Chronic renal failure | Uremia |
| Renal tumor in selected patients | Large renal tumors or cysts |
| | Solitary kidney |
| | Previous technical failure |
| | Atrophic kidney(s) |
| | **Absolute** |
| | Bleeding diathesis |
| | Anatomic abnormalities |
| | Uncooperative behavior |
| | Pregnancy |

Table 1. Indications and contraindications of kidney biopsy

## 5. Procedure

As mentioned earlier, percutaneous renal biopsy under ultrasound guidance is now the gold standard method to obtain renal tissue for the diagnosis of renal diseases. It is generally considered superior to other techniques because of its numerous advantages: it allows continuous visualization of both kidney and needle, can be done regardless of the renal function, avoids exposure to radiation, permits procedure to be performed at bedside and avoids the administration of nephrotoxic contrast media (Korbet, 2002). Several other biopsy techniques exist, such as laparoscopic, computed tomography (CT)-guided and transjugular renal biopsy. Here, we will focus mainly on ultrasound-guided techniques.
An adequate tissue sample (Figure 1) permitting an accurate diagnosis of a glomerular disease with light microscopy usually contains 8 to 10 glomeruli. It must include juxtamedullary glomeruli due to their preferential involvement in focal segmental glomerulosclerosis. In these focal lesions, at least 25 glomeruli may be required to have greater than 95% chance of finding evidence of such renal injury (Fogo, 2003).
In 1988, the American College of Physicians (ACP) stated the minimal requirements (Table 2) that a nephrology fellow must acquire to perform percutaneous renal biopsy safely (ACP, 1988). It is interesting to note that in a recent survey among 133 nephrology trainees, 75.3%

of them reported that they had little or no training, or some training but not enough to feel competent in doing renal biopsy independently (Berns, 2010).

| **Skills** |
|---|
| **Cognitive skills** |
| Knowledge of: |
| Indications and contraindications |
| When to use open renal biopsy |
| Renal and surrounding anatomy |
| Technique to use and position of the biopsy needle |
| Examining and handling tissue for histologic processing |
| Complications and how to detect and treat them |
| Medications required for the procedure |
| Role of the biopsy in determining treatment |
| Alternatives to the procedure |
| Ability to: |
| Provide medical monitoring and intervention |
| Communicate the risks, benefits, and results to the patient for purposes of informed consent |
| **Technical skills** |
| Ability to: |
| Choose appropriate biopsy needle |
| Use appropriate techniques to localize the kidney |
| Appropriately place biopsy needle and obtain tissue |

Table 2. Skills related to percutaneous renal biopsy (from ACP, 1988)

The patient should provide an informed consent before the procedure. No oral intake is usually permitted after midnight on the day of the procedure, except for a light meal if the procedure is planned late in the morning or early in the afternoon. A well-trained nephrologist or radiologist at the radiology department, or at bedside if needed, usually performs the procedure. An intravenous access is placed to insure adequate hydration. Vital signs have to be monitored throughout the procedure.

Kidney biopsies are usually performed with the patient in prone position, after the skin is properly disinfected and draped. This position provides the most rational approach to a retroperitoneal organ. It also brings the kidney closer to the posterior abdominal wall. Local anesthesia is usually carried out with lidocaine. Tissue biopsies are acquired from the lower pole of the kidney, next to the renal capsule, with the left kidney usually preferred for ergonomic reasons. The operator must be aware that subcapsular cortical samples have overrepresentation of sclerosis related to hypertension, aging and non-specific scarring (Fogo, 2003). Samples are obtained when the patient is holding his breath. One or two needle passes are routinely performed.

Another approach, commonly used to perform liver biopsy, is the transjugular renal biopsy. This technique is usually performed in academic centers by well-trained interventional physicians (nephrologists or radiologists) and should be reserved for high-risk patients with contraindications to percutaneous renal biopsy such as liver disease, bleeding diathesis and obesity. The main disadvantage of this technique is lower diagnostic yield, mainly because medulla needs to be traversed first before reaching the renal cortex. A recent retrospective study showed a good safety and efficacy of transjugular renal biopsy in 23 high-risk patients (Sarabu et al., 2010). An adequate tissue for histopathological diagnosis was obtained in 87% of patients. Three patients (13%) experienced bleeding requiring blood transfusion. Neither deaths nor embolization/nephrectomy were reported.

A supine antero-lateral position (SALP) for percutaneous biopsy has been suggested recently (Gesualdo et al., 2008). It can be an interesting and useful alternative to the prone position for obese patients. This technique is also less invasive than a transjugular biopsy, and certainly provides a better diagnostic yield due to a direct access to the distal cortex. High-risk patients with a BMI >30 and/or respiratory difficulty underwent a SALP biopsy and were compared with low-risk (BMI ≤30 and/or no respiratory difficulty) patients receiving ultrasound-guided renal biopsy in either the prone position or SALP, for a total of 110 patients. There were a significantly better comfort compliance and less breathing difficulties for SALP patients. Post-procedure bleeding complications were minor in all three groups. The authors concluded that SALP may therefore be considered seriously for patients who otherwise would have been submitted to more invasive procedure.

### 5.1 Optimal depth

Pasquariello and colleagues (Pasquariello et al., 2007) published a novel approach to calculate the optimal depth needed to decrease significantly hemorrhagic complications, as well as tissue sample inadequacy. All 126 percutaneous native kidney biopsies, using a 14-gauge automated biopsy gun under sonographic guidance, were performed with optimal depth previously calculated. Adequacy rate of specimens for diagnosis and complication rate were compared with retrospective data obtained for 123 biopsies. Incidence of bleeding complications was significantly reduced using the theoretical calculation of optimal depth, together with an adequate sampling permitting an accurate diagnostic evaluation from renal tissue. Depth where pushing the trigger was calculated by a mathematical formula defined below (1).

$$\text{Optimal depth} = BW/H - 0.5 \quad (1)$$

BW represents the body weight expressed in hectograms and H the height expressed in centimeters.

### 5.2 Real-time versus blind ultrasound

Biopsy procedure can be performed under real-time or blind ultrasound-guided technique. Real-time method implies continuous visualization of the kidney for exact localization of the biopsy site (Figure 2). Blind method requires a sonographic localization of the kidney only before needle insertion. A proper needle placement is thereafter assessed by appropriate tissue resistance and observation of the respiratory excursion of the needle. A study by Maya and colleagues (Maya et al., 2007) showed that real-time ultrasound-guided technique provided a superior yield of kidney tissue and resulted in fewer bleeding complications. This retrospective study of 129 patients showed a higher mean number of glomeruli per biopsy in the sonographic-guided group compared to the blind biopsy group (18 ± 9 versus 11 ± 9), and fewer large hematomas requiring intervention (0% versus 11%).

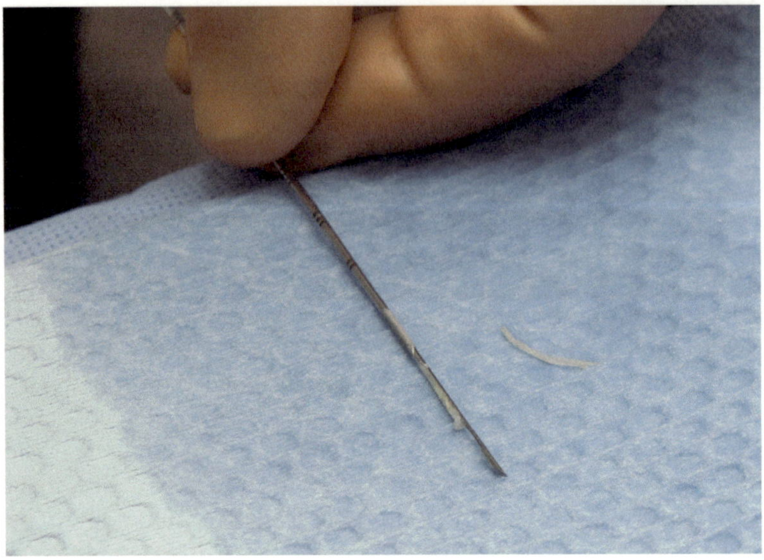

Fig. 1. Adequate tissue sampling

### 5.3 Outpatient observation versus hospitalization

The low occurrence rate of bleeding complications with percutaneous kidney biopsies performed under real-time ultrasound led to elective procedures in an outpatient setting using standardized protocols. Overnight hospitalization would not be therefore needed, reducing the overall cost of elective renal biopsies.

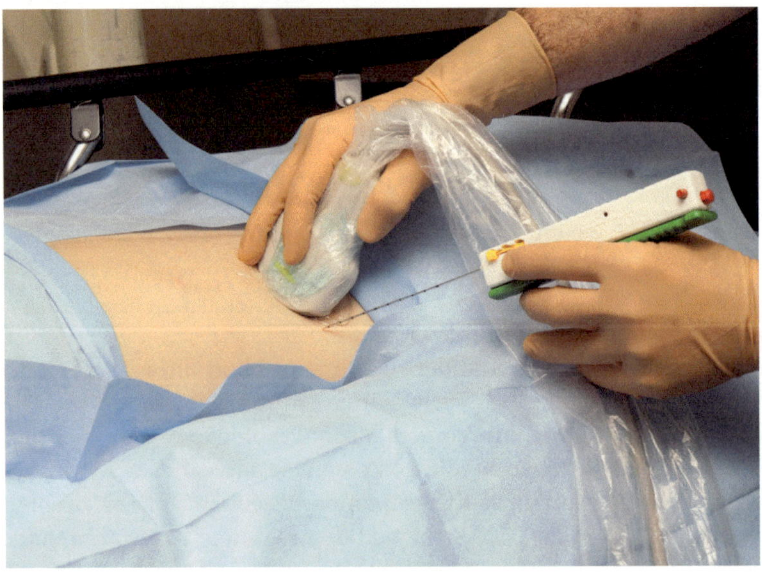

Fig. 2. Real-time ultrasound biopsy in prone position

A recent study by Maya and Allon (Maya & Allon, 2009) confirmed the safety and effectiveness of such an approach. During a 20-month period, 100 patients underwent a

percutaneous renal biopsy under real-time ultrasound guidance with a 16-gauge spring-loaded biopsy gun. A majority of patients (91%) required only one or two needle passes, reflecting the technical advantage of the real-time ultrasound guidance. A color Doppler ultrasound was performed immediately after the procedure to exclude active bleeding. In this series, no patient experienced serious complications related to the biopsy. Only four patients were hospitalized because of an >4% decrease in their hematocrit. Neither blood transfusion nor selective embolization was needed for these patients. Nonetheless, one can argue that such an approach should be reserved for highly selected patients who do not need urgent renal biopsy in the setting of acute kidney injury or bleeding disorders.
Common sense should therefore prevail regarding the decision to hospitalize or not a patient after biopsy. It is mainly an institution-based decision. At our hospital, we prefer to hospitalize all patients overnight after the biopsy.

## 6. Needle

Several types of needles have been used during medical history to perform percutaneous renal biopsy. In 1951, Iversen and Brun (Iversen & Brun, 1951) described a percutaneous native kidney biopsy technique using an aspiration needle. Later, Kark and Muehrcke (Kark & Muehrcke, 1954) published a technique whereby cutting needles were employed, such as the Franklin-Vim-Silverman and the Tru-Cut (Baxter, Deerfield, IL) needles. The automated biopsy-gun (Figure 3) became popular in the nineties based on its potential benefits in reducing bleeding complications, for shorter actual time the needle resides in the kidney, and the fact that it requires less dexterity by the operator (Madaio, 1990). A randomized prospective trial comparing the two methods showed adequate tissue sampling, but the extent of bleeding was more severe in the free-hand biopsy group (D. Kim et al., 1998).

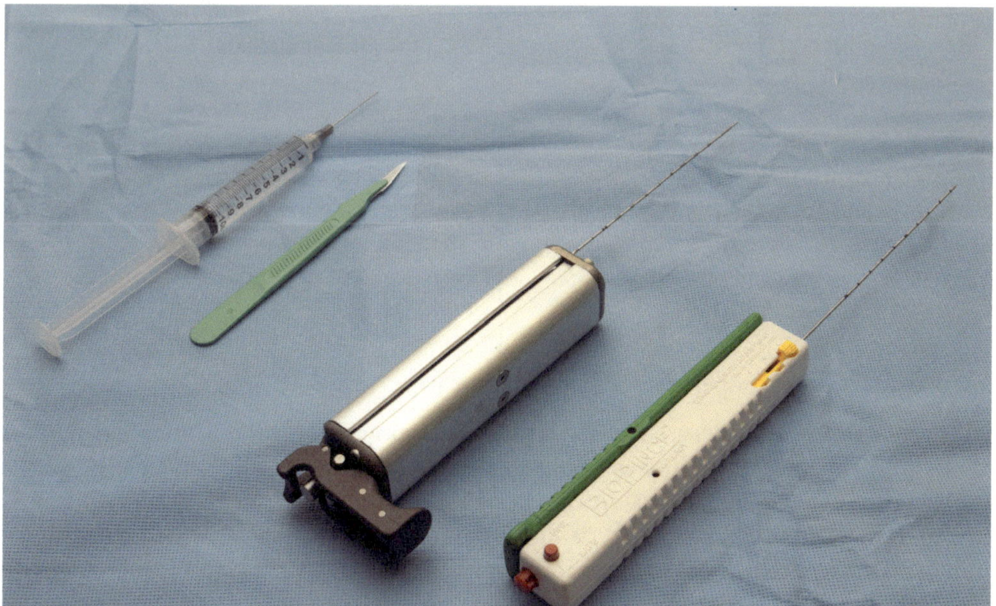

Fig. 3. Automated biopsy-gun

A number of different needle sizes are available for percutaneous biopsy techniques, ranging from 14 to 18 gauge (G). Needle gauge has a huge impact on the sample obtained. Eighteen- or 19-G needles are often unable to give a good specimen, and provide inadequate representation of vessels. In past years, there were concerns in the literature regarding bleeding risk with the use of larger needles. However, recent data (Tung et al., 1992; Song & Cronan, 1998; Nicholson et al., 2000; Manno et al., 2004) refuted such beliefs by showing that larger gauge needles provided better adequacy in tissue sampling and were not associated with higher complication rates. More specifically, a study (Nicholson et al., 2000) comparing 14, 16, and 18-G needles in renal transplants demonstrated an improved diagnostic value with increased needle size and no significant difference in macroscopic hematuria between the three groups. Nevertheless, the use of 14-G needle may create more pain. Overall, utilization of 16 G needle appears to be the best compromise between patient comfort and histopathological diagnostic yield.

## 7. Complications

Complications associated with percutaneous renal biopsy can be categorized as minor (gross hematuria and silent hematoma), major (hematoma requiring transfusion and/or embolization) or catastrophic (loss of functional mass and death) (Mendelssohn & Cole, 1995). Percutaneous renal biopsies using aspiration technique were associated with severe complications, mainly hemorrhage, with mortality rates of nearly 0.07% in large series reported in the fifties (Schwarz et al., 2005).

| Complications | Rate of occurrence |
|---|---|
| **Minor** | |
| Gross hematuria | 0 to 6% (Maya et al. 2009) |
| Silent hematoma | 33.3% (Manno et al. 2004) |
| **Major** | |
| Hematoma requiring transfusion and/or embolization | 1.2 % (Manno et al. 2004) |
| **Catastrophic** | |
| Loss of functional mass | 6 per 10 000 (Schow et al. 1992) |
| Death | 7 per 10 000 (Schow et al. 1992)<br>Close to zero (Mendelssohn et al. 1995) |

Table 3. Complications of percutaneous renal biopsy

Two main technical advances have resulted in safer procedures: the ultrasound guidance and the automated core biopsy system (automated biopsy-gun). Rates of serious complications were as low as <1% in recent series, with an overall risk of kidney function loss of 6 per 10 000 and a mortality risk of 7 per 10 000 (Schow et al., 1992). Nonetheless, complications more commonly reported are transient gross hematuria and hematoma with a frequency ranging between 0% to 6% (Maya & Allon, 2009). A literature review published in 1995 supports the opinion that the risk of catastrophic complications using the actual biopsy methods is close to zero (Mendelssohn & Cole, 1995). These differences observed in complication rates may result from patient selection, biopsy technique, needle gauge, operator experience and number of needle passes.

Despite the fact that percutaneous biopsy can be now considered as a procedure with almost no catastrophic complications if it is performed with standard techniques, it is always associated with minor complications that the attending physician must be aware of. There is obviously a transient damage to the collecting system and to the structures surrounding the kidney. This generates bleeding, creating symptoms such as hematuria and a drop in hemoglobin level (see below). Microscopic hematuria is normally seen in all patients who undergo a kidney biopsy (Altebarmakian et al., 1981), but is generally clinically insignificant and revolves spontaneously within 24 to 48 hours. On the other hand, macroscopic hematuria is seen less frequently, complicating up to 5 to 10% of patients (Marwah & Korbet, 1996). It is also generally clinically insignificant and self resolving in 48 hours. It can be severe, resulting in a significant loss of blood. It should also raise concerns for a concomitant hematoma or arteriovenous fistula, requiring further investigation and monitoring.

Normally, a fall in hemoglobin level is observed after a percutaneous renal biopsy, with a decrease ≥1 g/dL reported in 20.8% of patients in a recent Japanese study (Ishikawa et al., 2009). A perinephric hematoma of more than 2 cm was associated with a significantly greater decrease in Hg level in this study. This drop is usually caused by several factors including local bleeding at the biopsy site (e.g. hematoma, hematuria), hemodilution secondary to hydration with intravenous fluids, recumbency and stimulation of anti-diuretic hormone secretion by pain; and it is not a good predictor of post-biopsy outcome.

Subcapsular perinephric hematoma is certainly more common than previously noted in older retrospective studies where post-procedure sonography was not routinely performed. A recent series of patient showed that hematoma was seen in 33.3% of patients, with a mean surface area of 289.6 $mm^2$ (Manno et al., 2004). These hematomas were clinically silent in 90.4% of subjects, with 2.5% complaining of lumbar pain. It appears that there was no association between post-biopsy bleeding and the surface area of the hematoma. Another series reported hematomas in more than 86% of cases, and older studies using computerized tomography (CT) scanning also showed an incidence of 90%, depending on the timing of the evaluation. Furthermore, the clinician must be aware of an extremely rare complication that may be associated with a perinephric hematoma: the laceration of a lumbar artery passing over the lower pole of the kidney (K.T. Kim et al., 1991).

Arteriovenous fistulas are also clinically silent complications of percutaneous renal biopsy. Angiography-based imaging studies reported an incidence of about 10%. The majority (over 90%) resolved spontaneously a year later, requiring no invasive procedure. They rarely become a symptomatic aneurysm that causes high output cardiac failure, hypertension, hematuria and renal failure (by arterial steal). Due to the gravity of the potential complications related to arteriovenous fistulas, they should be monitored with Doppler ultrasound every 3 to 6 months (Korbet et al., 2002).

In summary, there are numerous complications related to percutaneous kidney biopsy ranging from silent hematomas to uncontrolled bleeding with hemorrhagic shock. Clinicians must therefore be aware of these adverse events and investigate rapidly patients who present signs of clinical deterioration. This argues for an overnight observation of the patient after the procedure, with adequate monitoring of his vital signs, degree of hematuria and abdominal pain.

### 7.1 Predictors of bleeding complications

Determining the predictors of bleeding complications related to percutaneous kidney biopsy has always been a matter of debate in the literature over the last decades, despite the fact that this procedure is routinely and frequently performed worldwide. There are scant prospective data regarding which baseline conditions (e.g. bleeding time, age) can affect significantly the outcomes. A recent Italian prospective study tried to answer this important question (Manno et al., 2004). The authors analyzed baseline characteristics and outcomes of 471 consecutive native kidney percutaneous ultrasound-guided biopsies. Univariate and multivariate analysis of predictors of post-biopsy bleeding complications demonstrated a strong association between post-procedure bleeding and female gender, higher baseline partial thromboplastin time and age, as bleeding tends to occur less in older patients. Surprisingly, no association was made between bleeding time and post-biopsy bleeding. Patients with complications had exactly the same bleeding time than patients without any complications, but all patients with abnormal bleeding time received 8-D-arginine vasopressin (DDAVP), showing afterwards a normalization of their bleeding time prior to biopsy. Only 11 patients had increased bleeding time prior to biopsy, two with moderate von Willebrand factor deficiency and nine with moderate renal failure. Moreover, there was also no impact of the histologic diagnosis on the occurrence of post-biopsy bleeding.

| Predictors of post-biopsy bleeding | Factors not associated with post-biopsy bleeding |
|---|---|
| **Manno et al. 2004** | **Manno et al. 2004** |
| Younger age | Blood pressure |
| Female gender | Body weight |
| Elevated partial thromboplastin time | Serum creatinine |
| **Ishikawa et al. 2009** | Proteinuria |
| Perirenal hematoma ≥2.0 cm assessed immediately after biopsy | Needle gauge |
| PT-INR ≥1 | **Waldo et al. 2009** |
| Mean blood pressure ≥105 mmHg | Absence of hematoma 1 h post-biopsy |
| Steroid use | **Ishikawa et al. 2009** |
| | Age |
| | Creatinine ≥2.0 mg/dL |

Table 4. Predictors of post-biopsy bleeding

A recent retrospective study of 317 patients tried to find predictors of overt bleeding after renal biopsy (Ishikawa et al., 2009). More than 86% of patient presented a perirenal hematoma after biopsy, a majority with a diameter of less than 2 cm. A hematoma ≥2 cm was associated with a greater decrease in hemoglobin levels. The authors determined by multivariate analysis the clinical predictors of bleeding (Hb decrease ≥1.0 g/dL). Perirenal hematoma, prothrombin time-international normalized ratio (PT-INR), mean blood pressure and steroid use were found to be related to overt bleeding (Table 4). Of these factors, perirenal hematoma ≥2cm immediately after the biopsy was the strongest predictor, with a risk of severe anemia increased to about eight times. Post-biopsy ultrasound may therefore be a useful tool to discriminate patients with the highest risk of bleeding complications. However, a recent investigation studying the presence of a hematoma 1 hour post-biopsy as a predictor of major complications was not conclusive (Waldo et al., 2009). The absence of hematoma was predictive of an uncomplicated post-biopsy evolution, with a negative predictive value of 95%.

### 7.2 Role of bleeding time in predicting bleeding complications

Utilization of bleeding time prior to the renal biopsy procedure remains controversial. Bleeding time is used frequently by nephrologists before biopsy, mainly for historical reasons, as a predictor of bleeding in spite of no clear evidence supporting its role.

On the one hand, a widespread consensus among hematologists supports the fact that it is not a useful predictor of the risk of hemorrhage after a surgical procedure, especially if there is absence of a clinical history of bleeding disorder. Bleeding time could indeed be altered in several conditions including technique variability related to the operator, drugs (e.g. beta-blockers, antibiotics) and various clinical states such as liver disorders and diabetes mellitus (Mattix & Singh, 1999). No study linking the bleeding risk of performing kidney biopsies with abnormal bleeding time has been published. Furthermore, an article describing the position of the College of American Pathologists and the American Society of Clinical Pathologists concluded that bleeding time can be a test useful for testing the response to DDAVP in uremic patients, but it is not a predictor of the bleeding risk in these patients (Peterson et al., 1998).

On the other hand, recent data has shown that prolongation of the bleeding time is not without risk. It was found that the risk of post-biopsy hematoma increased by 21 % for each minute of bleeding time prolongation, conferring a two times greater risk of bleeding in patients in which such a rise was seen (Stratta et al., 2007). More recent data demonstrated the same increased risk of major bleeding complications in patients with prolonged bleeding time (Waldo et al., 2009). Moreover, a prospective study of liver biopsies performed without correcting the bleeding time prior to the procedure showed five times higher bleeding complications (Boberg et al., 1999).

DDAVP seems to enhance the release of von Willebrand factor from endothelial cells into plasma. It also increases release of factor VII and adenosine triphosphate by platelets, as well as the uptake of serotonin. Studies have shown a normalization of the bleeding time by DDAVP infusion. Administration of this drug systematically regardless of bleeding time values appears to be cost-ineffective, considering that approximately 80% of patients had normal bleeding times, and it could be related to serious side effects such as hypertension and hyponatremia (Mattix & Singh, 1999; Korbet, 2002). However, a recent randomized controlled trial showed a significant advantage of a systematic DDAVP administration in patients without a significant renal impairment (Manno et al., 2011).

## 8. Role of percutaneous biopsy in renal tumors

Percutaneous renal biopsies also have a smaller role in the management of renal tumors in adults. Indeed, surgical resection permits a clear pathological diagnosis, as well as generally curing the patient from his/her malignancy. This is based on the fact that carcinomas represent 90% of all renal solid masses in adults when tumor size is greater than 40 mm on imaging studies (Lebret et al., 2007).

Nevertheless, partial or total nephrectomies can be spared for renal masses less than 40 mm in size. A study from a French group showed that renal biopsy prior to surgical resection of a renal mass should be reserved for patients in whom imaging was not able to make an accurate diagnosis (Lebret et al., 2007). It mainly consisted of equivocal lesions that lacked one or more radiological criteria for malignant lesions, or were less than 40 mm. In this single institution series of 432 patients, 119 percutaneous biopsies were performed in 101 patients. A diagnosis of benign lesions was made in 20% biopsies together with 9 malignant lesions not requiring surgery (lymphoma and metastasis) (Table 5). Thus, 30.4% of patients were not candidates for nephrectomy.

Performing such technique in patients with renal cancer is not without risk. In fact, biopsy tract seeding has been reported in 0.01% of cases in a large series (Smith, 1991, as cited in Lebret et al., 2007). This can be prevented by using coaxial system. In the series described above, no cancer seeding was reported, making percutaneous biopsy a safe procedure in the hands of well-experienced interventional physicians.

| Histological findings | % of lesions |
|---|---|
| **Malignant** | |
| Renal cell carcinoma | 59 |
| Transitional cell carcinoma | 48 |
| Metastasis | 3 |
| Lymphoma | 7 |
| **Benign** | <1 |
| Oncocytoma | 20 |
| Angiomyolipoma | 13 |
| Renal abscess/xanthogranulomatosus | 3 |
| pyelonephritis | 4 |
| **Inconclusive** | 21 |
| Normal parenchyma | 10 |
| Necrotic tissue | <1 |
| Inflammatory tissue | 10 |

Table 5. Histological findings in renal masses (from Lebret et al. 2007)

Despite the fact that surgical resection remains the standard approach for patients with renal tumors, percutaneous biopsy could also be an alternative for particular cases. Fine needle aspiration of a renal mass can also be reserved for patients who would not be able to tolerate surgery, mainly elderly patients, and those with comorbid conditions.

## 9. Conclusion

Ultrasound-guided percutaneous renal biopsy is a safe procedure with a central role in the diagnosis of parenchymal kidney diseases. Real-time ultrasonography and automated biopsy-gun are the major technical improvements permitting the procedure to be performed with safety and effectiveness. It is accomplished in a hospital setting by well-trained radiologist or nephrologist. With recent technical advances, bleeding complications are quite rare, allowing a shorter observation period (6 to 8 hours) after the procedure in highly selected elective patients.

Areas of uncertainty however still exist. Predictors of bleeding complications are difficult to define clearly. Age, female gender and elevated prothrombin time seem to correlate with an increased risk of post-biopsy bleeding. Ultrasound undertaken immediately after the biopsy procedure can be helpful to determine if the patient is at a risk of bleeding and should be observed for longer period. The role of bleeding time remains controversial to predict overt bleeding mainly due to the fact that no prospective data are available to guide the clinical practice.

Randomized controlled trials would therefore be needed to evaluate certain important questions mainly related to post-procedure bleeding. As approximately 1 to 2 million bleeding time tests are performed annually, it would be interesting to clarify its usefulness as a predictor of post-biopsy bleeding.

## 10. Acknowledgements

We wish to thank the staff of the Hôpital Maisonneuve-Rosemont radiology department.

## 11. References

Altebarmakian, V. K. et al. (1981). Percutaneous kidney biopsies. Complications and their management. *Urology*, Vol. 18, No. 2, (August 1981), pp. 118-22, ISSN 0090-4295

American College of Physicians. (1988). Clinical competence in percutaneous renal biopsy. Health and Public Policy Committee. *Ann Intern Med*, Vol. 108, No. 2, (February 1988), pp. 301-3, ISSN 0003-4819

Berns, J. S. (2010). A survey-based evaluation of self-perceived competency after nephrology fellowship training. *Clin J Am Soc Nephrol*, Vol. 5, No. 3, (March 2010), pp. 490-6, ISSN 1555-905X

Boberg, K. M. et al. (1999). Is a prolonged bleeding time associated with an increased risk of hemorrhage after liver biopsy? *Thromb Haemost*, Vol. 81, No. 3, (March 1999), pp. 378-81, ISSN 0340-6245

Conlon, P. J., Kovalik, E., & Schwab, S. J. (1995) Percutaneous renal biopsy of ventilated intensive care unit patients. *Clin Nephrol*, Vol. 43, No. 5, (May 1995), pp. 309-11, ISSN 0301-0430

Fogo, A. B. (2003). Approach to renal biopsy. *Am J Kidney Dis*, Vol. 42, No. 4, (October 2003), pp. 826-36, ISSN 1523-6838

Gesualdo, L. et al. (2008). Percutaneous ultrasound-guided renal biopsy in supine antero-lateral position: a new approach for obese and non-obese patients. *Nephrol Dial Transplant*, Vol. 23, No. 3, (March 2008), pp. 971-6, ISSN 1460-2385

Gwyn, N. B. (1923). Biopsies and the Completion of certain Surgical Procedures. *Can Med Assoc J*, Vol. 13, No. 11, (November 1923), pp. 820-3, ISSN 0008-4409

Ishikawa, E. et al. (2009). Ultrasonography as a predictor of overt bleeding after renal biopsy. *Clin Exp Nephrol*, Vol. 13, No. 4, (August 2009), pp. 325-31, ISSN 1437-7799

Iversen, P. & Brun, C. (1951). Aspiration biopsy of the kidney. *Am J Med*, Vol. 11, No. 3, (September 1951), pp. 324-30, ISSN 0002-9343

Kark, R. M. & Muehrcke, R. C. (1954). Biopsy of kidney in prone position. *Lancet*, Vol. 266, No. 6821, (May 1954), pp. 1047-9, ISSN 0140-6736

Kim, D. et al. (1998). A randomized, prospective, comparative study of manual and automated renal biopsies. *Am J Kidney Dis*, Vol. 32, No. 3, (September 1998), pp. 426-31, ISSN 1523-6838

Kim, K. T. et al. (1991). Embolic control of lumbar artery hemorrhage complicating percutaneous renal biopsy with a 3-F coaxial catheter system: case report. *Cardiovasc Intervent Radiol*, Vol. 14, No. 3, (May-June 1991), pp. 175-8, ISSN 0174-1551

Korbet, S. M. (2002). Percutaneous renal biopsy. *Semin Nephrol*, Vol. 22, No. 3, (May 2002), pp. 254-67, ISSN 0270-9295

Lebret, T. et al. (2007). Percutaneous core biopsy for renal masses: indications, accuracy and results. *J Urol*, Vol. 178, No. 4, (October 2007), pp. 1184-8, ISSN 0022-5347

Madaio, M. P. (1990). Renal biopsy. *Kidney Int*, Vol. 38, No. 3, (September 1990), pp. 529-43,. ISSN 0085-2538

Manno, C. et al. (2011). Desmopressin Acetate in Percutaneous Ultrasound-Guided Kidney Biopsy: A Randomized Controlled Trial. *Am J Kidney Dis*, Vol. 57, No. 6, (February 2011), pp.850-855, ISSN 0272-6386

Manno, C. et al. (2004). Predictors of bleeding complications in percutaneous ultrasound-guided renal biopsy. *Kidney Int*, Vol. 66, No. 4, (October 2004), pp. 1570-7, ISSN 0085-2538

Marwah, D. S. & Korbet, S. M. (1996). Timing of complications in percutaneous renal biopsy: what is the optimal period of observation? *Am J Kidney Dis*, Vol. 28, No. 1, (July 1996), pp. 47-52, ISSN 0272-6386

Mattix, H. & Singh, A. K. (1999). Is the bleeding time predictive of bleeding prior to a percutaneous renal biopsy? *Curr Opin Nephrol Hypertens*, (November 1999), Vol. 8, No. 6, pp. 715-8, ISSN 1062-4821

Maya, I. D. & Allon, M. (2009). Percutaneous renal biopsy: outpatient observation without hospitalization is safe. *Semin Dial*, Vol. 22, No. 4, (July-August 2009), pp. 458-61, ISSN 1525-139X

Maya, I. D. et al. (2007). Percutaneous renal biopsy: comparison of blind and real-time ultrasound-guided technique. *Semin Dial*, Vol. 20, No. 4, (July-August 2007), pp. 355-8, ISSN 0894-0959

Mendelssohn, D. C. & Cole, E. H. (1995). Outcomes of percutaneous kidney biopsy, including those of solitary native kidneys. *Am J Kidney Dis*, Vol. 26, No. 4, (October 1995), pp. 580-5, ISSN 0272-6386

Nicholson, M. L. et al. (2000). A prospective randomized trial of three different sizes of core-cutting needle for renal transplant biopsy. *Kidney Int*, Vol. 58, No. 1, (July 2000), pp. 390-5, ISSN 0085-2538

Pasquariello, A. et al. (2007). Theoretical calculation of optimal depth in the percutaneous native kidney biopsy to drastically reduce bleeding complications and sample inadequacy for histopathological diagnosis. *Nephrol Dial Transplant*, Vol. 22, No. 12, (December 2007), pp. 3516-20, ISSN 0931-0509

Peterson, P. et al. (1998). The preoperative bleeding time test lacks clinical benefit: College of American Pathologists' and American Society of Clinical Pathologists' position article. *Arch Surg*, Vol. 133, No. 2, (February 1998), pp. 134-9, ISSN 0004-0010

Sarabu, N. et al. (2010). Safety and Efficacy of Transjugular Renal Biopsy Performed by Interventional Nephrologists. *Semin Dial*, (December 2010), ISSN 1525-139X

Schow, D. A., Vinson, R. K., & Morrisseau, P. M. (1992). Percutaneous renal biopsy of the solitary kidney: a contraindication? *J Urol*, Vol. 147, No. 5, (May 1992), pp. 1235-7, ISSN 0022-5347

Schwarz, A. et al. (2005). Safety and adequacy of renal transplant protocol biopsies. *Am J Transplant*, Vol. 5, No. 8, (August 2005), pp. 1992-6, ISSN 1600-6135

Song, J. H. & Cronan, J. J. (1998). Percutaneous biopsy in diffuse renal disease: comparison of 18- and 14-gauge automated biopsy devices. *J Vasc Interv Radiol*, Vol. 9, No. 4, (July-August 1998), pp. 651-5, ISSN 1051-0443

Stratta, P. et al. (2007). Risk management of renal biopsy: 1387 cases over 30 years in a single centre. *Eur J Clin Invest*, Vol. 37, No. 12, (December 2007), pp. 954-63, ISSN 0014-2972

Tung, K. T., Downes, M. O. & O'Donnell, P. J. (1992). Renal biopsy in diffuse renal disease--experience with a 14-gauge automated biopsy gun. *Clin Radiol*, Vol. 46, No. 2, (August 1992), pp. 111-3, ISSN 0009-9260

Waldo, B. et al. (2009). The value of post-biopsy ultrasound in predicting complications after percutaneous renal biopsy of native kidneys. *Nephrol Dial Transplant*, Vol. 24, No. 8, (August 2009), pp. 2433-9, ISSN 1460-2385

2

# Renal Biopsy in the Pediatric Patient

Isa F. Ashoor, Deborah R. Stein and Michael J. G. Somers
*Division of Nephrology*
*Children's Hospital Boston*
*Harvard Medical School, Boston, Massachusetts*
*USA*

## 1. Introduction

Renal biopsy in children can be performed either by percutaneous, laparoscopic, or open surgical approaches. As reported in a recent large pediatric series (Hussain et al., 2010), the percutaneous approach is by far the most commonly utilized, with the open approach typically reserved for situations in which percutaneous biopsy may be relatively contraindicated or there is the need for a large wedge of tissue. Increasingly, more centers are reporting successful experience with laparoscopic approaches as an alternative to open surgical biopsies (Caione et al., 2000; Luque Mialdea et al., 2006; Mukhtar et al., 2005).

Native renal biopsy should be performed in a child when kidney disease is suspected and treatment decisions require confirmation, when staging or characterization of a known kidney disease is warranted, or when the disease diagnosis is known but the utility of further treatment is questioned. In contrast to adults, renal insufficiency in children is more often secondary to sequelae from congenital or structural anomalies rather than acquired diseases. As a result, loss of renal function is not unexpected and tends to progress more slowly. Typically, children with such well-defined renal anomalies do not undergo biopsy even as renal function declines, unless a new entity is thought to be present.

On the other hand, children presenting with an acquired kidney condition, especially with rapidly changing renal function or lack of response to empiric therapy, do require renal biopsy to allow for accurate diagnosis and tailoring of therapeutic intervention. Moreover, while relatively common medical conditions such as hypertension and diabetes mediate much of the chronic kidney disease seen in adults, these conditions are rarer in children and less likely to impact renal health in the pediatric patient, leading to a need for clinicians to actually identify why kidney disease has arisen in the child.

In contrast to many adults, children and adolescents typically require significant conscious sedation or even general anesthesia for successful renal biopsy. Consequently, the risks of both the procedure and sedation/anesthesia must be considered when determining whether to do the biopsy. There are several medical conditions that often preclude biopsy. Although each case must be individually considered and there may be an occasion when the information garnered at biopsy outweighs the potential risk, the following situations are often considered contraindications or relative contraindications for pediatric biopsy:

Contraindications for biopsy:
- Severe bleeding disorders such as hemophilia
- Known abdominal malignancy
- Multiple renal cysts or renal tumor preventing sampling of renal parenchyma
- Compromised skin or skin infection overlying biopsy entry site
- Uncontrolled hypertension, increasing the risk of post-operative bleeding

Relative Contraindications:
- Massive ascites
- Severe hydronephrosis

While some have challenged the safety of performing renal biopsy in a child with a solitary kidney, current complication rates have decreased to such a degree that, if warranted for diagnostic reasons and if being performed by experienced clinicians utilizing medical imaging to visualize the kidney during biopsy, this is generally not considered to be a contraindication.

## 2. Nuts and bolts: Logistics of planning and preparation for the biopsy procedure

If no ultrasound has been obtained in the past or if there is concern that there may have been an interval change in the kidney or urinary tract anatomy since the last imaging study, a renal ultrasound is performed to assess for anomalies such as hydronephrosis, to confirm location and number of kidneys, and to assess renal size prior to the biopsy. The point of the ultrasound is to identify any anatomic reason why biopsy would be contraindicated or that would alter the approach to the biopsy.

A complete blood count (CBC), coagulation panel including prothrombin time (PT) and partial thromboplastin time (PTT), as well as a sample for type and screen to be held in the blood bank are obtained, typically within 72 hours of the procedure. The CBC allows baseline hematologic parameters to be ascertained in case there is concern regarding bleeding or infection post-procedure and also confirms an acceptable platelet count prior to an invasive procedure. The PT/PTT identifies any tendency toward a coagulopathy that may increase the chances of a bleeding complication. Although transfusion post-biopsy is rare, having a blood type and screen in the blood bank will expedite this process if it is necessary, and especially if it is urgently required.

Informed consent is obtained from either the parent/guardian or the patient if the patient is of legal age. The consent process must include explaining the risks of the procedure, however rare, including bleeding, infection, and the potential need for surgery to control bleeding or perform nephrectomy. In children less than 18 years of age who are cognitively capable of understanding the rationale for the biopsy procedure, in addition to informed consent from the parent or legal guardian, there is utility in obtaining assent from the child. This documents that the patient was also involved in the decision to proceed with the biopsy and underscores the need to keep the patient involved in a developmentally appropriate fashion with the process.

Prior to the biopsy, the patient will need to fast for some period of time, depending on whether sedation or anesthesia is being utilized and institutional protocols. Most children should tolerate this period of time without the need for supplemental intravenous hydration, but individual circumstance and clinical status must be reviewed to determine if the usual period of fasting is likely to cause any untoward consequence; for instance, a child with diabetes insipidus or a child with a severe urinary concentrating defect would require special hydration plans.

## 3. Nuts and bolts: Sedation or anesthesia for the pediatric renal biopsy

Local standards and individual clinician preference have the greatest impact on the type of sedation or anesthesia for pediatric patients undergoing percutaneous renal biopsy. The overwhelming majority of children are offered intravenous conscious sedation or some sort of general anesthesia, with very few patients declining such measures and opting for local anesthesia injected at the biopsy site alone. In rare cases of children with serious contraindication or objection to sedation or anesthesia, "verbal sedation" has been used, with the child talked through the procedure with the help of a child life specialist trained in this approach (Hussain et al., 2003).

Case series from North American centers show that general anesthesia is most often reserved for infants or very small children where lack of cooperation during the procedure is a concern as well as in children whose airways may be at risk with sedation alone (Birk et al., 2007; Simckes et al., 2000; Sweeney et al., 2006). This approach is not necessarily the case worldwide and, in fact, a recent audit in the United Kingdom (Hussain et al., 2010) showed 6 of 11 centers routinely using general anesthesia for pediatric kidney biopsies.

Intravenous "conscious" sedation, sometimes termed "deep" procedural sedation, is usually administered by a nurse or physician who has acquired expertise in various sedation techniques and certification in pediatric advanced life support (Cravero et al., 2006; Mason et al., 2009). The patients should receive continuous cardiorespiratory monitoring throughout the procedure. A variety of agents may be utilized and the protocols are institution specific or dependent on local resources.

Our institution has successfully employed a radiologist-supervised ketamine sedation protocol for many solid organ biopsies (Mason et al., 2009). In this protocol, children receive an IV Ketamine bolus (2 mg/kg) over a 5-minute period with concomitant administration of 0.005 mg/kg of IV glycopyrolate. The bolus of ketamine is immediately followed by a continuous infusion of 25-150 mcg/kg/min of ketamine for the duration of the procedure. Patients older than 5 years also receive 0.1 mg/kg of midazolam hydrochloride (maximum = 3mg) before the initial bolus of ketamine. There have been no major adverse events reported with this protocol and both patient and family satisfaction rates have been high.

Other published sedation protocols employ a combination of meperidine (1 mg/kg–maximum 50 mg) and diazepam (0.2-0.4 mg/kg), with ketamine reserved for additional sedation if necessary (Hussain et al., 2003); midazolam 0.1 mg/kg with additional ketmaine where required (Mahajan et al., 2010); or intravenous propofol (1 mg/kg/dose titrated to effect) and fentanyl (1 μg/kg/dose) (Birk et al., 2007). Again, local practice and clinician familiarity and expertise with certain medications tend to influence the type of sedation provided most successfully and is more critical than the use of any specific medication or combination of medications.

Local anesthesia may be achieved by applying a topical anesthetic cream (EMLA, lidocaine 2.5% and pritocaine 2.5% or Ametop tetracaine 4%) (Hussain et al., 2003) or local infiltration with 1% lidocaine. At our center, for local infiltration with lidocaine, 9 mls of lidocaine are mixed with 1 ml of 8.4% sodium bicarbonate; this approach seems to decrease complaints of burning at the site of infiltration, and this is employed regardless of the type of sedation utilized.

The majority of percutaneous renal biopsies performed under sedation are done outside the operating room, usually in an interventional radiology suite, a procedure area with access to ultrasound imaging, or in ward treatment rooms (Davis et al., 1998; Hussain et al., 2003; Mason et al., 2009). Although there were initial concerns about providing sedation in such settings for invasive procedures, our own experience and that of others have shown few safety concerns. The Pediatric Sedation Research Consortium reported a large series of 30,037 sedation encounters from 26 centers, with data submitted on a variety of pediatric procedures performed under sedation or anesthesia outside the operating room (Cravero et al., 2006). This study demonstrated the overall safety of such procedures, with no deaths and only one cardiopulmonary resuscitation event. The most commonly encountered adverse event in this cohort was more than 30 seconds of oxygen desaturation to less than 90% by transcutaneous monitoring, and this only occurred in 1.5% of cases. Needless to say, the safety and success of such programs depend on consistently following well-developed protocols, the presence of certified providers throughout the procedure, and readily available anesthesia services to handle unexpected complications.

## 4. Nuts and bolts: Performing the renal biopsy

As discussed above, institutional practice and resources often guide the location for pediatric biopsies. For instance, in our center, biopsies are performed in an Interventional Radiology suite with either nurses providing conscious sedation by protocol or Pediatric Anesthesiologists providing general anesthesia. The use of sedation versus anesthesia typically depends on the age of the patient, developmental and emotional factors, and any co-morbid medical conditions. For instance, a very young child with nephrotic syndrome and significant volume overload will likely warrant general anesthesia whereas a mature adolescent undergoing a transplant biopsy may need little other than local anesthesia over the biopsy site.

Biopsies are performed under sterile conditions. As a result, it is important for the individual performing the biopsy to follow standard protocol for a sterile invasive procedure including aseptic technique and wearing appropriate gowns, gloves, masks, and eye protection.

Obtaining an adequate sample is crucial for any renal biopsy, but is even more imperative in children undergoing biopsy where the logistics of the procedure may be more complicated. Availability of a dissecting microscope to view each core obtained to assess tissue adequacy is extremely useful to guide the number of cores needed. Presence of either a pathologist or nephrologist experienced in identifying renal tissue under dissecting microscope is obviously essential and should allow some estimation of tissue adequacy.

For a native renal biopsy, the child is placed in a prone position and typically the left kidney is imaged to discern an acceptable biopsy site. In a transplant patient, the child will be supine and the area immediately over the allograft is imaged. The skin overlying the area most appropriate for biopsy needle introduction is marked during this process. Generally, a site in the lower pole of the kidney is selected, away from the renal hilum and large vessels.

At this point, prior to proceeding further with the procedure, a pause or "time-out" is worthwhile, with the individual performing the procedure reviewing aloud the patient's name, medical diagnosis, planned procedure including site of biopsy, and confirming that informed consent has been obtained. All others in the procedure area should then verbally identify themselves and their role in the procedure, for instance "Jane Jones, RN performing sedation" or "John Smith, attending radiologist" so that there is both acknowledged consensus of the procedure to be done by all involved and understanding of the specific roles of all the individuals present in the area.

The biopsy area is cleaned thoroughly with a betadine solution, and all areas outside the sterile field are covered with sterile drapes. A local anesthetic such as lidocaine is injected at the marked skin site. An initial wheal is made and then deeper infiltration performed, following the anticipated path of the biopsy needle. A superficial dermatotomy is made over the wheal, and the biopsy needle is advanced through this area.

Typically, most pediatric renal biopsies are now done with ultrasound guidance. If desired, this allows use of a needle guide that helps to position the path of the biopsy needle along the desired biopsy tract. It also allows for continuous monitoring of the position of the needle during the procedure and allows for ready identification of structures such as bowel or large vessels that must be avoided. Optimally, the individual performing the biopsy has been trained in biopsy sonography as well, so that the same individual is controlling the imaging and the needle placement; otherwise, there needs to be continuous communication between the individual advancing the biopsy needle and the sonographer to be sure that both agree as to the needle position and the target.

Local practice and available resources will determine the biopsy devices and needles used, most of which are readily available from medical vendors. For most percutaneous pediatric renal biopsies at our center, we use an 18-gauge needle and an automated biopsy device or "gun" that is loaded with the needle. The desired "throw" -- or length of the biopsy needle that gets propelled into the kidney when the device is engaged -- depends on the size of the child and the size of the kidney being biopsied. For most children, a throw of approximately 2 centimeters allows for a safe biopsy with sufficient tissue but, in especially young children or with small kidneys, a shorter throw may be needed to avoid the renal hilum or other surrounding structures.

The needle is advanced to the selected site in the lower pole renal cortex under continuous ultrasound guidance. Once the needle reaches the renal capsule, it is advanced slightly further to enter kidney tissue. The biopsy device is then "fired" which allows the inner hollow-core biopsy needle to deploy, cutting a piece of kidney tissue. The cutting needle is then automatically ensheathed by an outer protective core. The entire biopsy needle device is withdrawn from the kidney and the protective sheath withdrawn to expose the tissue core. The biopsy sample is carefully transferred onto a saline-soaked gauze by rolling the needle onto the gauze, and then the core is examined by the pathologist or nephrologist under a dissecting microscope for quick estimation of tissue adequacy. During this time following needle extraction, the physician performing the biopsy or another designee applies pressure to the biopsy site.

This procedure is repeated until adequate renal tissue has been obtained for the biopsy indication, depending on the patient's medical condition and the studies to be performed on the tissue. Typically, for native kidney biopsies, we obtain three cores of tissue to allow for sufficient tissue for light microscopy, immunofluorescence, and electron microscopy. For transplant biopsies, two cores are generally obtained since fewer studies are usually done. As always, the size and adequacy of tissue cores obtained will specifically define the number of cores needed for any patient. If adequate tissue is not obtained after three to five passes of the needle, then there must be consideration of the risk of ongoing passes into the kidney versus the benefits of obtaining more kidney tissue at this point in time.

At completion of the entire biopsy procedure, pressure is applied externally over the biopsy site for a minimum of 5 minutes. A post-biopsy ultrasound with Doppler imaging is then performed to evaluate for any hematoma or active bleeding. If bleeding is observed, pressure is maintained until there is evidence of stable imaging with no expanding hematoma or determination is made that there needs to be some other intervention. The dermatotomy site is covered with a sterile dressing that may be removed the following day. This dressing is observed for any bleeding or drainage while it is in place.

## 5. Open renal biopsy in children

Rarely, an open renal biopsy is appropriate in children. Common indications for open renal biopsy are listed in Table One. Some clinical scenarios where open biopsy is more common include when attempts at a percutaneous biopsy have failed, when a wedge resection is required for pathologic diagnosis, or when there is a bleeding disorder but the biopsy is paramount to treatment decisions. Open biopsy is performed typically by a general surgeon, urologist, or transplant surgeon in an operating room. Open renal biopsy will usually result in exposure to general anesthesia or more prolonged sedation with longer post-procedure recovery times, hence increasing health care delivery costs.

- Failed percutaneous renal biopsy
- Percutaneous renal biopsy deemed unsafe:
  - Uncontrolled hypertension
  - Bleeding disorder
- Solitary native kidney with specific concerns for percutaneous approach
- Anatomic abnormalities complicating percutaneous approach:
  - Horseshoe kidney
  - Pelvic kidney
- Intraperitoneal renal allograft with specific concerns for percutaneous approach
- Donor implantation biopsy at time of transplant
- Biopsy performed concurrent with other surgical intra-abdominal procedure
- Morbid obesity

Table 1. Common Indications for Open Renal Biopsy

There may be center-specific variation in the use of open biopsy depending on local experience and expertise. Similarly, there may be changes in local practice regarding specific clinical scenarios that may come to decrease the need for open renal biopsy. For instance, several centers have published their experiences transitioning from open to percutaneous biopsies of solitary kidneys and transperitoneal allografts (Mendelssohn & Cole, 1995; Vidhun et al., 2003). In cases that may be considered higher risk for percutaneous approach, most clinicians think it judicious to pay special attention to coagulation parameters, blood pressures and serum creatinine in determining the optimal approach for renal biopsy (Davis et al., 1998; Simckes et al., 2000). Similarly, in situations where a clinician is performing a higher risk percutaneous biopsy, it would be warranted to ensure in advance that there is availability of interventional radiology or surgical support services for unexpected complications.

## 6. Laparoscopic renal biopsy

Within the last decade, there has also been increased utilization of laparoscopic approach as an alternative to traditional open biopsy. This approach has been well-established in morbidly obese adults where the body habitus precludes percutaneous approach (Mukhtar et al., 2005, as cited in Shetye et al., 2003). Unfortunately, obesity rates in children are at an all-time high and show no signs of abating (Anderson & Whitaker, 2009; Broyles et al., 2010). Obesity is also a frequent complication of steroid therapy commonly used in treating various glomerular lesions and in maintenance immunosuppression for renal transplant recipients who may come to require biopsy. Furthermore, in the face of the obesity epidemic, we are increasingly recognizing the entity of obesity-related secondary focal segmental glomerulosclerosis presenting with heavy proteinuria (Fowler et al., 2009). Consequently clinicians may find an increasing population of obese children requiring biopsy whose body habitus prevents a percutaneous approach.

Mukhtar et al (Mukhtar et al., 2005) reported their experience with two morbidly obese children where initial attempts at percutaneous biopsy failed. The procedures were then carried out laparoscopically with no major complications, and both children were discharged home within 48 hours at significant cost savings compared to an open biopsy. Two larger case series from Italy and Spain (Caione et al., 2000; Luque Mialdea et al., 2006) also described successful experiences with laparoscopic renal biopsies in 20 and 53 pediatric patients, respectively. Children in those series ranged in age from 13 months to 19 years. The procedure was safe and successful in all but one patient in each series who required conversion to an open biopsy. The mean hospital stay in both cohorts was 48 hours or less.

## 7. Differences between native and transplant biopsies in children

In most children > 20 kg, transplanted kidneys are typically placed extraperitoneally in the lower abdomen within the iliac fossa. In smaller children, kidneys may need to be placed intraperitoneally. In most pediatric renal transplant recipients, transplanted kidneys are far more superficial than native kidneys and this must be kept in mind during biopsy to avoid improper sampling or damage to the vascular structures. Again, ultrasound guidance during the biopsy procedure will help to minimize these technical complications. In those children with intraperitoneal allografts, care must be taken to avoid bowel or other structures that may overlie the allograft.

Allograft biopsies are typically performed to evaluate for acute rejection, to assess for recurrence of diseases such as Focal Segmental Glomerulosclerosis (FSGS), to define new onset suspected glomerular disease, to assess extent of chronic allograft nephropathy, or to document infectious insults such as BK virus nephropathy. Some centers may perform interval "protocol" biopsies at set intervals to assess the allograft parenchyma. Processing and staining of the biopsy samples from transplanted kidneys depends on the biopsy indication (see section 10).

## 8. Post-biopsy monitoring in children

There are currently no standard guidelines established for post renal biopsy monitoring. The standard of care in adult patients has included bed rest with close observation for up to 24 hours (Whittier & Korbet, 2004). In their retrospective analysis of 750 adult patients who underwent native renal biopsy, Whittier and Korbet found an observation time of up to 24 hours to be optimal, with an observation period of 8 hours or less missing up to 33% of complications. There are, however, various clinical and social factors that impact any specific patient's circumstances and, as a result, the length of observation post-biopsy should be somewhat individualized.

In children, there are also wide variations in practice for post-biopsy monitoring. For instance, a survey of pediatric nephrologists in Japan (Kamitsuji et al., 1999) covering complications in 2,045 native percutaneous renal biopsies revealed that no center allowed discharge within 24 hours of the biopsy, with 67% of patients remaining in the hospital for at least 4-8 days. The patients in this cohort had similar complication rates to other pediatric series with shorter duration of observation, however, and the prolonged hospital stay was attributed to local practice.

Over the last two decades, with increasing safety of percutaneous renal biopsy, particularly when performed with an automated biopsy needle under real time ultrasound guidance, more centers are moving towards short post-biopsy monitoring times for both native and allograft renal biopsies in children. In fact, several centers in North America and Europe have implemented same day renal biopsy in ambulatory or day clinical care units as standard practice for low risk patients since the early 1990s (Birk et al., 2007; Hussain et al., 2003; Sweeney et al., 2006). This trend has been associated with significant cost savings compared to inpatient renal biopsies and comparable safety outcomes (Chesney et al., 1996; Hussain et al., 2003; Lau et al., 2009; Simckes et al., 2000). In addition, several centers in developing countries are reporting successful experiences with percutaneous renal biopsies in the ambulatory setting, where it was initially promoted for logistical reasons associated with limited inpatient bed space (Al Makdama & Al-Akash et al, 2006; Mahajan et al., 2010).

In most centers where pediatric renal biopsies are performed as an inpatient procedure, there is consensus regarding the utility of bed rest in the supine position for a period of 3-6 hours post biopsy. Patients are asked to save their urine for gross inspection and most centers allow the patient to stand to void if two consecutive post-biopsy urine samples are negative for gross hematuria. Vital signs are usually monitored every 15-30 minutes in the first 2 hours post biopsy and less frequently thereafter. Some centers provide intravenous hydration until patients are fully awake and able to drink. Most centers utilize acetaminophen for analgesia.

Local standards often dictate post biopsy laboratory investigations or imaging studies. In our institution, biopsies are performed by nephrologists trained in renal sonography in the presence of an interventional radiologist who can immediately assist if there is some question or concern for an adverse event. As noted above, immediate post-biopsy images are also obtained by ultrasound to assess for hematoma formation and to provide a post-biopsy baseline. Others employ routine post-biopsy ultrasound from 24 hours to two weeks following renal biopsy in all patients to detect peri/intra renal hematoma formation with consideration of Doppler studies to assess for arteriovenous fistula formation (Al Rasheed et al., 1990; Kamitsuji et al., 1999; Mahajan et al., 2010), though it is unclear whether this changes clinical care of the stable patient (Castoldi et al., 1994).

It is also our practice to observe patients for at least 6 to 8 hours post-procedure and to check a hemoglobin and hematocrit level at 4-6 hours post biopsy and again the next morning as long as there is no concern to warrant repeat laboratory work sooner. A hematocrit drop of greater than 5-7%, severe abdominal or flank pain, gross hematuria that does not clear or markedly improve within two to three voids, or any evidence of hemodynamic instability would prompt urgent renal imaging with an ultrasound to detect ongoing bleeding or expanding hematoma formation.

In those centers that perform percutaneous renal biopsies in the ambulatory setting without provision for hospital admission, the selection criteria for low risk patients generally include normal or controlled blood pressure, normal pre-biopsy hematocrit and coagulation studies, a competent care giver to monitor the patient after the procedure, and the family's willingness to stay within a reasonable distance of the hospital for the first night post-biopsy (Ogborn & Grimm, 1992). Following the biopsy, patients are typically monitored for 6-8 hours with strict bed rest for 1-3 hours. Patients are discharged home at the end of this observation period if their urine is free of gross hematuria, their vital signs are stable and they have no significant pain at the biopsy site (Birk et al., 2007; Hussain et al., 2003; Ogborn & Grimm, 1992; Simckes et al., 2000).

The value of routine post-biopsy imaging studies is controversial, with several studies suggesting the development of post biopsy perinephric hematomas is common and does not negatively impact patient outcomes or change the need for patient care in most cases (Castoldi et al., 1994; Vidhun et al., 2003). Detection of hematoma may also be a function of sensitivity of the imaging technique employed. For instance, data from CT scanning post biopsy reveals that perinephric hematoma is almost universal (Castoldi et al., 1994, as cited in Ralls et al., 1987). Castoldi et al further attempted to stratify hematomas according to size and correlate them with patient outcomes. In their retrospective analysis of 230 patients where 218 underwent post-biopsy sonography within 72 hours, the incidence of parenchymal, subcapsular, and perinephric hematomas combined was 42%. In the absence of clinical signs of bleeding, no short or long-term adverse effects were reported and, even in the presence of clinical signs of bleeding, serious complications only occurred in those with large hematomas. Large hematomas were defined as those having a thickness greater than 1 cm and length greater than 3 cm. Moreover, although these large hematomas were found in 20 patients (9% of their total cohort), only 7 of these patients had more than a 7% decrease in their post-biopsy hematocrit values. On the other hand, all hematomas with a thickness less than 2 cm in their study had a favorable clinical course.

Davis et al (Davis et al., 1998) evaluated the utility of monitoring the post-biopsy change in hemoglobin concentration to identify bleeding complications that were otherwise not clinically apparent. In their retrospective review of 177 percutaneous renal biopsies (137 native, 40 transplant), hemoglobin measurements were obtained at 4-10 hours and 15-24 hours post biopsy. In their study, using a drop in hemoglobin levels of more than 16% of baseline - for instance from 10 g/dl to 8.4 g/dl -- served as a sensitive (100%) and specific (98%) marker of major bleeding complication that required either transfusion or additional monitoring. The change in post-biopsy hemoglobin was not associated with the presence of gross hematuria or perinephric hematoma, which were considered minor complications in this study.

Children are allowed to return to school within one to two days of biopsy, though participation in physical education classes is usually avoided for one week. Children are also encouraged to avoid contact sports or vigorous activities that might result in direct trauma to the biopsy site for one week. Children are allowed to shower but immersion of the biopsy site in water is not recommended until the dermatotomy site is scabbed over, which typically occurs within 48 to 72 hours. In the immediate post-biopsy period, families are instructed to contact their pediatric nephrologist urgently for new onset gross hematuria, dysuria, pain at the biopsy site, or fever.

## 9. Complications post-biopsy

Percutaneous renal biopsy as performed in most pediatric centers today with ultrasound guidance and automated biopsy needles is an extremely safe procedure with few associated minor and major complications. Those complications are summarized in Table 2.

Various factors such as indication for biopsy, operator experience, needle type, and number of passes can affect the rate of post biopsy complications. In the large Japanese cohort of 2,045 percutaneous native renal biopsies (Kamitsuji et al., 1999), the rate of gross hematuria was very low and comparable between patients in whom an automated biopsy needle was used compared to the older Vim-Silverman needle in which the cutting core was advanced manually (2.7% vs. 3%). On the other hand, in a retrospective analysis of 177 percutaneous renal biopsies, Davis et al (Davis et el., 1998) noted a significantly higher rate of post-biopsy hematoma in those procedures performed with an automated biopsy needle (Meditech ASAP Automatic 15-G Core Biopsy System needle) compared to a non-automated device (14 G Franklin-Vim-Silverman needle or 15 G Trucut needle). However, the authors report the use of CT scan or ultrasound for post-biopsy imaging in the automated group compared to ultrasound only in the non-automated group, which might have led to increased detection of hematomas in the former because of CT's higher sensitivity, rather than actual difference related to the biopsy device. Simckes et al (Simckes et al., 2000) found a trend for the non-automated Trucut needle to be the least traumatic compared to the modified Franklin-Vim-Silverman and automated spring-loaded needles in their cohort. In comparison, Webb et al (Webb et al., 1994) reported significantly more total complications with the Trucut needle compared to the automated biopsy needle, though the difference in major complications was not significant. Most likely, clinical factors and operator experience play a larger role in post-biopsy hematoma formation that the biopsy device itself.

| Minor complications | Major complications |
|---|---|
| • Microscopic hematuria<br>• Self-limited gross hematuria<br>• Asymptomatic peri-nephric hematoma<br>• Asymptomatic decrease in Hb concentration<br>• Self-limited arteriovenous fistula<br>• Mild pain/ discomfort at biopsy site<br>• Inadequate biopsy tissue and/ or failed biopsy | • Persistent gross hematuria<br>• Symptomatic peri-nephric hematoma causing hemodynamic instability<br>• Significant decrease in Hb concentration requiring blood transfusion<br>• Hypotension<br>• Symptomatic arteriovenous fistula<br>• Inadvertent damage to adjacent organs (e.g. liver, intestine)<br>• Severe abdominal and/ or flank pain<br>• Urinary tract infection<br>• Urinary tract obstruction<br>• Acute Renal Failure<br>• Allograft loss<br>• Nephrectomy<br>• Death |

Table 2. Complications Post-Renal Biopsy

No difference has been reported in complication rates between using a 14-G Biopty gun needle or an automated 14-G Trucut needle, suggesting that needle size may influence the rate of complications more than needle type (Webb et al., 1994). Along those lines, Vidhun et al (Vidhun et al., 2003) have shown in renal allograft biopsies a higher incidence of perinephric hematoma (43% vs. 13.3%) and macroscopic hematuria (29% vs. 2.3%) with use of a 16-G versus an 18-G biopsy needle. Similar findings in native renal biopsies were also reported from a large Brazilian cohort (Piotto et al., 2008). As such, Birk et al (Birk et al., 2007) hypothesized that the slightly higher incidence of post-biopsy gross hematuria (8.4%) in their cohort of 43 renal transplant recipients compared to previously published reports (1.9-3.5%) was their use of a larger 16-G needle compared to an 18-G needle used elsewhere.

With regards to other factors, several retrospective analyses have shown no significant difference in complication rates whether the biopsy was performed as an outpatient or inpatient procedure (Hussain et al., 2003, 2010; Simckes et al., 2000), under general anesthesia or sedation (Durkan et al., 2006; Hussain et al., 2010; Webb et al., 1994), by a supervised trainee or by an attending physician or consultant (Durkan et al., 2006; Simckes et al., 2000), and between an intraperitoneal and extraperitoneal graft in the case of allograft percutaneous biopsies (Vidhun et al., 2003).

Interestingly, in native percutaneous biopsies, one author (Hussain et al., 2003) observed a trend for a higher incidence of gross hematuria post biopsy in those patients with a histological diagnosis of IgA Nephropathy/ Henoch-Schonlein Purpura. In the case of renal allografts, biopsies for urgent issues were noted to have a higher incidence of post biopsy hematoma compared to protocol biopsies (Vidhun et al., 2003). Increased number of passes was significantly associated with obtaining more adequate tissue for making a histological diagnosis (Durkan et al., 2006), but with a slightly increased but not significant trend towards hematoma formation (Simckes et al., 2000).

Through the decades, the safety of percutaneous renal biopsy has been verified in several large pediatric case series. Death is extremely rare. One early review (Al Rasheed et al., 1990, as cited in White, 1963) reported 17 deaths in more than 10,000 biopsies (0.17%). Similarly, another large review at that time reported a mortality rate of 0.12% in 4000 biopsies (Simckes et al., 2000, as cited in Dodge et al., 1962). On the other hand, Edelmann found no deaths in a review of reports published between 1971-1976 of more than 1,700 percutaneous biopsies in children (Simckes et al., 2000, as cited in Edelmann et al., 1992). This improved safety profile continues to be reported in more recent series from North American and various institutions in Europe and Asia (Al Makdama & Al-Akash, 2006; Birk et al., 2007; Hussain et al., 2010; Kersnik Levart et al., 2001; Mahajan et al., 2010) and likely is mediated by concomitant imaging at the time of biopsy decreasing the chances for catastrophic hemorrhage or damage to vital organs other than the kidney.

Given the use of different definitions and thresholds to report complications, it is worth noting, however, that rates of so-called minor and major complications post-biopsy are somewhat difficult to compare between individual centers. For example, one study included microscopic hematuria as a minor complication, a finding almost universally seen in all patients undergoing renal biopsy (Al Rasheed et al., 1990). Some studies include gross hematuria as a major complication, while others only include it if persistent and associated with hemodynamic instability and transfusion requirement. In their audit of UK centers, Hussain et al included 39 patients with gross hematuria in the major complication group while only 4 of them required blood transfusions (Hussain et al., 2010). Regardless of those differences, most recent series report "major" complication rates in the 0-5% range and "minor" complications rates in the 8-15% range, though most complications that are reported in either category are of little immediate or long-lasting clinical significance to the patient's well-being.

Similar low complication rates also can be found with allograft biopsies. Benfield et al (Benfield et al., 1999) reported data from 19 pediatric transplant centers on 86 children who underwent 212 allograft biopsies. There were a total of 9 complications (4.2%) with only 4 (1.9%) requiring intervention. No patient lost kidney function or required nephrectomy after graft biopsy. Vidhun et al (Vidhun et al., 2003) specifically analyzed complication rates in adult-sized renal allografts in children and reported an overall complication rate of 16.1%, consisting mostly of perinephric hematomas (13.4%), while the gross hematuria rate (2.7%) was similar to the cohort reported by Benfield. Most of those hematomas (81.4%) were small (< 1 cm), and no patient in that cohort required intervention related to post-biopsy complications.

## 10. Pathologic findings

The ultimate goal of the renal biopsy is to obtain sufficient tissue to make a diagnosis or guide therapy. Based on histologic assessment of the biopsy samples, therapeutic intervention may be initiated or altered and important prognostic information may be gained.

It is crucial to obtain sufficient tissue to allow proper assessment by the pathologist. In certain pediatric renal diseases, light microscopy may be the most critical element, such as in the child with steroid resistant nephrotic syndrome in which the differential is minimal change disease versus focal and segmental glomerulosclerosis. In others, such as IgA nephropathy, immunofluorescence studies play a vital role and, in some, such as idiopathic membranoproliferative glomerulonephritis, electron microscopy will be necessary to supplement light microscopy and immunofluorescence results. Table Three summarizes the key pathologic studies to obtain on biopsy samples based on suspected clinical diagnosis. Table Four lists the histopathologic changes typically seen in several pediatric renal diseases.

| Suspected or Known Disease | Light Microscopy | Immunofluorescence | Electron Microscopy |
|---|---|---|---|
| IgA Nephropathy Henoch-Schonlein Purpura | X<br>Defines extent and severity of process | X<br>Necessary for diagnosis | Suggested but not required |
| Systemic Lupus Erythematosus | X<br>Necessary to identify class/severity | X | X<br>Necessary to diagnose Class V (membranous) |
| Membranoproliferative Glomerulonephritis | X | X | X<br>Necessary for diagnosis |

| | | | |
|---|---|---|---|
| Thin Basement Membrane Disease<br>Hereditary Nephritis<br>Alport's<br>Nail Patella Syndrome | X | X | X<br>Necessary for diagnosis |
| Minimal Change Nephrotic Syndrome<br>Focal and Segmental Glomerulosclerosis | X | X | X |
| ANCA associated vasculitis<br>Anti-GBM disease<br>Rapidly progressive glomerulonephritis | X | X | ? May not be crucial |
| Transplant Biopsies* | X | X ** | |

*If suspected recurrent disease, see above disease categories for tissue processing recommendations.
** C4d crucial for diagnosis of acute antibody-mediated rejection

Table 3. Desired Pathology Studies Based on Suspected Diagnosis

| Disease | Light Microscopy | Immunofluorescence | Electron Microscopy |
|---|---|---|---|
| Nephritis | | | |
| IgA Nephropathy | Focal or diffuse mesangial hypercellularity | Mesangial IgA deposits | Focal mesangial proliferation with electron-dense subendothelial deposits |
| Henoch-Schonlein Purpura | Focal or diffuse mesangial hypercellularity, ± crescents | Granular IgA | Immune deposits |
| Systemic Lupus Erythematosus | | | |
| I: Minimal Mesangial | Normal | Mesangial immune deposits (Ig, C3, C4) | Normal |
| II: Mesangial Proliferative | Increased mesangial matrix | Mesangial immune deposits (Ig, C3, C4) | Few or no subepithelial or subendothelial deposits |
| III: Focal | Less than 50% of glomeruli involved | Mesangial deposits, few subepithelial and subendothelial deposits (Ig, C3, C4) | Focal, subendothelial deposits |
| IV: Diffuse | Nearly all glomeruli involved, wire-loop appearance-thickened BM | Mesangial deposits, few subepithelial and subendothelial deposits (Ig, C3, C4) | Endothelial cell proliferation Subendothelial immune complex deposition |

| | | | |
|---|---|---|---|
| V: Membranous | See membranous GN | Subepithelial Ig, C3, C4 | Subepithelial deposits |
| VI: Advanced Sclerosing | ≥90% of glomeruli globally sclerosed | | |
| Membranoproliferative Glomerulonephritis Type I | Mesangial and endothelial cell proliferation, thickened basement membrane due to extensive immune complex deposition, increased mesangial matrix<br>"Tram-track" or double-contour appearance of basement membrane (best seen with silver stain) | Granular IgG and C3 | Mesangial Proliferation with immune deposits, subendothelial electron dense deposits between layers of BM double contours |
| Membranoproliferative Glomerulonephritis Type II (Dense Deposit Disease) | See MPGN Type I | C3 linear or double-contoured along BM | Subepithelial deposits-Electron dense deposits in ribbon-like pattern |
| Thin Basement Membrane Disease | Normal | Normal | Diffuse thinning of BM |
| Alport's | Early: Normal<br>Late: Sclerosis | Negative | Split basement membrane |
| Post-Infectious Glomerulonephritis | Enlarged glomeruli<br>Endocapillary proliferation<br>Obliteration of capillary loops<br>Increased mesangial cells<br>"Exudative proliferative GN" | Irregular granular C3, IgG, and others<br>• Starry sky: fine granular C3, IgG (early in disease)<br>• Mesangial: mesangial C3 (week 4-6) | Acute: subepithelial humps, disappear by 6th week<br><br>Garland type: dense deposits along capillary loops, subepithelial |
| Interstitial Nephritis | Cellular infiltrates in interstitium | Negative | Interrupted BM with thickened areas |
| Hemolytic Uremic Syndrome | Thrombosis of glomeruli, arterioles | Negative | No deposits |
| **Nephrotic Syndrome** | | | |
| Minimal Change Nephrotic Syndrome | Normal | Negative | Marked foot process effacement |
| Focal and Segmental Glomerulosclerosis | Segmental sclerosis of glomeruli | Negative (may be positive for mesangial C3, IgM) | Foot process effacement, early hyaline deposition |
| Membranous Nephropathy | All glomeruli affected<br>Thickened capillary walls<br>Membrane "spikes" | Granular IgG or C3 | Thickened basement membrane<br>Electron dense subepithelial immune deposits<br>Spikes |

| | | | |
|---|---|---|---|
| Rapidly Progressive Glomerulonephritis | | | |
| ANCA associated vasculitis | Endocapillary proliferation, some mesangial proliferation, urinary space open, focal necrosis, crescents Proliferation of podocytes and epithelial cells, proliferation of cells around Bowman's capsule leads to crescent formation | Negative | No deposits |
| Anti-GBM disease | Endocapillary proliferation, some mesangial proliferation, urinary space open, focal necrosis, crescents<br><br>Proliferation of podocytes and epithelial cells, proliferation of cells around Bowman's capsule leads to crescent formation | Anti-glomerular basement membrane antibodies (IgG) Linear pattern | No deposits |
| Transplant Biopsies | | | |
| Acute Cellular Rejection | Tubulitis Endothelialitis | | |
| Humoral Rejection | | C4d positive staining | |
| Calcineurin Inhibitor Toxicity | Concentric hyalinosis Interstitial Fibrosis | + Arteriolar IgM | Necrosis, smooth muscle cell injury |

Table 4. Histopathology Based on Diagnosis and Type of Tissue Study

## 11. Conclusion

Renal biopsy in children is a safe procedure, typically performed percutaneously with ultrasound guidance and conscious sedation, and with an 8 to 24 hour period of post-procedure observation. Biopsy allows diagnosis of new renal conditions, assesses health of the renal parenchyma by defining the extent of injury and potential for recovery, and provides the pediatric clinician with valuable information to tailor further diagnostic or therapeutic interventions. Surgical renal biopsy by open technique or laparoscopic approach is less commonly required for the child with an isolated renal condition. The ability to rely on percutaneous biopsy simplifies the typical procedure, decreases patient time spent hospitalized or under supervised observation, and ultimately provides economy of health care costs. More importantly, by allowing for precise histopathologic diagnosis rather than clinical assessment alone, the use of renal biopsy as needed in children helps to expand the understanding of the impact and course of certain pediatric renal diseases, their response to therapy, and their prognosis.

## 12. References

Al Makdama, A., and S. Al-Akash. 2006. Safety of percutaneous renal biopsy as an outpatient procedure in pediatric patients. Ann Saudi Med 26 (4):303-5.

al Rasheed, S. A., M. M. al Mugeiren, M. B. Abdurrahman, and A. T. Elidrissy. 1990. The outcome of percutaneous renal biopsy in children: an analysis of 120 consecutive cases. Pediatr Nephrol 4 (6):600-3.

Anderson, S. E., and R. C. Whitaker. 2009. Prevalence of obesity among US preschool children in different racial and ethnic groups. Arch Pediatr Adolesc Med 163 (4):344-8.

Benfield, M. R., J. Herrin, L. Feld, S. Rose, D. Stablein, and A. Tejani. 1999. Safety of kidney biopsy in pediatric transplantation: a report of the Controlled Clinical Trials in Pediatric Transplantation Trial of Induction Therapy Study Group. Transplantation 67 (4):544-7.

Birk, P. E., T. D. Blydt-Hansen, A. B. Dart, L. M. Kaita, C. Proulx, and G. Taylor. 2007. Low incidence of adverse events in outpatient pediatric renal allograft biopsies. Pediatr Transplant 11 (2):196-200.

Broyles, S., P. T. Katzmarzyk, S. R. Srinivasan, W. Chen, C. Bouchard, D. S. Freedman, and G. S. Berenson. 2010. The pediatric obesity epidemic continues unabated in Bogalusa, Louisiana. Pediatrics 125 (5):900-5.

Caione, P., S. Micali, S. Rinaldi, N. Capozza, A. Lais, E. Matarazzo, G. Maturo, and F. Micali. 2000. Retroperitoneal laparoscopy for renal biopsy in children. J Urol 164 (3 Pt 2):1080-2; discussion 1083.

Castoldi, M. C., R. M. Del Moro, M. L. D'Urbano, F. Ferrario, M. T. Porri, P. Maldifassi, G. D'Amico, and F. Casolo. 1994. Sonography after renal biopsy: assessment of its role in 230 consecutive cases. Abdom Imaging 19 (1):72-7.

Chesney, D. S., B. H. Brouhard, and R. J. Cunningham. 1996. Safety and cost effectiveness of pediatric percutaneous renal biopsy. Pediatr Nephrol 10 (4):493-5.

Cravero, J. P., G. T. Blike, M. Beach, S. M. Gallagher, J. H. Hertzog, J. E. Havidich, and B. Gelman. 2006. Incidence and nature of adverse events during pediatric sedation/anesthesia for procedures outside the operating room: report from the Pediatric Sedation Research Consortium. Pediatrics 118 (3):1087-96.

Davis, I. D., W. Oehlenschlager, M. A. O'Riordan, and E. D. Avner. 1998. Pediatric renal biopsy: should this procedure be performed in an outpatient setting? Pediatr Nephrol 12 (2):96-100.

Durkan, A. M., T. J. Beattie, A. Howatson, J. H. McColl, and I. J. Ramage. 2006. Renal transplant biopsy specimen adequacy in a paediatric population. Pediatr Nephrol 21 (2):265-9.

Fowler, S. M., V. Kon, L. Ma, W. O. Richards, A. B. Fogo, and T. E. Hunley. 2009. Obesity-related focal and segmental glomerulosclerosis: normalization of proteinuria in an adolescent after bariatric surgery. Pediatr Nephrol 24 (4):851-5.

Hussain, F., M. Mallik, S. D. Marks, and A. R. Watson. 2010. Renal biopsies in children: current practice and audit of outcomes. Nephrol Dial Transplant 25 (2):485-9.

Hussain, F., A. R. Watson, J. Hayes, and J. Evans. 2003. Standards for renal biopsies: comparison of inpatient and day care procedures. Pediatr Nephrol 18 (1):53-6.

Kamitsuji, H., K. Yoshioka, and H. Ito. 1999. Percutaneous renal biopsy in children: survey of pediatric nephrologists in Japan. Pediatr Nephrol 13 (8):693-6.

Kersnik Levart, T., A. Kenig, J. Buturovic Ponikvar, D. Ferluga, M. Avgustin Cavic, and R. B. Kenda. 2001. Real-time ultrasound-guided renal biopsy with a biopsy gun in children: safety and efficacy. Acta Paediatr 90 (12):1394-7.

Lau, K. K., G. L. Berg, and L. Butani. 2009. Financial implications of pediatric outpatient renal biopsies: a single-center experience. J Nephrol 22 (1):69-74.

Luque Mialdea, R., R. Martin-Crespo Izquierdo, L. Diaz, A. Fernandez, D. Morales, and J. Cebrian. 2006. [Renal biopsy through a retroperitoneoscopic approach: our experience in 53 pediatric patients]. Arch Esp Urol 59 (8):799-803.

Mahajan, V., D. Suri, A. Saxena, and R. Nada. 2010. Should ultrasound guided percutaneous renal biopsy in children be done in a day care setting? Indian J Nephrol 20 (1): 21-4.

Mason, K. P., H. Padua, P. J. Fontaine, and D. Zurakowski. 2009. Radiologist-supervised ketamine sedation for solid organ biopsies in children and adolescents. AJR Am J Roentgenol 192 (5):1261-5.

Mendelssohn, D. C., and E. H. Cole. 1995. Outcomes of percutaneous kidney biopsy, including those of solitary native kidneys. Am J Kidney Dis 26 (4):580-5.

Mukhtar, Z., H. Steinbrecher, R. D. Gilbert, and P. V. Deshpande. 2005. Laparoscopic renal biopsy in obese children. Pediatr Nephrol 20 (4):495-8.

Ogborn, M. R., and P. C. Grimm. 1992. Pediatric renal biopsy in the ambulatory care environment. Pediatr Nephrol 6 (3):311-2.

Piotto, G. H., M. C. Moraes, D. M. Malheiros, L. B. Saldanha, and V. H. Koch. 2008. Percutaneous ultrasound-guided renal biopsy in children - safety, efficacy, indications and renal pathology findings: 14-year Brazilian university hospital experience. Clin Nephrol 69 (6):417-24.

Simckes, A. M., D. L. Blowey, K. M. Gyves, and U. S. Alon. 2000. Success and safety of same-day kidney biopsy in children and adolescents. Pediatr Nephrol 14 (10-11): 946-52.

Sweeney, C., D. F. Geary, D. Hebert, L. Robinson, and V. Langlois. 2006. Outpatient pediatric renal transplant biopsy--is it safe? Pediatr Transplant 10 (2):159-61.

Vidhun, J., J. Masciandro, L. Varich, O. Salvatierra, Jr., and M. Sarwal. 2003. Safety and risk stratification of percutaneous biopsies of adult-sized renal allografts in infant and older pediatric recipients. Transplantation 76 (3):552-7.

Webb, N. J., J. K. Pereira, P. G. Chait, and D. F. Geary. 1994. Renal biopsy in children: comparison of two techniques. Pediatr Nephrol 8 (4):486-8.

Whittier, W. L., and S. M. Korbet. 2004. Timing of complications in percutaneous renal biopsy. J Am Soc Nephrol 15 (1):142-7.

# 3

# Skin Biopsy as Alternative for Renal Biopsy in Acute Renal Failure and Suspected Cholesterol Emboli Syndrome

Martijn B. A. van Doorn and Tijmen J. Stoof
*Dermatologists, Department of Dermatology, VU Medical Centre, Amsterdam The Netherlands*

## 1. Introduction

A 74-year old man with complaints of malaise was diagnosed with acute renal failure of unknown cause and was referred to our outpatient clinic because of bluish-red maculae in a reticular pattern on his forefeet and toes of unclear duration. Six weeks prior to the onset of his general symptoms he had undergone an endovascular aorta repair (EVAR) procedure. A lesional skin biopsy was taken and revealed multiple cholesterol emboli. The cholesterol emboli syndrome is a complication of atherosclerosis caused by cholesterol crystal embolization. These cholesterol crystals originate from atherosclerotic plaques of the large arteries and can migrate to various organs like the kidneys and the skin where they occlude small arteries causing ischemia and tissue damage. Often precipitating factors like vascular procedures, cardiac or aorta surgery, or treatment with anticoagulant or thrombolytic drugs can be identified. With our cutaneous findings an invasive renal biopsy could be avoided.

## 2. Case

A 74-year old man was referred to our Dermatology outpatient clinic by a nephrologist because of non-painful bluish-red discoloration of his feet and toes of unclear duration. He had been suffering from general malaise for some days and the laboratory results in the emergency department had revealed acute renal insufficiency of unknown cause. Six weeks prior to the emergence of symptoms he was treated for an aneurysm of the infrarenal aorta with a so-called EVAR (Endovascular Aneurysm Repair or Endovascular Aortic Repair) procedure.

On physical examination we observed livid-erythematous maculae in a reticular pattern on the distal end of both feet and toes (figure 1). The pulsations of the tibialis posterior and dorsalis pedis arteries were present, and there was a normal capillary refill.

Laboratory results showed a creatinine of 601 μmol/L, urea of 359 mmol/L, an erythrocyte sedimentation rate (ESR) of 70 mm/hour, a white blood cell (WBC) count of 8.4 $x10^9$/L, with eosinophils of $0.59x10^9$/L, and thrombocytes of $161x10^9$/L.

We performed a 3 mm lesional skin biopsy (from a blanched area) which showed compact hyperkeratosis and a normally structured epidermis and dermis. However, in the dermis we observed a small artery with some intimal hyperplasia containing a number of needle-shaped

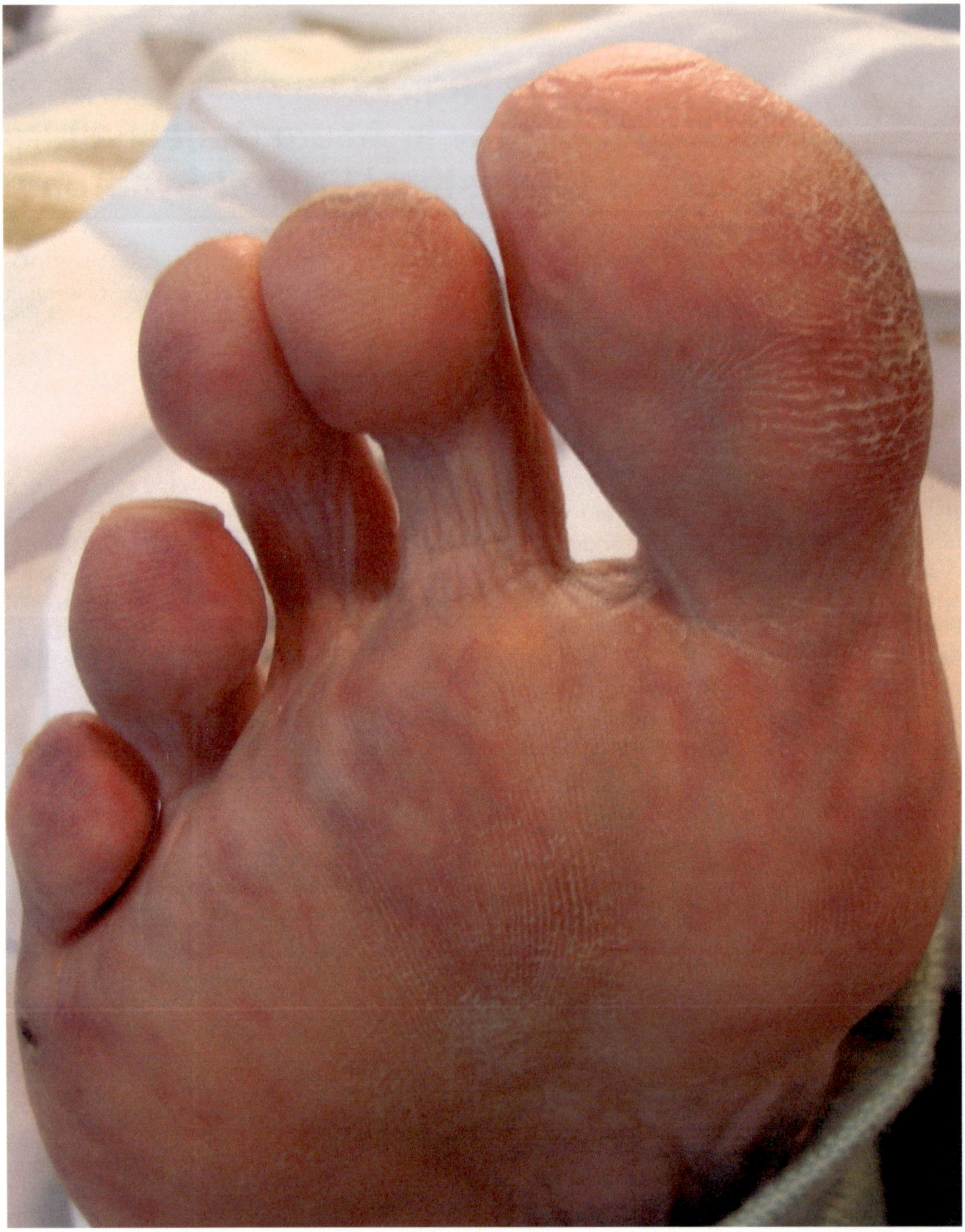

Fig. 1. Livid-erythematous maculae in a reticular pattern on the plantar surface of the distal forefoot and toes.

spaces which occluded the lumen (figure 2). Herewith a histological diagnosis of cholesterol emboli syndrome was made.

## 3. Discussion

The cholesterol emboli syndrome (or cholesterol embolization syndrome) is a complication of atherosclerosis as a result of cholesterol crystal embolization. These cholesterol crystals originate from atherosclerotic plaques in the larger arteries and can migrate to various organs like the skin, the kidneys, gastro-intestinal system and central nervous system. Because these small crystals are hydrophobic and low in weight they can travel swiftly through the blood vessels until they strand in the arterial bifurcations or when the calibre of the arterial lumen decreases. This means that they will usually occlude small peripheral arteries leading to localized ischaemia which can result in (sometimes severe) end-organ damage. The cholesterol emboli syndrome primarily affects patients above 60 years of age with two or more risk factors for atherosclerosis.(1, 2)

The incidence of the syndrome in the general population, is low. For example, in the Dutch population, an average rate of 6.2 cases per million people per year has been reported.(3) However, in high risk patients, such as those undergoing cardiac catheterization, incidence rates up to 1.4% have been reported.(4)

In post-mortem studies, cholesterol emboli were observed in up to 20% of patients older than 60 years of age with a history of atherosclerotic disease.(5) Considering the relatively low rate of the clinical diagnosis of cholesterol emboli (even in high risk patients groups), it thus appears that the diagnosis is frequently missed.

Since the disintegration of (ulcerated) atherosclerotic plaques in the arterial vessel wall is the cause of cholesterol embolization, affected patients generally have severe (but sometimes subclinical) atherosclerotic disease. Although the syndrome may appear spontaneously without any clearly established predisposing etiological factor, there are three distinctive clinical settings that are known to increase the risk for cholesterol embolization. The first is prior arterial or coronary catheterisation (as for our patient) and cardiac or aorta surgery, which may disrupt an atherosclerotic plaque, leading to emboli within hours to several weeks of the procedure. The second is prolonged treatment with anticoagulant drugs, which slowly dissolves the clot that strengthens the brittle atherosclerotic plaque exposing eroded areas of the plaque to the shear stress of the arterial blood flow. The anticoagulant drug-induced syndrome of cholesterol emboli usually occurs within 1 to 2 months of initiating therapy. This 'warfarin blue toe syndrome' is not limited to anticoagulation with warfarin and can occur after treatment with other (classes of) anticoagulant drugs. The third setting in which cholesterol embolization can occur is when thrombolytic therapy is initiated for acute myocardial infarction or stroke. In this case, the embolization process may occur within hours to days of thrombolytic therapy.(6) A summary of the most common predisposing factors for cholesterol emboli syndrome is presented in table 1.(1, 7-10)

In our case the referring nephrologist made a provisional diagnosis of acute renal insufficiency due to cholesterol embolization related to the prior EVAR procedure after excluding all other possible causes. When performing an EVAR procedure of the infra-renal aorta, the catheters usually reach above the renal artery branches.

Manipulation with the endovascular catheter and stent in this area can cause small fragments (emboli) to detach from a friable atherosclerotic plaque in the arterial wall. The nephrologist sought support for his provisional diagnosis in the accompanying skin symptoms since the emboli can also migrate to the peripheral small arteries in the skin resulting in the typical reticular vascular pattern. With the demonstration of cholesterol emboli in a skin biopsy a more invasive ('gold standard') renal biopsy could be avoided.

In the cholesterol emboli syndrome the clinical symptoms may include fever, weight loss, myalgias, altered mental status and a rapid onset of arterial hypertension. Transient ischemic attacks, strokes, renal failure, gastrointestinal ulcerations and hemorrhagic pancreatitis may also occur. Patients with extensive organ involvement can have significant morbidity, and may even die from complications of the embolization process.(6) Generally, the primary site of cholesterol embolization is the kidney, followed by the skin and gastrointestinal tract.(3) Skin manifestations are present in 35 to 100% of patients and are often the first clinical symptom of the cholesterol emboli syndrome. Their clinical presentation is variable ranging from the symmetrical livedo reticularis, acrocyanosis, ulcerations, and purpura to severe leg and/or foot pain and focal digital ischaemia ("blue toe syndrome")(11). Findings of a relatively large English case study included: livedo reticularis (49%), multiple sites of peripheral gangrene (35%), cyanosis (28%), ulceration (17%), nodules (10%) and (retiform) purpura (9%).(5) Because these figures originate from a review article that also included patients in whom the diagnosis was made post-mortem (41%), it probably underestimated the true incidence of cutaneous findings in patients suffering from the cholesterol emboli syndrome.(6) This point is corroborated by a study of eight patients with acute renal insufficiency of unknown cause, whose history suggested cholesterol emboli. On careful examination, all eight were found to have prior unrecognized livedo reticularis, which on histological sections confirmed the diagnosis of cholesterol emboli.(12) In two of these patients, the livedo reticularis was visible in the standing position, but disappeared when the patients were placed in the supine position. Retiform purpura are usually a purpuric accentuation of the livedo reticularis pattern, and therefore may have been included as livedo reticularis in some reports. This may explain the relatively low observation rate of retiform purpura in the study by Falanga et al. Livedo reticularis is ususally found in the lower extremities but upper extremity lesions may also occur if the atherosclerotic plaque is located in the aortic arch.(6)

The skin manifestations are often (but not always) painful and peripheral pulsations are generally intact. Elevations in the ESR, serum creatinine, BUN and amylase and transient elevations of creatine kinase, leukocytosis, thrombocytopenia as well as decreased complement levels are frequent associated findings, but are not always present.(5, 13) Peripheral blood eosinophilia is common, occurring in up to 80% of confirmed cases, and may be related to generation of the complement component C5.(13) Other reported laboratory findings include heme-positive urine and/or stool.

The acute onset of peripheral livedo reticularis (and even more so if retiform purpura are also present) should raise the suspicion of cholesterol or oxalate embolization. The occurrence of oxalate emboli is rare and recognized histologically as birefringent yellow-brown crystal depositions in and around arteries of deep reticular dermis and subcutis. Oxalate crystal embolization is an uncommon event, usually occurring in association with

primary hyperoxaluria. Primary hyperoxaluria is caused by a rare metabolic disorders of increased oxalic acid production or increased intestinal absorption. Hyperoxalemia will eventually lead to calcium oxalate deposition in various tissues.(14, 15) The history of kidney stones in a patient with sudden-onset livedo reticularis or retiform purpura should point in the direction of hyperoxaluria as a key diagnostic possibility. In addition to emboli from acute bacterial or fungal endocarditis (which are generally inflammatory in nature), cutaneous emboli or thrombi have been occasionally reported in patients with atrial myxomas, marantic endocarditis, crystal globulins and hypereosinophilic syndrome. Emboli resulting from these disorders may produce retiform purpura, but cutaneous manifestations may vary.(6) Other differential diagnoses one should consider include (small vessel) vasculitis (kidney and skin involvement) and perniones ("chilblains").(16)
A lesional (large) skin biopsy or elliptical excision of a blanched area of the livedo reticularis is diagnostic in 92% of cases, provided the sample includes tissue from the mid- to deep reticular dermis.(1) Areas of retiform purpura usually provide excellent diagnostic findings in punch biopsy specimens and should be the first choice for biopsy when present.(6) Frozen sections show birefringent cholesterol crystals and with the Schulz staining blue-green coloured crystals can be observed.(17) However, in fixated material the cholesterol crystals are dissolved during the laboratory workup and the negative image remains in the form of needle-shaped optical empty spaces (figure 2), often in association with thrombi.(18) Neutrophils, eosinophils and mononuclear cells may be present in the arterial wall within 24-48 hours in an experimentally produced cholesterol embolus. This is followed by the invasion of multinucleated histiocytes within 3 to 6 days, and sometimes intimal fibrosis. Lesions of different ages can be observed in the same patient, which is consistent with repeated showers of emboli.(6)
The cholesterol emboli syndrome is associated with a very high mortality rate (up to 80%).(1, 2) The prognosis depends on the degree of organ damage and severity of the underlying vascular condition. Treatment with aspirin appears to have a beneficial effect and in patients suffering from aortal atherosclerosis regression of the atherosclerotic plaque size was observed upon treatment with statins.(19) Furthermore, discontinuation of anticoagulation, initiation of anticoagulation in patients with severe renal damage, corticosteroid therapy, and infusion of the prostacyclin analogue iloprost have all been proposed as being effective in sporadic patients, but no therapeutic gold standard exists.(13, 18, 20) Additional measures include supportive treatment like hydration, antihypertensive therapy and haemodialysis.(21) Our patient needed long term haemodialysis; after approximately one and half year spontaneous recovery of renal function occurred, allowing discontinuation of haemodialysis.

## 4. Conclusion

In summary, we believe that in all patients presenting with the classical triad of peripheral livedo reticularis, acute renal failure, and eosinophilia, the cholesterol emboli syndrome should be suspected. An invasive vascular procedure or recent initiation of anticoagulant or thrombolytic treatment in the months preceding onset of symptoms is an important diagnostic clue. A proper (large) lesional skin biopsy can confirm the diagnosis and therewith a more invasive renal biopsy can be avoided.

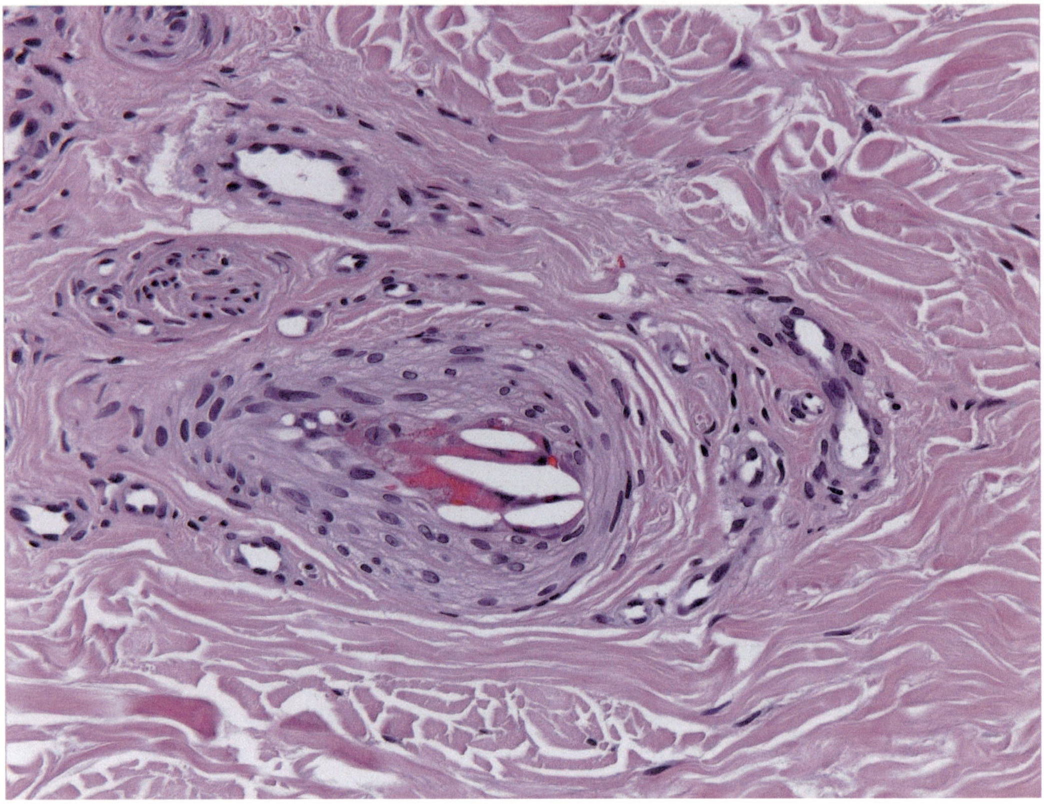

Fig. 2. Histological slide showing a small dermal artery branch with needle-shaped optical empty spaces as a result of the cholesterol crystals that dissolved during tissue processing (HE 20x).

| |
|---|
| The cholesterol emboli syndrome should be suspected if the following items apply:<br>• confirmed atherosclerotic lesions in large vessels<br>• history of potential triggering predisposing factors (see below)<br>• typical clinical presentation, including renal failure, livedo reticularis or ulceration of the toes with intact peripheral arterial pulsations<br>• exclusion of small vessel vasculitis<br>• exclusion of diseases causing infective emboli (e.g. endocarditis)<br>• typical histopathological findings; evidence of cholesterol crystals (optical empty spaces) in the lumen of small arteries accompanied by an inflammatory cell infiltrate<br><br>Potential predisposing factors for the cholesterol emboli syndrome:<br>• angioplasty<br>• vascular surgery<br>• any invasive vascular procedure (including angiography)<br>• prolonged anticoagulant therapy<br>• fibrinolytic therapy |

Table 1. Diagnosis of the cholesterol emboli syndrome

## 5. References


[1] Fine MJ, Kapoor W, Falanga V. Cholesterol crystal embolization: a review of 221 cases in the English literature. *Angiology* 1987 Oct,38(10), 769-784.

[2] Hyman BT, Landas SK, Ashman RF, Schelper RL, Robinson RA. Warfarin-related purple toes syndrome and cholesterol microembolization. *Am J Med* 1987 Jun,82(6), 1233-1237.

[3] Moolenaar W, Lamers CB. Cholesterol crystal embolization in the Netherlands. *Arch Intern Med* 1996 Mar 25,156(6), 653-657.

[4] Fukumoto Y, Tsutsui H, Tsuchihashi M, Masumoto A, Takeshita A. The incidence and risk factors of cholesterol embolization syndrome, a complication of cardiac catheterization: a prospective study. *J Am Coll Cardiol* 2003 Jul 16,42(2), 211-216.

[5] Falanga V, Fine MJ, Kapoor WN. The cutaneous manifestations of cholesterol crystal embolization. *Arch Dermatol* 1986 Oct,122(10), 1194-1198.

[6] Bolognia et al. Disorders of occlusion by emboli. Dermatology. Second ed. Mosby, Elsevier, 2009.

[7] Bittl JA. Cholesterol embolization syndrome: unifying principles. *Catheter Cardiovasc Interv* 2000 Nov,51(3), 326-327.

[8] Funabiki K, Masuoka H, Shimizu H, et al. Cholesterol crystal embolization (CCE) after cardiac catheterization: a case report and a review of 36 cases in the Japanese literature. *Jpn Heart J* 2003 Sep,44(5), 767-774.

[9] Hirano Y, Ishikawa K. Cholesterol embolization syndrome: how to recognize and prevent this potentially catastrophic iatrogenic disease. *Intern Med* 2005 Dec,44(12), 1209-1210.

[10] Meyrier A. Cholesterol crystal embolism: diagnosis and treatment. *Kidney Int* 2006 Apr,69(8), 1308-1312.

[11] Nijhof IS, Majoie IM, Dijkhorst-Oei LT, Bousema MT. [Blue toe syndrome; a sign of end-arterial occlusion]. *Ned Tijdschr Geneeskd* 2007 Jun 9,151(23), 1261-1267.

[12] Chaudhary K, Wall BM, Rasberry RD. Livedo reticularis: an underutilized diagnostic clue in cholesterol embolization syndrome. *Am J Med Sci* 2001 May,321(5), 348-351.

[13] Lawson JM. Cholesterol crystal embolization: more common than we thought? *Am J Gastroenterol* 2001 Dec,96(12), 3230-3232.

[14] Marconi V, Mofid MZ, McCall C, Eckman I, Nousari HC. Primary hyperoxaluria: report of a patient with livedo reticularis and digital infarcts. *J Am Acad Dermatol* 2002 Feb,46(2 Suppl Case Reports), S16-S18.

[15] Spiers EM, Sanders DY, Omura EF. Clinical and histologic features of primary oxalosis. *J Am Acad Dermatol* 1990 May,22(5 Pt 2), 952-956.

[16] Peat DS, Mathieson PW. Cholesterol emboli may mimic systemic vasculitis. *BMJ* 1996 Aug 31,313(7056), 546-547.

[17] Pennington M, Yeager J, Skelton H, Smith KJ. Cholesterol embolization syndrome: cutaneous histopathological features and the variable onset of symptoms in patients with different risk factors. *Br J Dermatol* 2002 Mar,146(3), 511-517.

[18] Kang K, Botella R, White CR, Jr. Subtle clues to the diagnosis of cholesterol embolism. *Am J Dermatopathol* 1996 Aug,18(4), 380-384.

[19] Sharifkazemi MB, Zamirian M, Aslani A. Blue toe syndrome. *J Cardiovasc Med (Hagerstown )* 2007 Nov,8(11), 975-976.

[20] Elinav E, Chajek-Shaul T, Stern M. Improvement in cholesterol emboli syndrome after iloprost therapy. *BMJ* 2002 Feb 2,324(7332), 268-269.
[21] Belenfant X, Meyrier A, Jacquot C. Supportive treatment improves survival in multivisceral cholesterol crystal embolism. *Am J Kidney Dis* 1999 May,33(5), 840-850.

# Part 2

# Biopsy Handling, Processing and Pathologic Interpretation

# 4

# Renal Biopsy Interpretation

Sakineh Amoueian and Armin Attaranzadeh
*Mashhad University of Medical Sciences*
*Iran*

## 1. Introduction

The kidney is a mysterious organ that makes urine from Shiraz wine (1). It has a role in excreting waste products, regulating body fluids and balancing soluble ions.
The focus of this chapter is the gross anatomy and histology of the kidney renal biopsy techniques and diferential diagnosis of the important renal disease and interpretation of these.

## 2. Anatomy

The kidneys are two bean shape organs within peritoneum located between12th thoracic rib to 3rd lumbar vertebrae. A space named perirenal, with fatty tissue, surrounds each kidney (2). In the anterior, there are the pancreas, duodenal loop, ascending and descending colon, and the hepatic, splenic, and proximal superior mesenteric arteries. In the posterior, there is fat but no organs. The kidneys exhibit craniocaudal movement of 1.9 to 4.1 cm during respiration (4). Each organ weights 125 to 170 gr in males and 115 to 150 gr in females(4). Both together represent 0.04% of total body weight. Kidney weight correlates best with body surface area, whereas age, sex, and race do not influence it (5). The dimensions of the kidney are 11-12 cm (length), 5-7.5 cm (width) and 2.5-3 cm (thickness). Renal volume can increase or decrease by 15% to 40% with major fluctuations in blood pressure, intravascular volume, or interstitial expansion by edema (6). The renal artery divides into anterior and posterior arteries which in turn give off segmental arteries, which supply the apical, upper, middle, lower and posterior segmental regions of the parenchyma (7). After branching to anterior and posterior divisions at the hilus, the main renal artery gives off interlobar (between lobes and extend to corticomedullary junction), arcuate (between cortex and medulla) and interlobular arteries (extend cortex to capsule) respectively. Afferent arterioles are branched from interlobular arteries which make glomerulus and efferent arterioles after glomerulus, forms peritubular or interstitial capillaries around tubules. Efferent arterioles form vasa recta which supplies the outer and inner medulla (8). Multiple anastomoses between capillaries within the lobule create a capillary meshwork. The vasa recta and peritubular capillaries form interlobular veins and with a similar pattern as arteries leave the kidneys as renal veins (8).
On the cut surface of kidney, there is a pale outer region (cortex) and a darker inner region (medulla) .The medulla is divided to 18 pyramids. Each pyramid base is located at the corticomedullary junction, and apex has 20-70 small openings representing the distal ends of

collecting ducts (9). The renal cortex forms a 1.0-cm layer beneath the renal capsule and extends down between the renal pyramids forming the columns of Bertin (10).
Renal lobe is composed of a pyramid with its surrounding cortical parenchyma (11). The renal pelvis is an extension of upper ureter. A detailed anatomy description of kidney is provided elsewhere (12).

## 3. Nephrons

The functional and basic unit of the kidney is the nephron which is composed of renal corpuscle (glomerulus and Bowman's capsule), and cylindrical epithelial-lined tubular component (proximal tubule, Henle`s loop and distal tubule).
Tubular part of the nephron has complex spatial and topographic relationship with its microvasculature and demonstrates sequential variation in its cellular constitution depending on the function (10). The glomeruli are located in cortex. There are two main groups of nephrons: those with a short loop of Henle and those with long loop. The length depends on the glomerulus location. The superficial and midcortical nephrons have short loops (85%) and the juxtamedullary and some deep midcortical ones, have long loops (15%) (10). Henle`s loop is located in the medulla and is connected proximally to proximal tubule just after glomerulus, and distally to distal tubule. These two groups of tubules are located in the cortex. The distal tubule then connects to collecting ducts ending in renal papilla. The Henle`s loop and collecting ducts are arranged in radial form from papilla to cortex. The number of Nephrons depends on weight at birth and age , meaning that in low birth weight is the nephrons weight less than normal with increased risk of hypertension (13). The estimated number of nephrons is 400-800 thousands (14). Even a broader range of 227000-1825000 has been reported (15).

## 4.Kidney histology

### 4.1 Glomerulus

Malpigi first described the glomerulus and demonstrated its relation with the renal vasculature (16). Latter, Bowman showed and presented glomerulus, in detail (17,18). Glomerulus is used to refer to the glomerulus tuft and Bowman's capsule. Bowman's capsule is the dilated part of the proximal tubule (19). Glomerulus is a vascular tuft lined by endothelium and is supported by a mesangium that contains cells and a matrix material and glomerular capillary loop basal lamina. The term GBM (glomerular basement membrane) is used for capillary loop components observable by light microscopy that includes cellular elements, podocyte and endothelial cells and the matrix component of basal lamina (10). Bowman's capsule (BC) is a thick connective tissue barrier between the glomerular filtrate within Bowman's space and the interstitium (20). It is approximately spherical and lined along its inner surface by parietal epithelial cells.
The vasculature unit is covered by epithelial cells which form the visceral layer of Bowman's capsule. There is another epithelial layer named parietal epithelium that is continuous with visceral layer and make a pouch space between the two layers and surrounds the glomerular vascular tuft. The glomerulus has a round figure and 200 μm diameter (21). There are some variations in size depending physiologic conditions (22). Lobularity of glomerulus is not prominent in normal kidney.
Cellularity assessment of glomerulus mesangium is obtained in sections of 2-4 μm thickness. The normal mesangial cell number is one or two cells per matrix area (10). Generally there are less than 4 cells in mesangial region of far from vascular pole.

Endothelial cells have eosinophilic cytoplasm and round to oval nucleoli which project into capillary lumen. Their surfaces have a negative charge (23). Endothelial cells completely line the inner surface of the glomerular capillary loops and have fenestrated regions and nonfenestrated regions. The fenestrations are round to oval and measure approximately 70 to 100 nm in diameter. These fenestrations are open and lack a diaphragm (10). Many molecules are produced by endothelial cells that function in the immune response and coagulation system, and also mediate vasoconstriction and vasodilatation (24).

The mesangium supports glomerulus capillary tuft which regulate glomerular filtration by contraction properties (25). These cells have a phagocytic function that clears debris from this region (26). The mesangial matrix is structurally similar to basement membrane of glomerulus. This can be seen by Periodic Acid Schiff (PAS) and silver staining.

Endothelial cells and visceral epithelial cells have a common basement membrane of 310-380 nm thickness (27). It is thicker in males than females and has variation depending physiologic conditions (28).

Visceral epithelial cells are located outside of glomerulus capillary wall, bulging to Bowman's space between the two epitheliums. They have eosinophilic cytoplasm and processes that surround glomerulus and capillaries and divide to foot processes afterwards. The processes have contraction function related to actin, myosin and α-actinin in their cytoplasm (28). The foot processes are arranged on basement membrane with a 25-60 nm distance from each other and called filtration split . These cells have a negative charge (29).

The parietal epithelium of Bowman's space is simple squamous layer. These cells have 0.1-0.3 µm height which increases around nucleus region. The epithelial cells have a basement membrane on Bowman's capsule.

Golgi observed a unit named juxtaglomerular apparatus in vascular pole of glomerulus (30). The juxtaglomerular apparatus is a complex structure composed of specialized epithelial cells, the macula densa, vascular components (including portions of the afferent and efferent arterioles), and extraglomerular cells known as lacis cells (31,32). Rennin and angiotansin II are produced in these cells (33). The macula densa consists of a plaque of specialized tubular cells, polarized to the glomerular side of the tubule and projecting into the lumens that are taller than collecting tubules cell with an apical nucleus, and short surface microvilli, but lack lateral interdigitation characteristic of other cells of the thick ascending limb (10).

### 4.2 Proximal tubule

This unit is about 14 mm long and is composed of a convoluted and a straight portion (21). The convoluted part forms some coils near its glomerulus in the cortex and then goes to medulla and forms straight part. In histologic section of cortex, the major part of tissue is composed of proximal convoluted tubules. In biopsy sections, collapsed lumens of these tubules are seen (34). Proximal tubule cells are cuboid or short columnar with eosinophilic cytoplasm, often granular and a round nucleus in the center .

These cells have many mitochondria located at the cell base. In apex of cells, there is a brush like border which can vary in different parts of proximal tubules.

The proximal tubules' task is reabsorbtion of the majority (60%) of glomerular ultrafiltrate. This includes sodium, chloride, glucose, amino acids, bicarbonate and water.

### 4.3 Henle`s loop

Between proximal and distal tubule, there is a U-shape unit named Henle`s loop. Resting on medulla, Henle's loop can be long or short depending on the glomerulus location. Their cells are flat, 1-2 μm thick with nuclei bulged into lumen and with attenuated cytoplasm with no brush border which creates a resemblance to the endothelial lining of a capillary . Henle`s loop have a role in concentration of urine. The transporting of water and chloride sodium in this loop is passive.

### 4.4 Distal tubule

This unit connects to ascending part of Henle`s loop and is composed of thick part of the loop, distal convoluted tubule and macula densa as described in juxtaglomerular apparatus. The thick part of Henle`s loop has cuboidal cells with eosinophilic cytoplasm and round nuclei, often bulging into lumen .These cells have many mitochondria with active transport of materials especially sodium chloride. In contrast to proximal tubule, these cells have less height, less eosinophilic property and no brush border.

After this part, distal convoluted tubule begins which is the terminal part of distal tubules. These cells are similar but taller than thick ascending cells and have round nuclei, without brush border and indistinct lateral cell border and less eosinophilic than proximal tubules. Their lumen is often open . Their function is reabsorbtion of chloride sodium.

In the end of distal convoluted tubules, a transitional segment begins which connects these tubules to the collecting duct system.

Most nephrons connect to initial collecting tubules (35). About 40% of nephrons connect to arcades which have three nephron attachments and every cortical collecting tubule, connects to 11 nephrons (9). The collecting duct system has t similar cells to distal convoluting tubules and cortical collecting ducts.

### 4.5 Collecting duct

This unit begins near the end of distal convoluted tubules in the cortex and goes to the tip of papilla. This system has three part in cortex, outer medulla and inner medulla which are covered by different epithelial cells (36).

The cortical part has cuboidal cells with round central nucleus, distinct lateral cell border, open lumen and no brush border .There are two distinct cells in this unit: principal cells and intercalated cells, which are difficult to differentiate in light microscope, but the former has a clear cytoplasm.

Principal cells function, is potassium secretion into the cortical collecting duct.

Intercalated cells are darker than principal cells and are interspersed in lining of collecting duct. They have many mitochondria and also carbonic anhydrase II enzyme. The cortical part of collecting duct involves in acidification of urine (37). The outer medullary part of collecting duct is lined by similar cells to cortical part, only taller. This part is also involved in urine acidification. In the last part of collecting duct, named inner medullary collecting duct, there is an increase in diameter and height of epithelial cells as the duct is descending (38). It means that cuboidal cells gradually turn to columnar cells. This part plays a role in urine concentration.

### 4.6 Other parts of kidney tissue

The kidney artery distribution was introduced in the first pages of this chapter. Interstitium of the kidney is about 5-20% of cortex (39). This part is composed of extracellular matrix and interstitial cells, but cannot be seen in light microscopy (40). This part is increased in medulla and reaches 10-40% of medulla (41). In this region, it could be seen as gelatinous

appearance. The interstitial cells are involved in producing extracellular matrix and some endocrine substances such as those function as antihypertensive (42).
Lymphatic vessels are not prominent in light microscope view. They are originated close to interlobular arteries and make arcuate and interlobar lymphaticvessels which drain into lymph vessels locates at kidney hilus. The lymphatic vessels are believed that exist only in cortex (43,44).
The kidney nerves are originated from celiac plexus (45) and accompany vessels in cortex and medulla (46).

## 5. Renal biopsy techniques

Renal biopsy has an important role in diagnosis, prognosis, and response to therapy.
The first renal biopsy was taken about one century ago in the United States. Widespread introduction of renal biopsy for clinical use, began in 1950s (47). Renal biposy has been used to identify pathologic changes in different clinical conditions and recognize renal diseases with similar manifestations.

## 6. Requisition/referral form

In every medical center it should be a form designed for pathologic specimens. Over the biopsy procedure this form should be completed by the physician and sent to pathology laboratory. Minimum informations required in these forms include patient's full name, date of birth, sex, race, date of biopsy, clinical problem(s), type of insurance, address, phone number, emergency situation, fixative fluid, biopsy location and side, physician's name and phone.
Specimens should be labeled with patient's name and a second identifier like father's name or date of birth.

## 7. Biopsy technique

Renal biopsies are taken by nephrologists or radiologist by True-cut or biopsy gun under local anesthesia. It is performed in prone position for native kidneys and in supine position for transplanted kidneys. Nowadays, biopsies can be obtained by ultrasound or computed tomography guided (47). The use of biopsy gun, guided by ultrasound has more safety and yield (48,49,50).
Each glomerulus has a 200-250 μm diameter, therefore, the needle should be selected properly. 14-guage, 16-guage, and 18-guage needles have internal diameter of 900-1000, 600-700, 300-400 μm, respectively. It is better to use 16 or 14 guage needle as the use of 18 guage needle can result in narrower and fragmented tissue.
In renal mass biopsies, the 18-21 gauge needles can be used (51).
Biopsies from subcapsular region show nonspecific sclerosis. The optimum location for biopsy is juxtamedullary, because these glomeruli are the earliest ones involved in focal segmental glomerulosclerosis (52).
Other renal biopsy techniques include transjugular retrograde approach by catheter (53,54), laparascopic techniques (55), and open laparatomic biopsy.

## 8. Risks

There is little discomfort experienced by patients in renal biopsies although it is a painful procedure. The most common complication, is microscopic hematuria (almost all patients).

Gross hematuria is occurred in 5-7% of patients (56). There are some other complications including perinephric hematuria, arteriovenous fistula(57), ileus, renal pelvic rupture and entrance into neighbor organs. Other complications are the need for transfusion (less than 1%), renal loss (less than 0.1%), and death (very rare) ((47,58,59). Ultrasound guided biopsy and automatic biopsy devices are helpful techniques, but do not decrease the complications (57,59). Overall, renal biopsy is considered a safe medical approach (47,60,61).

## 9. Gross inspection

The specimen should be handled and processed with great care. It should be moved by a wooden stick like toothpick and forceps use is forbidden because of crush artifact (62). After renal biopsy is obtained, it should be placed in a drop of saline and examined under microscope for its color and appearance.

The reddish pin points or hemispheres on tissue surface are the glomeruli, which are not observable in conditions such as fibrosis and hypercellular bloodless glomeruli, (63). The biopsy should not be dried after taking the tissue and should be divided as soon as possible. The cylindrical tissue should be divided and fixed in proper solutions for light microscopy, immunofluorescence study and electron microscopy. Longitudinal sectioning is not advised, because the needle diameter is changed to narrower ones.

A cutting protocol for needle biopsy in the first sample is cutting 1-2 mm of each end side and fixing in glutaraldehyde for electron microscopy, two third of the remaining tissue from cortical side for light microscopy , and one third of the tissue from cortical side for immunofluorescence study (63). If there is a second sample, similar cutting is done for electron microscopy, but one third of cortical side is taken for immunofluorescence study and two third of medullary side for light microscopy (62).

Repeated biopsies, need only light microscopy sample (52).

If the specimen is small, immunofluorescence study might be omitted and if it is very small, it is better to process entire sample for electron microscopy(63)

The renal biopsies are studied in 4-5 μm sections using different stains. The main staining material for the biopsies is Hematoxilin & Eosin Other stains commonly used in renal biopsies are: Periodic Acid Schiff, Methenamin silver, Masson trichrome, Congo red and reticulin.

## 10. Fixatives

For light microscopy, neutral buffered formaldehyde is used. It is suitable for immunohistochemical study and also molecular procedures (62). Bouin`s fluid, mercury based fixatives such as Zenker`s, and Karnowsky`s fixatives have better morphology preservation properties (63), yet they need additional handling precautions, and are not suitable for immunohistochemistry and molecular studies (62).

Methacaren, a modified Carnoy fixative, provides good fixation for light microscopy as well as electron microscopy (64).In processing, the tissue is better to be wrapped in a wet thin paper like lens paper.

In emergency evaluation, the fixative and also processing is done by microwave devices.

For electron microscopy, 2-3% glutaraldehyde fluid is suitable. It should be cool and buffered and be made in the last 3 months. Immunofluorescence samples do not need any fixative and should be delivered and frozen in Michel`s media for frozen sections.

## 11. Sectioning and staining

After histologic processing and paraffin embedding, the tissues are sectioned by microtome. These sections are prepared as thin as 3 μm or less for light microscopy. Thicker sections in needed in congo red and Immunohistochemistry staining.

The most helpful stains for light microscopy are Hematoxiline and Eosine (H&E), methenamine silver, Periodic Acid Schiff (PAS), trichrome, congo red and reticulin.

H&E highlights the cells well, while methenamine silver shows basement membrane and matrix of connective tissues. In PAS staining, there is good highlighting of cells and basement membrane. Trichrome staining is suitable for basement membrane, fibrosis, and deposit assessment. Congo red is recommended for amyloid discovering while elastin stains such as reticulin are helpful in vascular lesions.

Table 1 provides a comparison of the characteristics of tissues provided by three different stains (8).

| | PAS | trichrome | silver |
|---|---|---|---|
| Basement membrane | red | Deep blue | black |
| Mesangial matrix | red | Deep blue | black |
| Interstitium collagen | - | Pale blue | - |
| Cell cytoplasm | - | Rust/orange-granular | - |
| Immune complex deposits | -/+ | Bright red-orange homogeneous | |
| fibrin | Weakly + | Bright red-orange fibrillar | - |
| amyloid | - | Light blue-orange | - |
| Tubular casts | red | Light blue | Gray to black |
| Insudative lesions | -/+ | Bright red-orange homogeneous | - |

Table 1.

## 12. Specimen adequacy

There is a question of how much tissue is necessary for diagnosis of renal disease. In diffuse glomerular diseases, such as amyloidosis and membranous glomerulopathy, one glomerulus is enough for diagnosis. In focal diseases, considering the random distribution of abnormalities, the probability of finding any glomerulopathy is represented by bionial equation (65). For example, if we have 10 glomeruli and the disease exist in 10% and 35% of them, we will have 65% and 95% positive report in the biopsy, respectively.

Fogo mentioned 25 and 10 glomeruli are needed for most accurate diagnosis in light microscopy for native and transplanted kidneys respectively (52). In one study it was found that a specimen with at least 25 glomeruli is needed for the biopsies of chronic lesions of the kidney (66).

There is semi-quantification of pathologic findings including glomeruli number, percentage of affected glomeruli, mesangial matrix volume, inflammatory cell infiltrate, percentage of fibrosis and atrophy in different patients. Also quantification techniques in renal biopsy have been reported (67,68,69,70). These quantifications ha help in monitoring the patients

and their response to therapy as well as comparison of different biopsies and their correlation with clinical points.
Quantification methods require a standard protocol for processing and sectioning (70).

## 13. Differential diagnosis of renal lesions

Renal biopsies are done to determine tissue diagnosis, exclude other diagnostic possibilities, assessing the severity and activity of the lesion (grade), and the amount of irreversible scarring (stage) (63). There are some steps in renal biopsy evaluation with each step correlating to one the part of the kidney including glomeruli, tubules, Interstitium and vascular parts and correlate them with each other. Any changes in each part of the kidney may be associated with secondary changes in others. The maximum data about renal biopsies is provided by light microscopy, immunofluorescence study and electron microscopy (71,72,73).
In the future, genomics and proteomics studies will be used for the diagnosis of renal diseases. In glomerular evaluation, pathologists should diagnose the inflammation, glomerular basement membrane changes, scarring, spikes, fibrinoid exudates, hypercellularity and deposits.
In tubular parts, the focus should be on cellular injuries, regeneration, atrophy, cast, edema, fibrosis and crystals.
Interstitium pathology includes cellular infiltrate, edema, and fibrosis, while vascular part changes are inflammation, sclerosis, hyalinosis and thrombosis.
In overall inspection of biopsy, pathologists should know about the clinical status and chronicity of the disease. In the chronic nephron loss, there is compensatory of remained normal nephrons which leads to a mixture of hypertrophied functioning glomeruli and atrophic non-functioning nephrons (10).
The pathologist also should know that many diseases which affect the kidney, have different manifestations other than kidney.
Light microscopy is often the most important tool for detecting the primary site of injury, but to differentiate between the diseases with common manifestation , electron microscopy and immunofluorescence study are helpful (10).
In this section we used Heptinstal Renal Pathology tables and their respective authors.

## 14. Glomerular lesions

The clinical presentations of glomerular diseases are very different including proteinuria, hematuria, casts, nephritic syndrome, acute nephritis, renal failure (acute and chronic) and rapidly progressive nephritis. Clinical data about age and urine sediment (nephritic or nephritic), narrows differential diagnoses (74).
There are some reports on the relative frequency of renal disorders in biopsies (75). The complexity and variety of glomerular diseases is a challenge for nephropathologists (10).
Renal injuries could be categorized as acute or fibrosing. Active lesions include proliferation, necrosis, crescent, edema, and active inflammation. Fibrosing lesions include glomerulosclerosis, fibrosis, crescent, tubular atrophy, interstitial fibrosis and vascular fibrosis (76).
It should be remembered in the prognosis and monitoring of renal diseases that glomerular lesion can change over time. .

There is a standard terminology for glomerular involving lesions report which is stated by Jennette and et al (10,75).

**Focal**: less than 50% of glomeruli

**Diffuse**: more than 50% of glomeruli

**Segmental**: part of a glomerulus

**Global**: all of a glomerulus

**Mesangial hypercellularity**: 4 or more nuclei in mesangial region

**Endocapillary hypercellularity**: increased cellularity internal to the GBM composed of leukocytes, endothelial cells or mesangial cells.

**Extracapillary hypercellularity**: increased cellularity in Bowman`s space (more than one layer of parietal or visceral epithelial cells or monocyte/machrophage)

**Crescent:** extracapillary hypercellularity other than the epithelial hyperplasia of collapsing variants of FSGS

**Fibrinoid necrosis**: lytic destruction of cells and matrix with deposition of acidophilic fibrin-rich material

**Sclerosis**: increased collagenous extracellular matrix that is expanding the mesangium, obliterating capillary lumens or forming adhesions to Bowman`s capsule

**Hyaline**: glassy acidophilic extracellular material

**Membranoprolifrative**: combined capillary wall thickening and mesangial or endocapillary hypercellularity

**Lobular (hypersegmented)**: expansion of segments that are demarcated by intervening urinary space

**Mesangiolysis**: detachment of the paramesangial GBM from the mesangial matrix or lysis of mesangial matrix

Each of these terms could be categorized further according to some other parameters ((74,77,78,79,80,81 ,82,83):

*Focal glomerulonephritis*: is includes inflammatory lesions in less than 50% of glomeruli. the differential diagnoses are noted based on the age and are as follow:

<15 years:

- mild postinfectious glomerulonephritis
- IgA nephropathy
- thin basement membrane disease
- hereditary nephritis
- Henoch Schoenlein purpura
- mesangial prolifrative glomerulonephritis

15-40 years:

- IgA nephropathy
- thin basement membrane disease
- systemic lupus erythematous
- hereditary nephritis
- mesangial prolifrative glomerulonephritis

>40 years:

- IgA nephropathy

*Diffuse glomerulonephritis*: affects most or all of the glomeruli and differential diagnoses according to age are:

<15 years:

- postinfectious glomerulonephritis
- membranoprolifrative glomerulonephritis

15-40 years:

- postinfectious glomerulonephritis
- systemic lupus erythematous
- rapid progressive glomerulonephritis
- fibrillary glomerulonephritis
- membranoprolifrative glomerulonephritis

>40 years:

- rapid progressive glomerulonephritis
- fibrillary glomerulonephritis
- vasculitis
- postinfectious glomerulonephritis

*Nephrotic syndrome*: is associated with proteinuria and lipiduria and its differential diagnoses according to age include:

<15 years:

- minimal change disease
- focal segmental glomerulosclerosis
- mesangioprolifrative glomerulonephritis

15-40 years:

- focal segmental glomerulosclerosis
- minimal change disease
- membranous nephropathy
- diabetic nephropathy
- preeclampsia
- post infectious glomerulonephritis

>40 years:

- focal segmental glomerulosclerosis
- membranous nephropathy
- diabetic nephropathy
- minimal change disease
- IgA nephropathy
- amyloidosis
- light chain deposition disease
- benign nephrosclerosis
- postinfectious glomerulonephritis

In each pattern, the injuries should be written and overall the proper diagnosis should be made. The optimum approach to pathologic diagnosis of a glomerular disease is based on the presence of features indicative of specific disease and the absence of the features indicative of other disorders (10).

One of the first steps in evaluation of glomeruli is the distinction between the primary and the secondary lesions. The systemic diseases including systemic lupus erythematous, systemic vasculitis (e.g.Wegner granulomatousis), microscopic polyangitis, Henoch Schoenlein purpura, cryoglobulinemic vasculitis, diabetes mellitus, amyloidosis, monoclonal immunoglobulin deposition disease, hypertension, hepatitis B infection and etc. affect the kidney as well as the other organs.

In light microscopy evaluation, each part of glomerulus should be noted for normal and abnormal cellularity and extracellular materials.

In normal morphology of glomeruli, the diagnoses are minimal change disease and thin basement membrane nephropathy and electron microscopy and immunofluorescence would be helpful. Early stages of many glomerulopathies show normal features in light microscopy. If there are capillaries with thick walls, diseases such as membranous glomerulopathy, diabetic glomerulosclerosis, amyloidosis, immunoglobulin deposit disease, should be remembered.

Alteration of glomerular basement membrane is summarized here (82,83,84):

Where limited sclerosis of glomeruli is observed, focal segmental glomerulosclerosis, Alport's syndrome, and sclerotic phase of different glomerulopathies are differential diagnoses.

Hypercellularity may result from increase in mesangial, visceral epithelial, endothelial cells or infiltrate of leukocytes.

Mesangial hypercellularity is seen in mesangioprolifrative glomerulonephritis, postinfectious glomerulonephritis, and membranoprolifrative glomerulonephritis. Lobular pattern of glomeruli should remind membranoprolifrative glomerulonephritis with nodular expansion, fibrillary glomerulonephritis, and immunotactoid glomerulopathy.

Diffuse sclerosis is seen in end stages of glomerular, vascular or tuboluinterstitial diseases. It should be noted that many diseases may have no changes in morphology at the beginning of their evolution while other diseases such as lupus or IgA nephropathies may result in any of the changes.

On the other hand glomerulus lesions are categorized like the following (76,80)

**Sclerosis:**

- usual:
- collapsing:
- tip lesion of FSGS:
- secondary:

**Crescent:**

- according to cellular and degree of fibrous:
  - cellular:
  - fibrocellular:
  - fibrous:
- according to immune deposits:
  - mmune etiology:
  - pauci immune:

**Proliferation:**

- mesangial with nodules
  - diabetic nephropathy
  - light chain deposition disease
  - membranoprolifrative glomerulonephritis
  - amyloidosis
  - idiopathic nodular sclerosis
- mesangial without nodules
  - lupus nephritis
  - IgA nephropathy

  - chronic infection related glomerulonephritis
- mesangial without deposits
  - minimal change disease
  - focal segmental glomerulosclerosis
  - early diabetic nephropathy
- mesangial and endocapillary
  - membranoprolifrative glomerulonephritis
  - prolifrative lupus nephritis
  - cryoglobulinemia glomerulonephritis
  - postinfectious glomerulonephritis
  - fibrillary glomerulonephritis
  - immunotactoid glomerulopathy
  - dense deposit disease

**Unusual lesions:**

- foamy podocytes:
- foamy macrophages intraglomerular:

It should be remembered that each specific histological pattern in light microscopy could be seen in different diseases (10,74,77,80,81,83,84):

*No abnormality:*

- normal glomerulus
- no light microscopic changes
  - minimal change disease
  - thin basement membrane nephropathy
- early lesion of glomerulus (near in all diseases)

*Thick capillary walls only*

- membranous glomerulopathy
- thrombotic microangiopathy
- preeclampsia/eclampsia
- fibrillary glomerulonephritis with capillary predominance of deposits

*Thick walls with mesangial expansion without hypercellularity:*

- diabetic glomerulopathy
- membranous glomerulopathy with mesangial deposits
- amyloidosis
- monoclonal Ig deposition disease
- fibrillary glomerulonephritis
- dense deposit disease

*Focal segmental glomerulosclerosis:*

- minimal change disease
- healing of previous glomerular injuries
- hypertension
- hereditary nephritis
- chronic phase of focal glomerulonephritis

*Membranous injury:*

- drug assumption like gold, penicillamin, mercury
- systemic lupus erythematous

- chronic hepatitis B
- underlying malignancy

*Membranoprolifrative glomerulopathy:*

- membranoprolifrative glomerulonephritis
- diabetic glomerulonephritis
- thrombotic microangiopathy
- fibrillary glomerulonephritis
- immunotactoid glomerulopathy
- systemic immune complex disease
    - systemic lupus erythematous
    - infectious endocarditis
    - hepatitis C
    - complement dysregulation
    - chronic thrombotic microangiopathy
    - monoclonal immunoglobulin deposition disease

As it is emphasized before, clinical information is very important and differential diagnoses of diseases are possible based on those information.

*According to serologic studies* (74):

- antistreptococcal antibody: poststreptococcal glomerulonephritis
- anti nuclear antibody: lupus nephritis
- anti GBM antibody: anti GBM antibody disease
- circulating cryoglobulins: mixed cryoglobulinemia
- antineutrophil cytoplasmic antibody: Wegner`s granulomatousis

*According to decreased serum complement levels:*

- postinfectious glomerulonephritis
- lupus nephritis
- membranoprolifrative glomerulonephritis
- mixed cryoglobulinemia

*According to presence of acute renal failure:*

- idiopathic minimal change disease
- collapsing focal segmental glomerulosclerosis
- minimal change disease with acute interstitial nephritis of NSAIDs
- crescentic glomerulonephritis
- nephrotic syndrome secondary to monoclonal immunoglobulin deposition disease because of myeloma casts

In addition to light microscopy, immunofluorescence could be helpful in many normal morphology and also many conditions where there is thickening of membranous or expansion of mesangial. It can help to determine the location and pattern of deposits and composition of deposits.

Nowadays the routine antibodies which are used in immunoflourescent study are including IgG, IgA, IgM, kappa, lambda, c3, c4, c1q.

Some diseases may be dismissed without immunofluorescence or immunohistochemistry use, including light chain associated disease, IgA nephropathy, c1q nephropathy, anti GBM disease, humeral (c4d) transplant rejection, and fibronectin glomerulopathy.

In electron microscopy, basement membrane changes such as split, existence and pattern of deposits, fibrillary changes and also mesangial deposits can be diagnosed. Some diseases are detected only by electron microscopy studies including but not limited to fibrillary/

immunotactoid glomerulopathy, amyloidosis, cryoglobulinemia, monoclonal immunoglobulin deposition disease, collagenofibrotic glomerulopathy, fibrinogen glomerulopathy, Alport's syndrome, dense deposit disease, thin glomerular basement membrane nephropathy, lipoprotein glomerulopathy, and nail-patella syndrome. Electron microscopy can differentiate between these diseases due to specific texture of deposits (10).

## 15. Tubular lesions

Kidney tubules in cortex and medulla have different architecture and also different cell types. It is worth noting that cortical tubules have few interstitial tissues, compared to medullary region.

Many changes could be seen in different renal diseases. these alterations are categorized based on different point of views. Some of these are presented below.

First tubular changes introduced (10, 85):

*Acute tubular cell injury*

- acute tubular necrosis (often coagulation necrosis/ usually secondary to toxins or ischemia. Other changes in the cells are karyorrhexis, ballooning of cytoplasm, detachment from basement membrane, loss of brush border, thinning, luminal dilation, intraluminal different casts, especially cellular ones)
- hyaline droplet formation (small to large droplets in lysosomes of tubular epithelium because of altered permeability and absorption of proteins.)
- vacuolar change (fine and diffuse appearance)
- fatty change (cytoplasm with fine small vacuoles in base of epithelial cells in severe proteinuria or nephrotic syndrome with hyperlipidemia, Reyes` syndrome, poisoning with phosphorus or carbon tetrachloride. In non nephrotic syndrome, it is in favor of Alport's syndrome)
- foam cells
- hypokalemic nephropathy (coarse and irregular varied size vacuoles due to chronic loss of potassium like laxative abuse, rectosigmoid polyps)
- hydropic change ( in conditions with assumption of sucrose, manitol, dextrane, radio opaque materials, IVIG and cyclosporine A)
- pigmented in tubular epithelium
- intranuclear inclusions (usually in immunosupressed patients infected by CMV or polyoma virus and adenovirus and lead poisoning)

*Tubular casts* (principal histologic feature of light chain disease, myoglubolnuria, hemoglubolinuria, oxalate nephropathy, urate nephropathy, nephrocalcinosis and drug induced tubular lesions)

- hyaline: renal failure or low urine output
- WBC: tubulointerstitial inflammation
- epithelial cell or granular: acute tubular injury
- RBC: glomerular bleeding
- large hyaline fractured: light chain casts (often accompanied by giant cells and neutrophils)
- coarse granular acidophilic or red brick: myoglobulin or hemoglobulin *Tubular atrophy* (simplified epithelial cells with thickening of basement membrane)

*Tubulitis* (infiltration of inflammatory cells indicative of active tubulointerstitial inflammation or nephritis or allograft rejection)

*Tubular basement membrane changes* (in tubular atrophy, hereditary nephritis, diabetic nephropathy, monoclonal immunoglobulin deposit, dense deposit disease)

## 16. Interstitium lesions

As it was mentioned in previous chapter, interstitium occupies small portion of kidney tissue and is slightly larger in medullary region. This part of the kidney tissue becomes affected primarily or secondarily in renal diseases. In many lesions of glomeruli, tubular or vascular, interstitium also gets involved and shows pathologic features.
Interstitium is the main site that demonstrates pathologic findings in drug allergic reactions and pyelonephritis (10).
Two main lesions are acute and chronic interstitium nephritis with the former showing reversible infiltration of inflammatory cells accompanied with edema , and the latter showing irreversible fibrosis and atrophy of other compartments.
Acute phase can heal or result in chronic phase and scarring.
The lesions of interstitium that can be observed in light microscopy are listed here (5 with modification). No pathologic changes

- normal kidney
- no changes in the portion
- early disease

Expansion and edema (due to increased permeability of vessels)

- acute tubular necrosis
- thrombosis of renal vein
- nephrotic syndrome
- acute glomerulonephritis
- thrombotic microangiopathy

Expansion with eosinophilic material

- fibrosis (chronic disease)
- sickle cell anemia
- radiation
- amyloidosis

Expansion with leukocyte infiltration

- interstitial nephritis with polymorphonuclear cells (infections, drug induced, sepsis)
- lymphoplasmacytic (chronic nephritis, vasculitis, lupus nephritis, infections, rejection, drug induced)
- eosinophils (vasculitis, drug induced, lupus nephritis)
- epithelioid cells/granuloma (tuberculosis, sarcoidosis, drug induced, malakoplakia)

Foam cells

- Alport`s syndrome
- prolonged nephrotic syndrome

Hemorrhagia

- acute rejection
- vasculitis
- severe glomerulonephritis
- malignant hypertension

Expansion with neoplastic cells

- lymphoma/leukemia

- primary or secondary tumors

Crystals
- calcium carbonate
- calcium oxalate
- uric acid
- cholesterol

Fibrosis
- chronic phase of inflammation
- secondary to chronic lesions of other parts

It should be noted that in every pathologic changes in the interstitium, other parts should be examined carefully, as usually there are changes of overall kidney tissue.

## 17. Vascular lesions

Kidney vessels are susceptible to many damages. Many immune complexes reach the kidney through blood circulation and are filtered in glomeruli. Receiving about 20% of the cardiac output, the kidneys are constantly exposed to the damaging elements which circulate in blood.

The main injuries of vascular elements are listed here (5 with modification).

Vasculitis
- in systemic injury of vessels
- in local injuries of vessels due to toxins or infection or inflammation

Deposition of materials
- amyloidosis
- immune complexes
- arteriosclerosis

Hypertension induced injuries
- hypertrophy of media
- intimal thickening
- fibrinoid necrosis
- thrombotic microangiopathy
- fibrointimal hyperplasia

Endothelitis
- drug induced
- toxins

Thrombus
- secondary lesion to endothelitis; may cause anemia and thrombocytopenia

Emboli
- small parts of coagulated blood, fat or tumor cells usually in larger arterioles of the kidney

In summary, the importance of clinical characteristics and laboratory results in pathologic assessment of renal biopsies should be stressed. Proper diagnoses can be achieved using light microscopy, electron microscopy and immunofluorescence study of biopsies, in addition to integration of all clinical, laboratory and pathologic data. (10)

## 18. References

[1] Cotran R S,Komar V, robbins and cotran pathologic basis of disease.7th edit,saunders Co,2010;905-69.

[2] Stephen S. Sternberg . Histology for pathologists , second edition. Lippincott-Raven Publishers , Philadelphia, 2010;799-830
[3.] Suramo I, Paivansalo M, Myllyla V. Cranio-caudal movements of the liver, pancreas and kidneys in respiration. Acta Radiol Diagn (Stockh) 1984;25:129.
[4] Wald H. The weight of normal adult human kidneys and its variability. *Arch Pathol Lab Med 1937;23:493-500.*
[5] Kaisiske BL, Umen *AI.* The influence of age, sex, race, and body habitus on kidney weight in humans. *Arch Pathol Lab Med 1986;110:* 55-60.
[6] Hodson CJ. Physiological changes in size of the kidneys. Clin Radiol 1961;12:91.
[7] Graves FT. The anatomy of the intrarenal arteries and its application to segmental resection of the kidney. *Br J Surg* 1954;42: 132-139.
[8] Agnes B. Fogo MD , Michael Kashgarian ,Diagnostic Atlas of Renal Pathology: A Companion to Brenner and Rector's The Kidney,2005;
[9] Oliver 1. *Nephrons and kidneys: a quantitative study of development and evolutionary mammalian renal architectonics.* New York: Harper & Row; 1968.
[10] Jennette, J. Charles; Olson, Jean L.; Schwartz, Melvin M.; Silva, Fred G. Hepinstall's Pathology of the Kidney, 6th Edition, Lippincott Williams & Wilkins,2007;1-72.
[11] Hodson CJ. The lobar structure of the kidney. *Br J Urol 1972;44:* 246-261.
[12] Clapp WM, Abrahamson DR. Development and gross anatomy of the kidney. In: Tisher CC, Brenner BM, eds. *Renal pathology.* 2nd ed. Philadelphia: JB Lippincott; 1994:3-59.
[13] Manalich R, Reyes L, Herrera M, et al. Relationship between weight at birth and the number and size of renal glomeruli in humans: A histomorphometric study. Kidney Int 2000;58:770.
[14] Neugarten J, Kasiske B, Silbiger SR, et al. Effects of sex on renal structure. Nephron 2002;90:139.
[15] Hughson M, Farris AB 3rd, Douglas-Denton R, et al. Glomerular number and size in autopsy kidneys: The relationship to birth weight. Kidney Int 2003;63:2113.
[16] Malpighi M. *De viscerum structura exercitatio anatomica.* Bonn, Germany;1666.
[17] Bowman W. On the structure and use of the Malpighian bodies of the kidney, with observations on the circulation through that gland. *Philos Trans R Soc Land* 1842;132:57-80.
[18] Fine LG. William Bowman's description of the glomerulus. *Am J Nephrol1985;5:437-440.*
[19] Rouiller C. General anatomy and histology of the kidney. In: Rouiller C, Muller AF, eds. The Kidney: Morphology, Biochemistry and Physiology. New York: Lippincott, 1989:67.
[20] Mbassa G, Elger M, Kriz W. The ultrastructural organization of the basement membrane of Bowman's capsule in the rat renal corpuscle. Cell Tissue Res 1988;253:151.
[21] Dunnill MS, Halley W. Some observations on the quantitative anatomy of the kidney. *J Pathol1973;110:113-121.*
[22] Newbold KM, Howie *AI,* Koram A, Adu A, MichaelJ. Assessment of glomerular size in renal biopsies including minimal change nephropa, thy and single kidneys. *J Pathol1990;160:255-258.*
[23] Horvat R, Hovoka A, Dekan G, Poczewski H, Kerjaschki D. Endothelial cell membranes contain podocalyxin-the major sialoprotein of visceral glomerular epithelial cells. *J Cell Bioi 1986;102:* 484-491.

[24] Savage CO. The biology of the glomerulus: endothelial cells. Kidney Int 1994;45:314.
[25] Schlondorff D. The glomerular mesangial cell: an expanding role for a specialized pericyte. *FASEB J 1987;1:272-281.*
[26] Michael AF, Keane WF, Raij L, Vernier RC, Mauer SM. The glomerular mesangium. *Kidney Int* 1980;17:141-154
[27] Steffes MW, Barbosa J, Basgen JM, Sutherland DER, Najarian JS, Mauer SM. Quantitative glomerular morphology for the normal human kidney. *Lab Invest 1983;49:82-86*
[28] Drenckhahn D, Franke R. Ultrastructural organization of contractile and cytoskeletal proteins in glomerular podocytes of chicken, rat and man. *Lab Invest 1988;59:673-682.*
[29] Latta H, Johnston WH, Stanley TM. Sialoglycoproteins and filtration barriers in the glomerular capillary wall. *J Ultrastruct Res 1975;51:* 354-376.
[30] Golgi C. Annotazioni intorno all'istologia dei reni dell'uomo e di altri mammiferi e sull'istogenesi: dei canalicoli oriniferi. *Atti R Accad Na: Lincei Rendiconti 1889;5:337-342.*
[31] Christensen JA, Meyer DS, Bohle A. The structure of the human juxtaglomerular apparatus. A morphometric, lightmicroscopic study on serial sections. Virchows Arch A Pathol Anat Histol 1975;367:83.
[32] Barajas L. Anatomy of the juxtaglomerular apparatus. Am J Physiol 1979;237: F333.
[33] Cantin M, Gutkowska J, Lacasse J, et al. Ultrastructural immunocytochemical-localization of renin and angiotensin II in the juxtaglomerular cells of the ischemic kidney. *Am J Pathol1984;115:212-224.*
[34] Parker MV, Swann HG, Sinclair JG..The functional morphology of the kidney. *Tex Rep Bioi Med 1962;20:"424-458.*
[35] Jamison RL, Kriz W. *Urinary concentrating mechanism: structure and function.* New York: Oxford University Press; 1982.
[36] Madsen KM, Tisher CC. Structural-functional relationships along the distal nephron. *Am J Physiol1986;250:FI-FI5.*
[37] Lonnerholm G. Histochemical-demonstration of carbonic anhydrase activity in the human kidney. *Acta Physiol Scand 1973;88:455-468.*
[38] Madsen KM, Clapp WL, Verlander JW. Structure and function of the inner medullary collecting duct. *Kidney Int 1988;34:441-454.*
[39] Kappel B, Olsen S. Cortical interstitial tissue and sclerosed glomeruli in the normal human kidney, related to age and sex. A quantitative study. *Virchows Arch* [A] 1980;387:271-277.
[40] Bohman SO. The ultrastructure of the renal medulla and the interstitial cells. In: Cotran RS, ed. *Tubulo-interstitial nephropathies.* New York: Churchill Livingstone; 1983:1-34.
[41] Pfaller W. Structure function correlation in rat kidney. Quantitative correlation of structure and function in the normal and injured rat kidney. *Adv Anat Embryol Cell Bioi* 1982;70:1-106.
[42] Muirhead EE. Antihypertensive functions ofthe kidney. *Hypertension* 1980;2:444-464.
[43] Bell RD, Keyl MJ, Shrader FR, Jones EW, Henry LP. Renallymphatics: the internal distribution. *Nephron 1968;3:454-463.*

[44] Lemley KV, Kriz W. Structure and function of the renal vasculature. In: Tisher CC, Brenner BM, eds. *Renal pathology.* 2nd ed. Philadelphia: J8 Lippincott; 1994:981-1026.

[45] Mitchell 1 GAG. The nerve supply of the kidneys. *Acta Anat 1950;10:* 1-37.

[46] Gosling JA. Observations on the distribution ofintrarenal nervous tissue. *Anat Rec* 1969;163:8J-88.

[47]. Walker P.D. The Renal Biopsy. Arch pathol lab med 2009; 133,181-188.

[48] Burstein DM, Korbet SM, Schwartz MM. The use of the automatic core biopsy system percutaneous renal biopsies: a comparative study. *Am J Kidney Dis.* 1993;22:545–552.

[49] Nicholson ML, Wheatley TJ, Doughman TM, et al. A prospective randomized trial of three different sizes of core-cutting needle for renal transplant biopsy. *Kidney Int.* 2000;58:390–395

[50] Ori Y, Neuman H, Chagnac A, et al. Using the automated biopsy gun with real-time ultrasound for native renal biopsy. *IMAJ.* 2002;4:698–701.

[51] Nadel L, Baumgartner B.R, Bernardino M.E. Percutaneous renal biopsies: accuracy, safety, and indications. Urol Radiol 1986;1:67-71.

[52] Fogo A.B. Approach to Renal Biopsy. Am J of Kidney Dis 2003;42: 826-836.

[53] Thompson BC, Kingdon E, Johnston M, et al. Transjugular kidney biopsy. Am J Kidney Dis. 2004;43:651–662.

[54] Fine DM, Arepally A, Hofmann LV, Mankowitz SG, Atta MG. Diagnostic utility and safety of transjugular kidney biopsy in the obese patient. Nephrol Dial Transplant. 2004;19:1798–1802.

[55] Gimenez LF, Micali S, Chen RN, Moore RG, Kavoussi LR, Scheel PJ. Laparoscopic renal biopsy. Kidney Int. 1998;54:525–529.

[56] Wickre CG, Golper TA. Complications of percutaneous needle biopsy of the kidney. Am J Nephrol 1982;2:173.

[57] Burstein DM, Schwartz MM, Korbet SM. Percutaneous renal biopsy with the use of real-time ultrasound. Am J Nephrol 1991;11:195.

[58] Preda A, Van Dijk LC, Van Oostaijen JA, Pattynama PMT. Complication rate and diagnostic yield of 515 consecutive ultrasound-guided biopsies of renal allografts and native kidneys using a 14-gauge Biopty gun. *Eur Radiol.* 2003;13: 527–530.

[59] Whittier WL, Korbet SM. Timing of complications in percutaneous renal biopsy. *J Am Soc Nephrol.* 2004;15:142–147.

[60] Fraser I.R, Fairly K.F. Renal biopsy as an outpatient procedure. Am J of Kidney Dis 1995; 6: 876-8.

[61] Khajehdehi P, Junaid SMA, Salinas-Madrigal L, et al. Percutaneous renal biopsy in the 1990s: safety, value, and implications for early hospital discharge. Am J Kidney Dis 1999;34:92-7.

[62] Walker P.D, Cavallo T, Bonsib S.M. Practice guidelines for renal biopsiy. Modern pathol 2004; 17: 1555-63.

[63] Furness P.N. Renal biopsy specimens. J Clin Pathol 2000;53:433–438.

[64] Shibutani M, Uneyama C. Methacarn: a fixation tool for multipurpose genetic analysis from paraffin embedded tissues. Methods Enzymol 2002; 356:114-125.

[65] Corwin HL, Schwartz MM, Lewis EJ. The importance of sample size in the interpretation of the renal biopsy. Am J Nephrol 1988;8:85.

[66] Wang H.J, Kjellstrand1 C.M, Cockfield S.M, and Solez K.On the influence of sample size on the prognostic accuracy and reproducibility of renal transplant biopsy. Nephrol Dial Transplant 1998; 13: 165–172.
[67] Bohle A, Wehrmann M, Bogenschutz O, et al. The long-term prognosis of the primary glomerulonephritides: A morphological and clinical analysis of 1747 cases. Pathol Res Pract 1992;188:908.
[68] Kim KH, Kim Y, Gubler MC, et al. Structural-functional relationships in Alport syndrome. J Am Soc Nephrol 1995;5:1659.
[69] Mauer SM. Structural-functional correlations of diabetic nephropathy. Kidney Int 1994;45:612.
[70] Pesce C. Glomerular Number and Size: Facts and Artefacts. The anatom record 1998; 251:66–71.
[71] Lajoie G, Silva FG. Approach to the interpretation of renal biopsy. In: Silva FG, D'Agati VD, Nadasdy T, eds. Renal Biopsy Interpretation. Part II. Manual of Renal Biopsy Interpretation, 1st ed. New York: Churchill Livingstone, 1996: 63.
[72] Chapman JR. Longitudinal analysis of chronic allograft nephropathy: Clinicopathologic correlations. Kidney Int Suppl 2005: S108.
[73] Coppo R, D'Amico G. Factors predicting progression of IgA nephropathies. J Nephrol 2005;18:503.
[74] Rose B.D. Differential diagnosis of glomerular disease. Uptodate.com
[75] Jennette JC, Falk RJ. Nephritic syndrome and glomerulonephritis. In: Silva FG, D'Agati VD, Nadasty T, eds. Renal Biopsy Interpretation. New York: Churchill Livingstone, 1996: 71.
[76] Fogo A.B. Approach to Renal Biopsy. Am J of Kidney Dis 2003;42: 826-836.
[77] Couser W.G. Rapidly progressive glomerulonephritis: classification, pathogenetic, mechanisms, and therapy. Am J Kidney Dis 1998;11(6):449-464.
[78] Lai K.N, Li P.K, Lui S.F, Au T.C, Tam J.S, Tong K.L, Lai F.M. Membranous nephropathy related to hepatitis B virus in adults. N Engl J Med 1991;324(21):1457-63.
[79] Neugarten J, Baldwin D.S. Glomerulonephritis in bacterial endocarditis. Am J Med 1984;77(2):297-304.
[80] Haas M. Histologic subclassification of IgA nephropathy: a clinicopathologic study of 244 cases. Am J Kidney Dis 1997;29(6):829-42.
[81] Cameron J.S. Focal segmental glomerulosclerosis in adults. Nephrol Dial Transplant 2003;18[suppl 6]:vi45-vi51.
[82] Jahanzad I,Amoueian S,Attaranzadeh .Familial Lecithin cholestrol Acetyl transfrase deficiency:a case report.Archives of Iranian medical journal.2009.vol,No2, P179-81.
[83] Jahanzad I,Amoueian S,Attaranzadeh A,Alport's syndrome:Ultrastructural study of 26 suspected cases.Iranian journal of pathology.2008;vol 2,No 2.p178-180 .
[84] Jennette J.C. An algorithmic approach to renal biopsy interpretation of glomerular disease. First International Renal Pathology Conference ,nephropathology workshop of European Society of Pathology.Native Kidney Pathology - Glomerular diseases last updated at 2010-09-19 20:26:56
[85] D'Agati VD, Jennette JC, Silva FG. Diseases of the renal tubules. In: D'Agati VD, Jennette JC, Silva FG, eds. Non-neoplastic Kidney Disease. Washington: American Registry of Pathology, 2005: 517

# 5

# Diagnostic Algorithms in Renal Biopsy Interpretation Along with Case Samples

Şafak Güçer
*Hacettepe University, Faculty of Medicine Pediatric Pathology Unit Ankara Turkey*

## 1. Introduction

Despite significant advances in molecular analytical techniques impacting the diagnostic approach to the renal biopsy a systematic study of morphological findings is still a magic tool to provide valuable diagnostic and prognostic information in patients with renal disease in the light of history and laboratory findings.

## 2. Approach to renal biopsy interpretation with algorithms

Kidney has three main histological compartments including glomerular, vascular and tubulointerstitial. First, an approach should be performed to localize in which department the main injury occurs and to recognize the severity and extent of the renal injury in each department. Then, the type of injury is to be assessed such as active versus chronic. Active lesions includes cellular proliferation, crescents, edema, necrosis and acute inflammation while chronic lesions represent fibrosing conditions such as fibrous crescents, interstitial fibrosis, glomerulosclerosis, tubular atrophy or vascular sclerosis. (Walker, 2004, 2009; Kretzler, 2002; Fogo, 2003)

### 2.1 The native kidney biopsy lesions

### 2.1.1 Glomerular lesions

#### 2.1.1.1 No or minimal hypercellularity (Figure 1.)

The first step is to determine whether there is hypercellularity or not. No or minimal hypercellularity offers usually a limited differential diagnosis. Then, in such cases further investigations with immunofluorescence (IF) and electron microscopy(EM) are needed along with a detailed clinical history. If glomerular capillaries are abnormal three main categories are defined; glomerular capillary wall thickening, sclerosis/capillary wall collapse and luminal occlusion(Furness,2000;Lajoie&Silva,1996).

If the patient has nephrotic syndrome three main diagnosis are considered ; minimal change disease, membranous GN(early stage ) and also amyloidosis in which amyloid deposits can be very subtle to detect on light microscopy. However, these disorders can be easily differentiated by immunofluorescence and ultrastructural microscopic findings.

Minimal change diseases(MCD) is the most common cause of idiopathic nephrotic syndrome and characterized by absence of pathologic changes by light microscopy but diffuse effacement of foot processes of podocytes by EM. (Figs. 2,3) It is usually a primary disease but it may be secondary to malignant diseases and nonsteroidal anti-inflammatory drugs(Mubarak,2011,Zhang,2011). Proteinuria is generally massive, selective and mostly of abrupt onset.

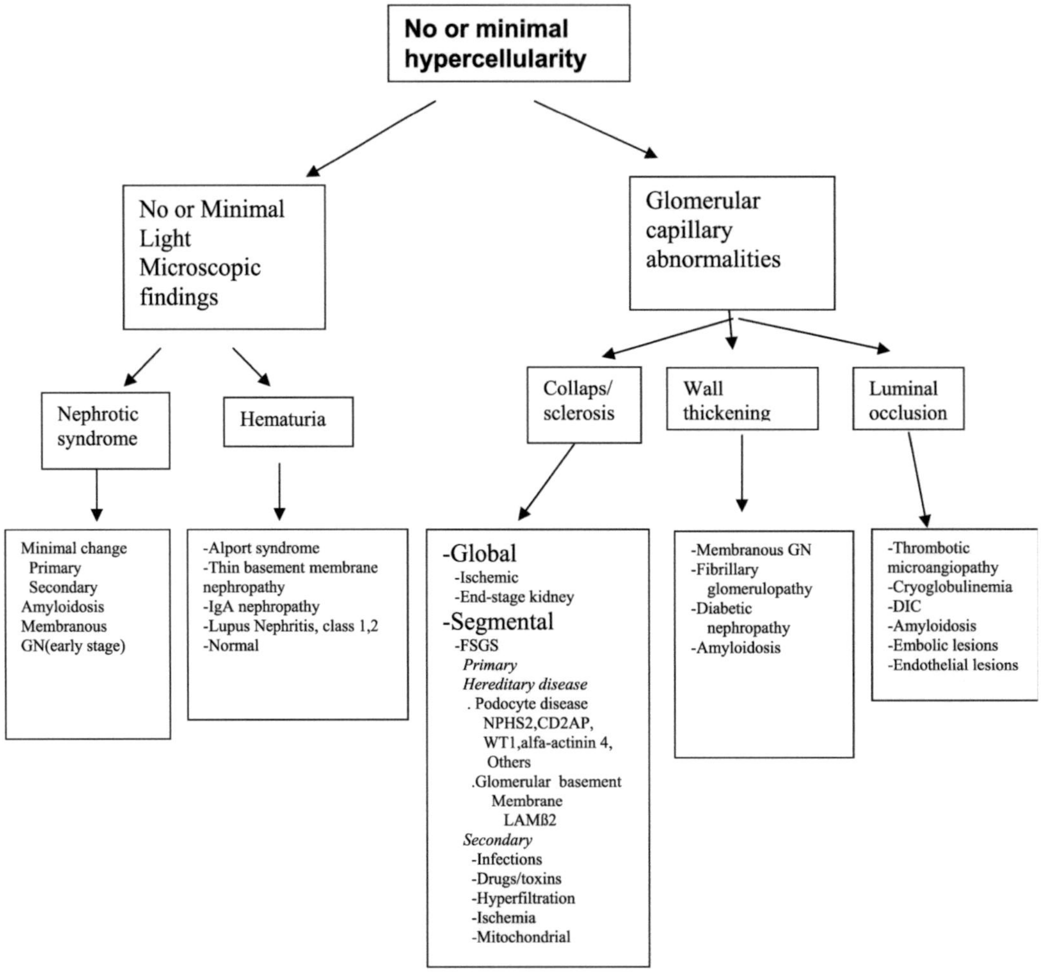


Fig. 1. An algorithm for interpretation of glomerular morphological changes with no or minimal hypercellularity.(GN:Glomerulonephritis, FSGS; Focal segmental glomerulosclerosis, NPHS2;(Podocin), CD2AP; CD-associated protein, WT1; Wilms' tumor1, LAMß2;Laminin ß2, DIC;disseminated intravascular coagulation)

**CASE 1.**

A 5 year-old-male was admitted to the hospital with the complaints of swelling of eyelids, legs and fatigue lasting for 2 months.
No family history for kidney disease or consanguinity between parents.
On physical exam: Blood pressure:100/60 mmHg , pretibial 4(+) pitting edema was noted.
Laboratory findings: Complete blood count and electrolytes were normal , ESR 33 mm/hr

BUN 10 mg/dl,Cr:0.3 m g/dl, Total protein/Albumin: 4.9/2 g/dl
Urinalysis: Density 1025, Proteinuria 80 mg/m2/hr, no glucose, sediment: 3-4 white blood cells.
Serum C3 ,C4 levels, ANA, Anti-DNA, viral markers were all normal.
Renal ultrasonography revealed unremarkable findings.
**Renal biopsy diagnosis**: Minimal change disease (Figs. 2,3)

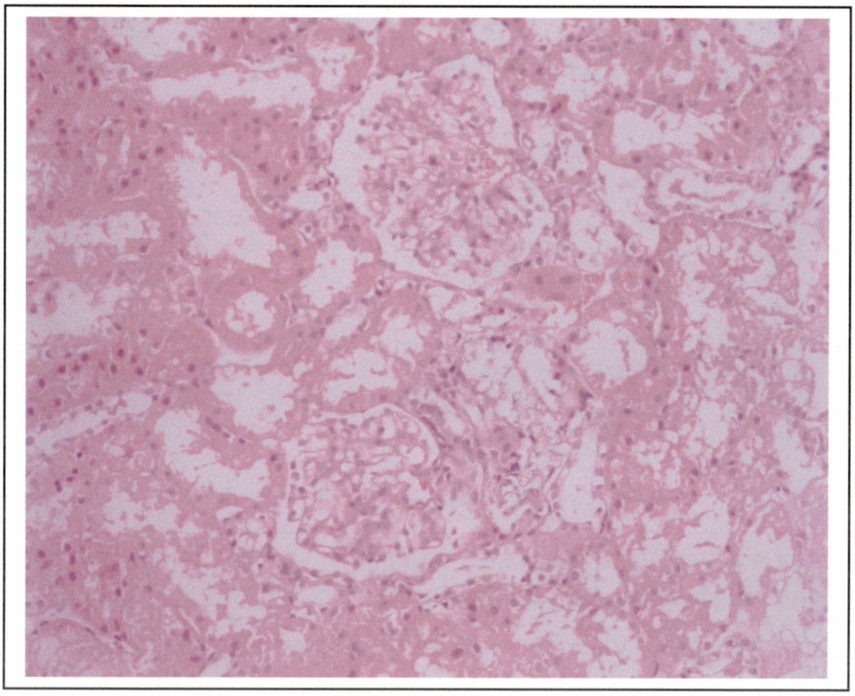

Fig. 2. Minimal change disease. Note the patent glomerular capillaries with normal amount of matrix and mesangial cells.(HEx100)

In cases with hematuria and glomerular basement membrane(GBM) thinning one should consider first Alport syndrome (AS) or thin basement membrane nephropathy(TBMN). Diagnosis of thinning should be made by comparison of age-matched controls. A cut-off value has been reported 250 nm in adults in most series. However, care must be taken to diagnose TBMN in children since GBM thickening increases with age(Kashtan, 2009).
A thinned GBM may be an early lesion in Alport syndrome. Children with Alport syndrome may show only diffuse GBM attenuation, making differentiation from TBMN a challenge.
However, in full-blown cases with AS there is also characteristic thickening of the glomerular basement membrane with splitting of the lamina densa, electron lucent areas and electron dense particles detected by EM. (Figs. 4,5)A progressive, high-frequency sensorineural deafness frequently detectable by audiometry in later childhood in boys with X-linked AS and both boys and girls with autosomal recessive AS and anterior lenticonus or perimacular retinal flecks are other characteristics of AS (Savige, 2003; Haas, 2009).

Thinning of lamina densa of GBM can be seen in normal children, IgA nephropathy, minimal change disease and in some forms of lupus nephritis. However, thinning in these disorders is mostly segmental whereas there is a diffuse involvement in patients with TBMN.

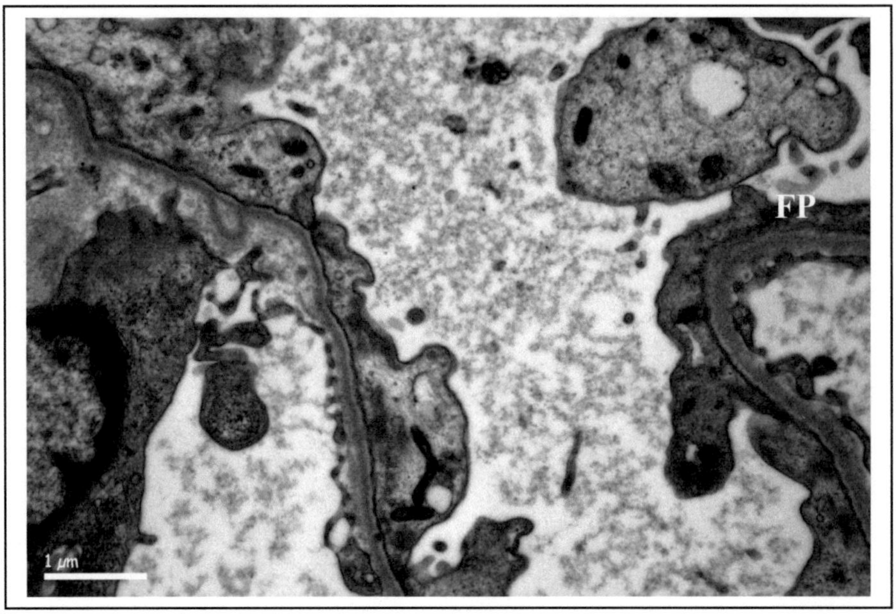


Fig. 3. Minimal change disease. Electron micrograph shows diffuse effacement of foot processes(FP).(Uranyl acetate and lead citratex10000)

A thickened GBM can be detected as a major feature in several glomerular diseases including membranous GN, membranoproliferative(mesangiocapillary) GN , fibrillary GN and diabetic nephropathy, thrombotic microangiopathy, Alport syndrome or transplant glomerulopathy. Aforementioned first three disorders have typical immunofluorescence microscopic findings while IF is expected to be negative in the others.

**CASE 2.**

A 7 year-old-male was admitted to the hospital with the complaints of dysuria and hearing problems. He had been suffering these symptoms for two years.

No consanguinity between parents but his grandmother died of chronic renal failure of unknown etiology.

Physical examination was unremarkable except a sensorineural hearing loss. Blood pressure:100/60 mmHg

Laboratory findings: Complete blood count and electrolytes were normal.

BUN 17.3 mg/dl,Cr:0.64 mg/dl, Total protein/Albumin: 6.9/3.6 g/dl

Urinalysis: Density 1025, Proteinuria 10 mg/m2/hr, no glucose, sediment: abundant red blood cells.

Serum C3 ,C4 levels, ANA, Anti-DNA,viral markers were all normal.

Renal USG revealed normal size and echogenicity in kidneys.

**Renal biopsy diagnosis:** Alport syndrome (Figures 4,5)

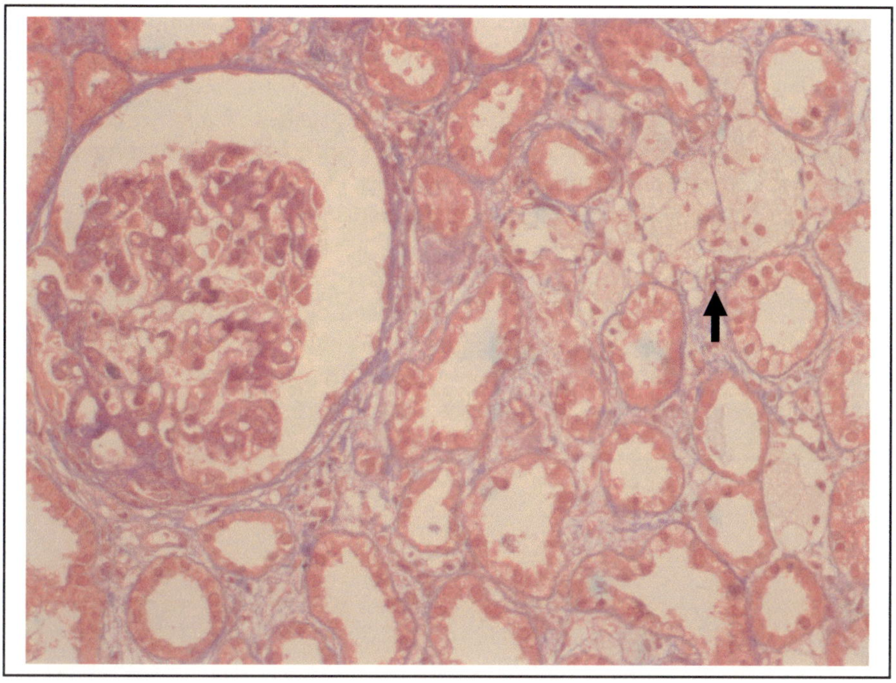

Fig. 4. Alport syndrome. Note mesangial matrix increment, adhesion to Bowman capsule, interstitial foam cells (arrow) and fibrosis in the interstitium. Trichromex200.

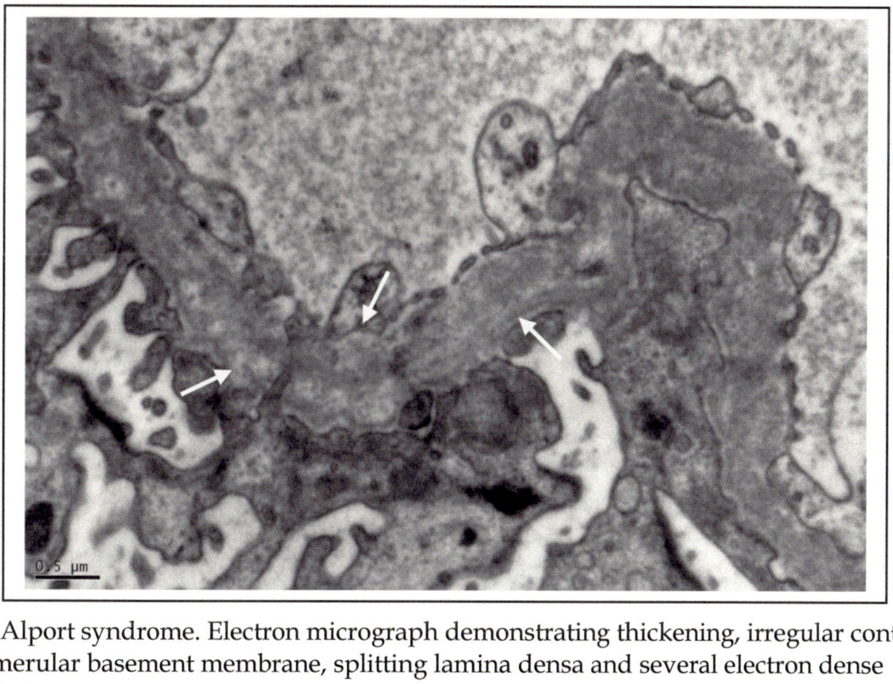


Fig. 5. Alport syndrome. Electron micrograph demonstrating thickening, irregular contours of glomerular basement membrane, splitting lamina densa and several electron dense granules(arrows). Uranyl acetate-Lead citrate x 30000.

In some cases, one may encounter unusual or rare lesions such as foamy podocytes and/or tubules with various storage material ,foam cells within the glomerular tuft or heavily deposited collagen Type III material detected by EM. These storage materials can be diagnostic clues of specific metabolic or hereditary diseases. Fabry disease is the most common which is characterized by foamy podocytes with myelin body type inclusions by EM in podocytes, corneal epithelium, endothelial cells, etc. (Fogo,2003).

If glomerular capillary collapse or sclerosis is the main lesion it can be global or focal. The former is usually the consequence of ischemia or a lesion of the end stage kidney. In fact, glomerulosclerosis is an end result of glomerular injury irrespective of cause.

Focal segmental glomerulosclerosis is a clinicopathological entity which is histologically characterized by segmental glomerulosclerosis in some glomeruli, or tuft collapse, segmental hyalinosis, mostly negative or IgM staining on immunofluorescence and effacement of foot processes on electron microscopy. (Figs. 6,7)

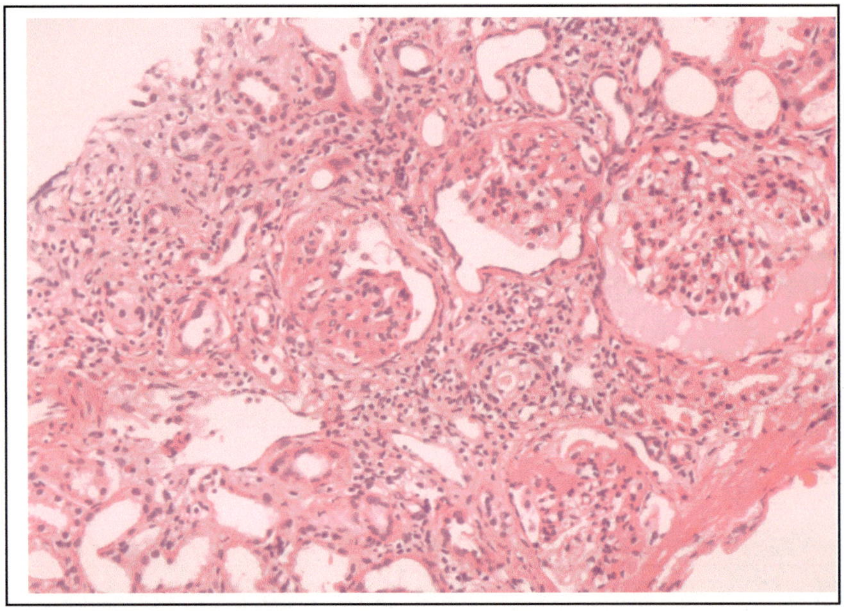

Fig. 6. Focal segmental glomerulosclerosis. The sclerotic lesion involves three glomeruli in a segmental pattern. There is also tubular atrophy with mononuclear inflammatory cell infiltration in the interstitium. (HEx100)

It may be etiologically classified as primary, hereditary disease associated or secondary to infections, drugs/toxins, hyperfiltration, ischemia and as a renal involvement of mitochondrial disease (Thomas, 2009; Gbadegesin, 2011; Baskın, 2011; Emma, 2011; Güçer,2005). (Figs. 8,9)

Data from the experimental and human studies has demonstrated that podocyte has a central role in the pathogenesis of FSGS. Identification of products of mutated genes located in the podocyte and its slit diagram has resulted in the recognition of the hereditary forms of FSGS, and NPHS2; (Podocin), CD2AP (CD-associated protein), WT1; (Wilms' tumor1), LAMß2; Laminin ß2 ACTN4 (Alfa-actinin4), TRPC6 (Transient receptor potential channel type6), PLCE1(Phospholipase Epsilon1), INF2(Inverted forming 2) and others are classified now genetic causes of FSGS and nephrotic syndrome (Gbadegesin,2011).

**CASE 3.**

A 8 year-old-female presented with the complaints of swelling of eyelids and face lasting for 3 months.

No family history for kidney disease or consanguinity between parents.

Physical examination revealed a high blood pressure of 160/90 mmHg and pretibial 3(+) pitting edema.

Laboratory findings: Complete blood count was normal, triglyceride 368 mg/dl, BUN 43 mg/dl,Cr:0.6 mg/dl, Total protein/Albumin: 3.7/1.2 g/dl

Urinalysis: Density 1010, Proteinuria 160 mg/m2/hr, no glucose, sediment: 8-10 white blood cells, 4-5 red blood cells and a few fine granular casts.

Serum C3 ,C4 levels, ANA, Anti-DNA, viral markers were all normal.

Renal USG revealed renal parenchymal disease with increased echogenity.

**Renal biopsy diagnosis:** Focal segmental glomerulosclerosis (Figs. 6,7)

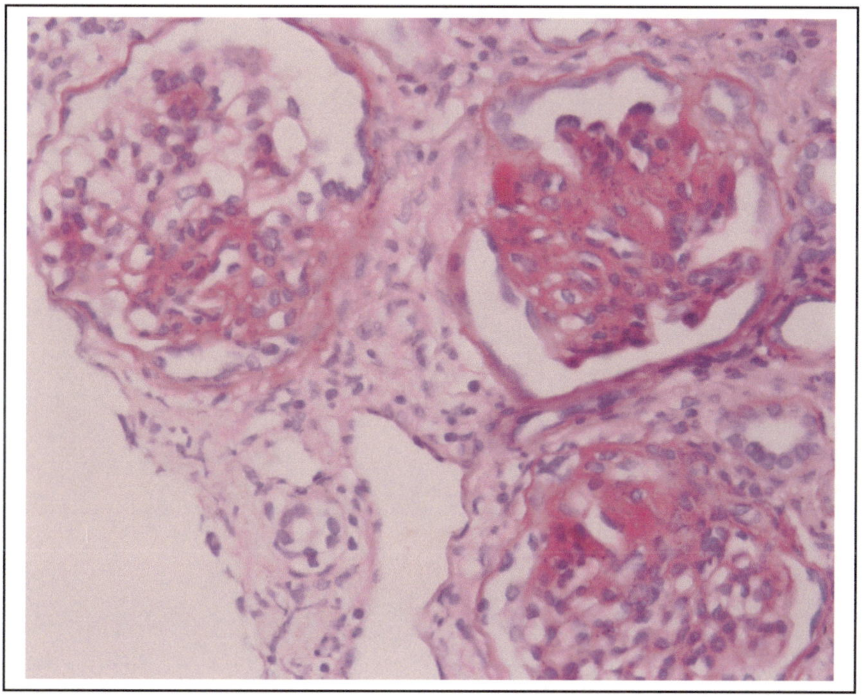

Fig. 7. Focal segmental glomerulosclerosis in 2 glomeruli and global sclerosis and Bowman capsule adhesions in the other. (PAS x200)

**CASE 4.**

A a 9 year-old girl admitted to the hospital because of hematuria and proteinuria lasting for two months.

She was initially diagnosed as mitochondrial disease by the findings of ptosis, ophthalmoplegia, failure to thrive, high serum lactate and pyruvate levels, ragged red fibers in muscle biopsy and the common 4.9 kb deletion in mtDNA.

She had been followed up for five years without any signs of other organ involvement before she developed hematuria and proteinuria.
On this admission, physical examination revealed failure to thrive, ptosis, hypo- and hyper-pigmented areas in both extremities.
Urinalysis showed 2+ proteinuria with normal blood biochemistry.
Urinary protein/creatinine ratio was 0.8, Hb 12 g/dl, WBC 7700/mm3 with normal complement components and β2 microglobulin levels.
**Renal biopsy diagnosis:** FSGS associated with mitochondrial disease(Figs.8,9)
Membranous glomerulonephritis(MGN) is mostly the disease of the adults and unusual in children. It can be primary or secondary to infections, drugs, systemic disease, malignant tumors etc. Patients may present with proteinuria, hypertension , hematuria or renal insufficiency. GBMs are the main site of injury and the characteristic pathologic features are thickened GBM along with a predominant IgG deposition of granular type. In early stages, GBM may show normal appearance and mild mesangial hypercellularity (Figs.10,11) (Cybulski,2011;Beck,2010).

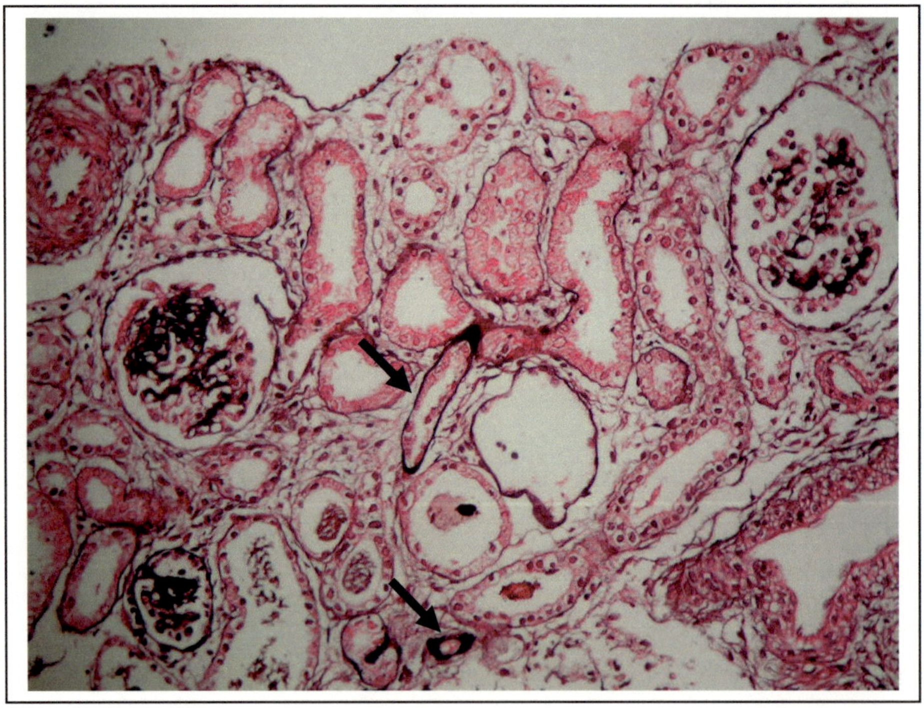

Fig. 8. Renal biopsy of Case 4 shows segmental sclerosis (arrow) in two glomeruli. Note focal atrophy of periglomerular tubules (arrows) and interstitial edema. HE&JSilverx100.

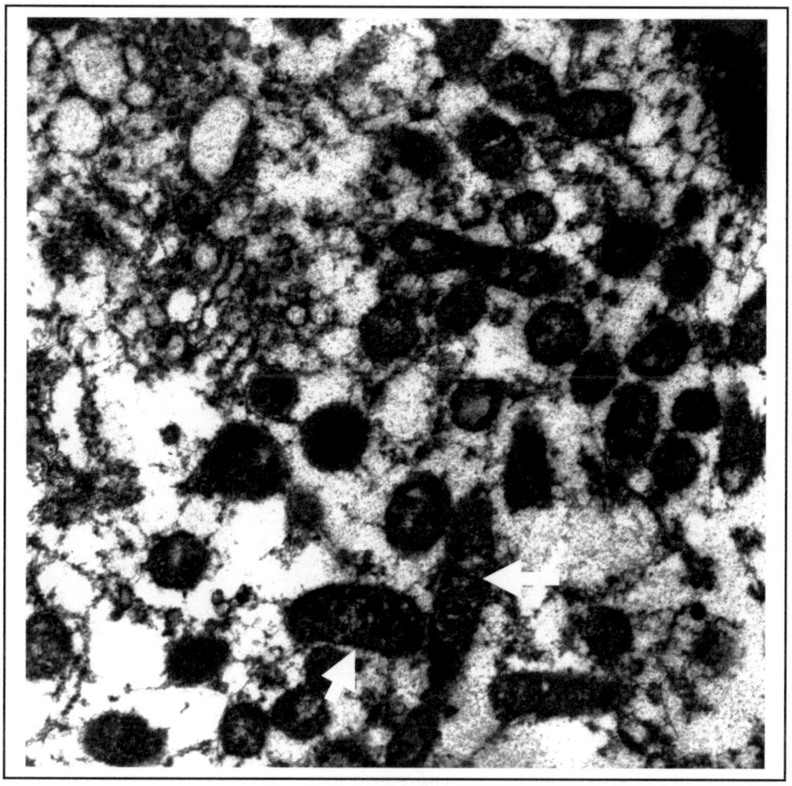

Fig. 9. Ultrastructural details of mitochondria in high magnification: Note increased matrix density and cristae formation. Vesicular structures (arrows) representing the increased cristae formation are evident. Uranyl acetate lead citrate x 20000.

**CASE 5.**

A 60 year old man was admitted with edema and hypertension lasting for one month.
No family history for kidney disease.
Physical examination revealed unremarkable findings except a high blood pressure of 170/100 mmHg and pretibial 2(+) pitting edema.
Laboratory findings: Complete blood count was normal, triglyceride 200 mg/dl, BUN 53 mg/dl, Cr 1.2 mg/dl, Total protein/Albumin 4/1.6 g/dl
Urinalysis: Density 1020, Proteinuria 3078 mg/ 24hrs, no glucose, sediment:, 10-15 red blood cells.
Serum IgA, IgG, IgM , C3 ,C4 levels, ANA, Anti-DNA, viral markers, CA 125,CA-19-9, CA-15-3 Rheumatoid factor, ASO and CRP were all normal.
**Renal biopsy diagnosis:** Membranous GN (Figs.10,11)
Renal amyloidosis must be included in differential diagnosis of proteinuria or nephrotic syndrome when the light microscopy gives no or minimal histopathological findings. Amyloid deposits in general appear as pink, homogenous and amorphous material in HE sections. Sometimes, the deposits may confine to the mesangium and be barely visible by light microscopy leading a misdiagnosis of minimal change disease. The diagnosis of amyloidosis is made by demonstration of apple-green birefringence under polarized light

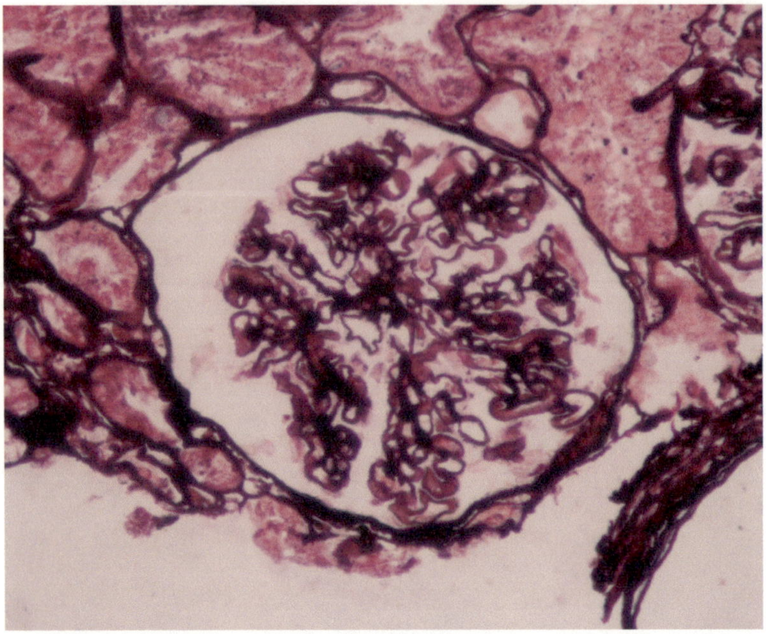

Fig. 10. Membranous GN. Early stage. A slight thickening of glomerular basement membrane. Jones Silver+HE.x400.

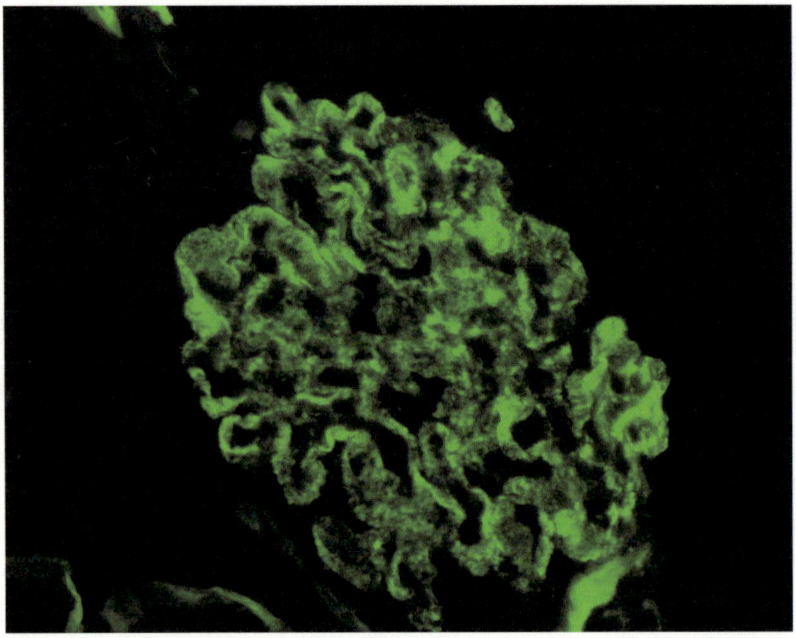

Fig. 11. Membranous GN. Granular type IgG staining of basement membranes in a glomerulus. Immunofluorescence microscopyx400.

in Congo-red stained sections which should be at least 6 microns in thickness.(Şen, 2010; Hopfer, 2011) (Figure 12,13).

**CASE 6.**

A 14 year-old-male was admitted to the hospital with the complaints of swelling of legs for 2 months. He had had recurrent fever and abdominal pain for 5 years.
No family history for kidney disease but $1^{st}$ degree consanguinity between parents.
On physical exam: Blood pressure:100/60 mmHg , pretibial 4(+) pitting edema was noted.
Laboratory findings: Complete blood count and electrolytes were normal ,
BUN 10 mg/dl,Cr:0.3 m g/dl, Total protein/Albumin: 3.9/1.89 g/dl
Urinalysis: Density 1010, Proteinuria 200 mg/m2/hr, no glucose, sediment: 1-2 white blood cells.
Serum C3 ,C4 levels, ANA, Anti-dsDNA, viral markers were all normal. MEFV mutation:M694V homozygote. Renal USG revealed minimal hyperechogenicity.
**Renal biopsy diagnosis**: Renal amyloidosis and familial Mediterranean fever(FMF) (Figs.12,13)

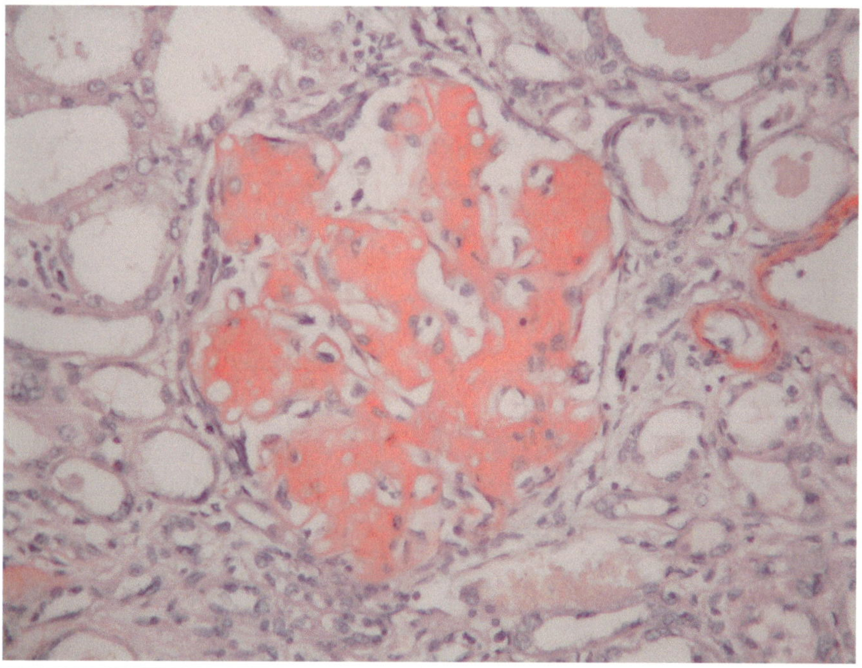

Fig. 12. Renal Amyloidosis. Diffuse nodular amyloid infiltration in a glomerulus. There is also vascular involvement (upper right).Congo red stain x200.

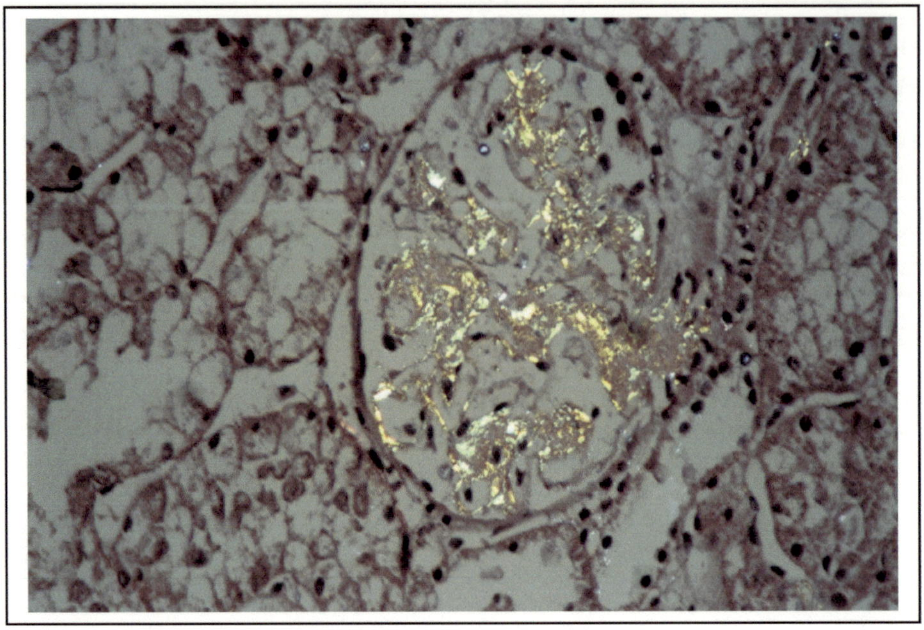

Fig. 13. Apple green birefringence of Congo red stained deposits under polarized light confirming the amyloid. Congo redx400

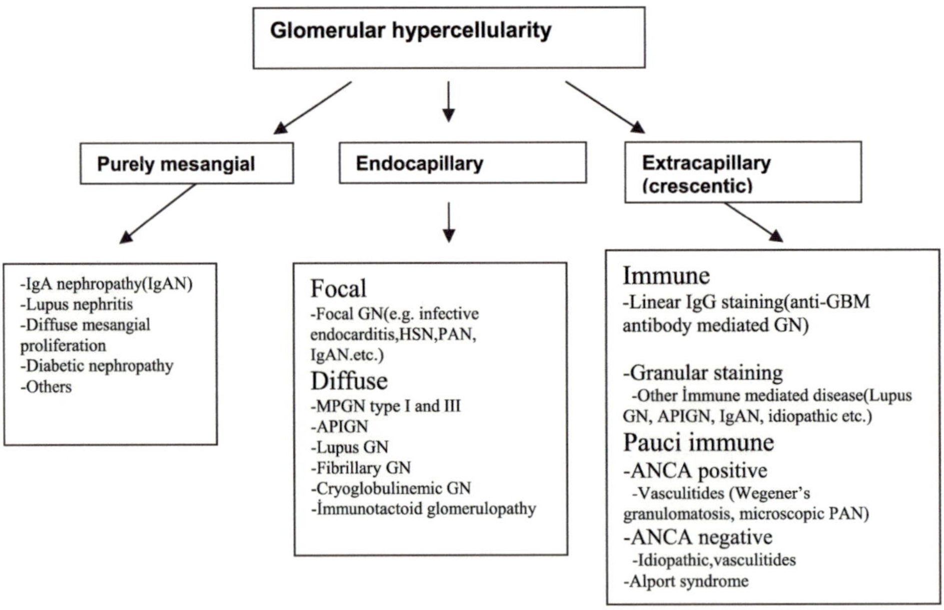


Fig. 14. An algorithm for interpretation of glomerular morphological changes with glomerular hypercellularity.(GN: Glomerulonephritis, MPGN: membranoproliferative GN, APIGN; acute postinfectious GN,ANCA; anti-neutrophil cytoplasmic autoantibodies,PAN; polyarteritis nodosa)

#### 2.1.1.2 Pure mesangial, endocapillary or extracapillary proliferative lesions

If the glomerular cellularity is increased the algorithm in Fig. 2 is used. At this point one should detect whether the glomerular hypercellularity is purely mesangial , endocapillary (occluding the capillary lumina) or extracapillary. Glomerular lesions may be focal or diffuse based on the percentage of involved glomeruli (i.e focal: the lesion involving less than 50% of number of glomeruli). Mesangial and Endocapillary proliferation may be segmental or diffuse while extracapillary proliferation may affect the glomerulus partially or globally.(Fogo, 2003; Lajoie & Silva,1996)
The differential diagnosis of mesangial proliferation depends on mainly immunofluorescence findings. IgA nephropathy is one of glomerular diseases which can present mesangial proliferation and is diagnosed by dominant or co-dominant IgA deposition in glomeruli by immunofluorescence microscopy and electron microscopy. (Cattran, 2009; Bellu, 2011)(Figs 15-17)

**CASE 7.**

A 20 year-old-male was admitted to the hospital with the complaints of flank pain and recurrent bouts of hematuria. He had a history of upper respiratory tract infection two days prior to the urinary symptoms.

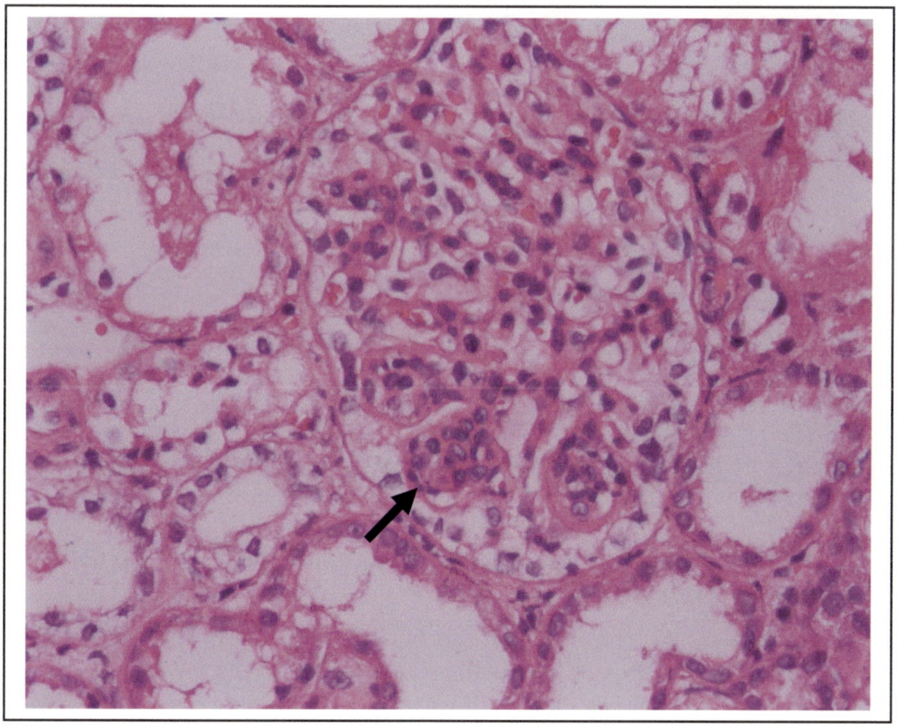

Fig. 15. Microphoto showing segmental endocapillary proliferation(arrow) a case with IgA nephropathy. HEx200.

No family history for kidney disease or consanguinity between parents.
On physical exam was unremarkable with a blood pressure of 100/60 mmHg .
Laboratory findings: Complete blood count and electrolytes were normal , ESR 30 mm/hr
BUN 20 mg/dl,Cr:0.8 m g/dl, Total protein/Albumin: 6.9/4 g/dl
Urinalysis: Density 1020, Proteinuria 30 mg/m2/hr, no glucose, sediment: abundant erythrocytes ,15-20 white blood cells and granular casts.
Serum C3 ,C4 levels, ANA, Anti-DNA, viral markers were all normal.
Renal USG revealed minimal increase in echogenicity and no evidence of urinary stone.
**Renal biopsy diagnosis**: IgA nephropathy (Figs. 15-17)

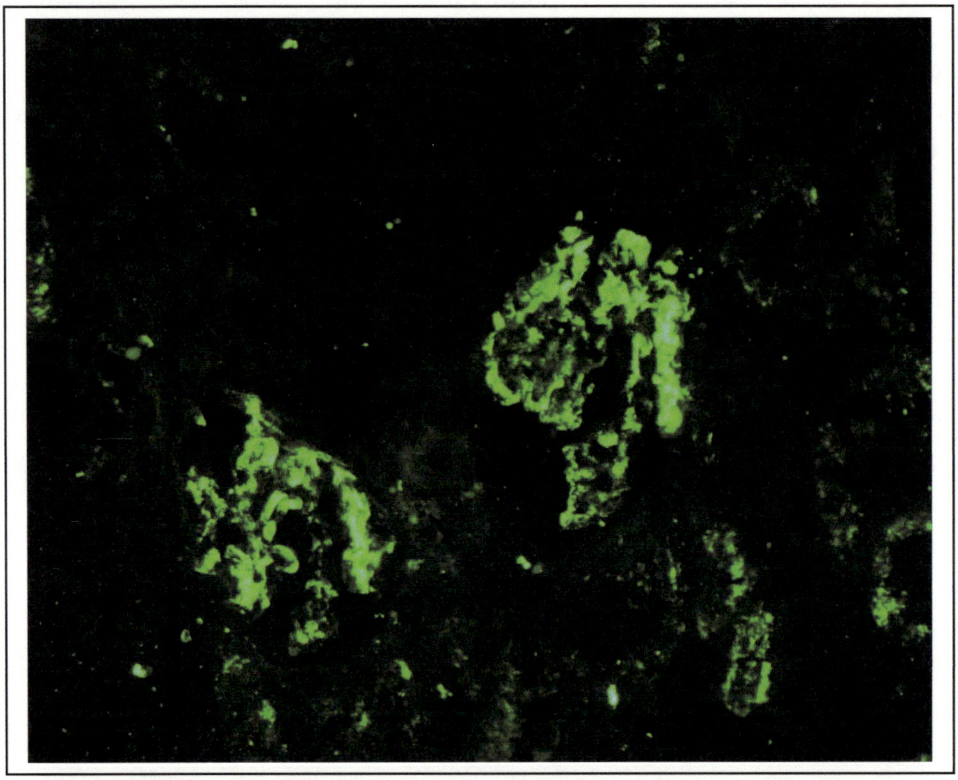

Fig. 16. IgA nephropathy. Mesangial distrubution of IgA deposits in two glomeruli. Immunofluorescence microscopy x200.

Mesangial and endocapillary proliferation can be seen together in membranoproliferative glomerulonephritis(MPGN) type 1, dense deposit disease(MPGN type 2), lupus nephritis, cryoglobulinemic GN, postinfectious GN, fibrillary GN or immunotactoid glomerulopathy. Then, immunofluorescence and electron microscopy are of vital importance for differential diagnosis. On the other hand, crescent formation not uncommonly associates to endocapillary proliferative ,necrotic or vasculitic lesions. The lesion is the consequence of capillary wall injury and proliferation of parietal epithelial cells. It can be categorized as

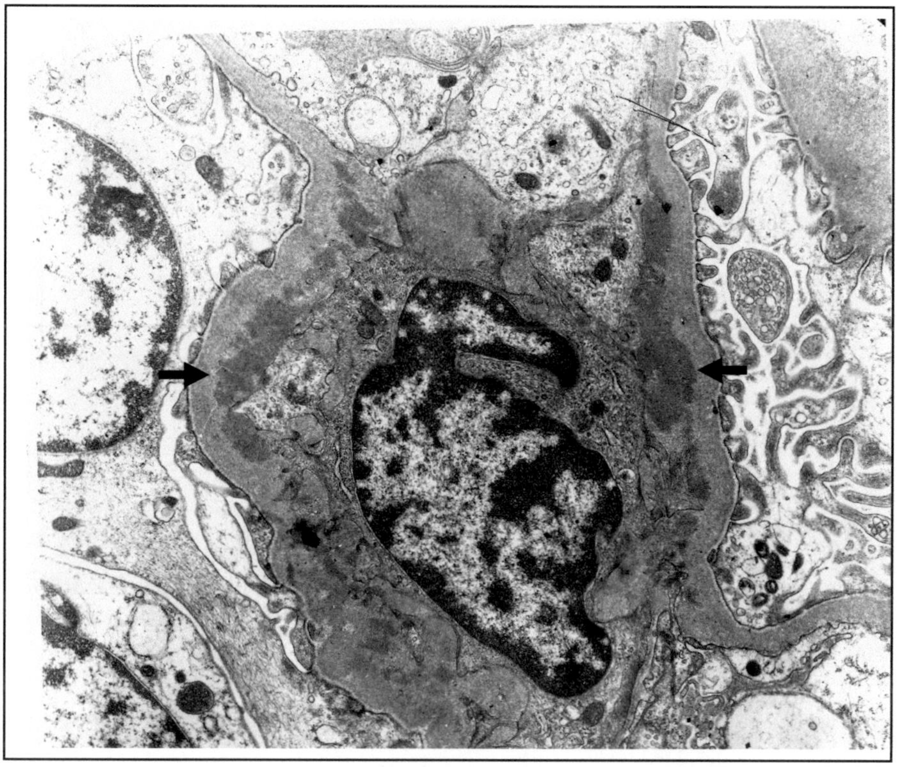

Fig. 17. IgA nephropathy. Electron microscopy shows immune deposits in the mesangial cell(arrows) uranyl acetate lead citrate x 8000.

immune mediated(lupus nephritis, acute postinfectious , anti GBM nephritis, IgA nephropathy etc.) or pauci-immune (Wegener's granulomatosis, microscopic PAN etc.)(Alchi,2010;Colucci,2011;Nasr,2008).(Figures 19-22)

**CASE 8.**

A 17 year-old-male presented with the complaints of hematuria and swelling of whole body. No family history for kidney disease or consanguinity between parents.

On physical exam was unremarkable except a blood pressure of 160/100 mmHg and pretibial 1+ edema.

Laboratory findings: Complete blood count and electrolytes were normal , CA 7.8 mg/dl,P 5.2 mg/dl, BUN 40 mg/dl,Cr:1.2 mg/dl, Total protein/Albumin: 4.14/2.7 g/dl

Urinalysis: Density 1027, Proteinuria 500 mg/24hrs, no glucose, sediment: abundant erythrocytes and white blood cells with fine granular casts.

Serum C3 40 mg/dl, ,C4 12.1mg/dl, ANA, Anti-DNA, viral markers were all normal.

Renal USG revealed minimal increase in echogenicity and no evidence of urinary stone.

**Renal biopsy diagnosis**: Membranoproliferative glomerulonephritis(MPGN) type 1 (Figs.15-17)

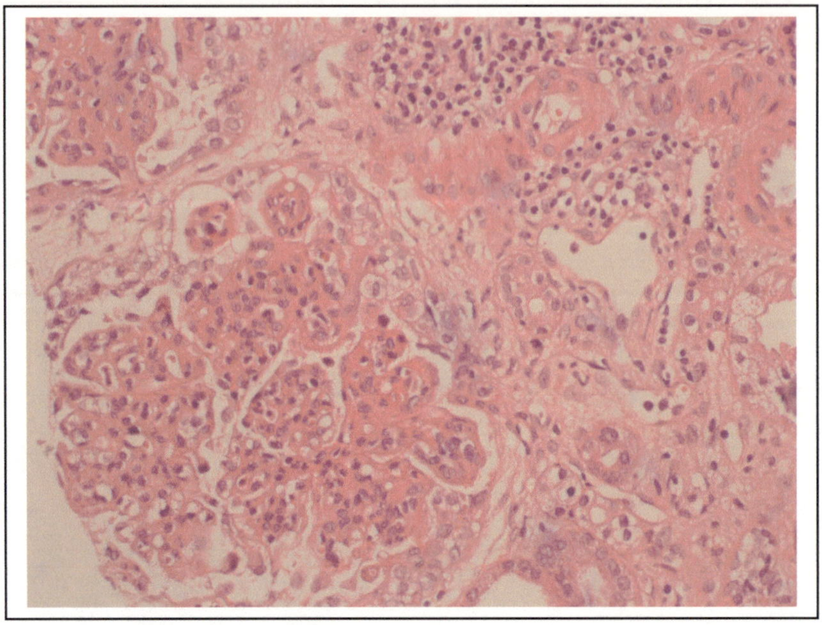

Fig. 18. Membranoproliferative glomerulonephritis. Note endocapillary proliferation, lobulation and thickening of glomerular capillary walls. A mononuclear inflammatory cell infiltration with tubular atrophy in the interstitium is also seen. HEx200.

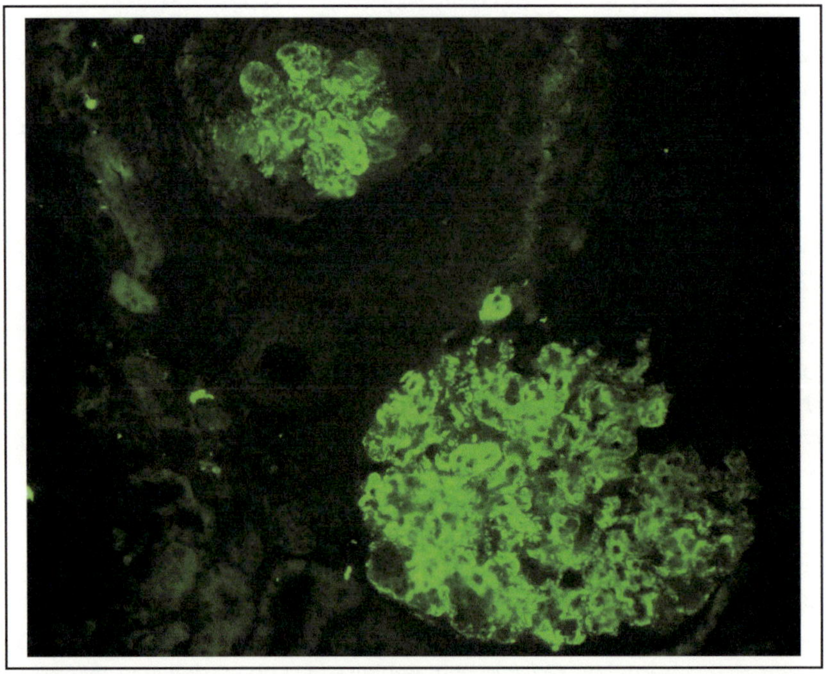

Fig. 20. Membranoproliferative type 1 GN. Granular frame-like staining of C3 the basement membrane and mesangium in 2 glomeruli. Immunofluorescence microscopyx200.

**CASE 9.**

A 15 year-old-male presented with the complaints of hematuria, oliguria and swelling of his face and eyelids. He suffered a throat infection 10 days prior to admission. No family history for kidney disease or consanguinity between parents.

On physical exam was unremarkable except a blood pressure of 160/100 mmHg and pretibial 1+ edema.

Laboratory findings: Complete blood count and electrolytes were normal , BUN 98 mg/dl,Cr:9.34 mg/dl, Total protein/Albumin: 6.14/3.2 g/dl

Urinalysis: Density 1018, Proteinuria 1200 mg/24hrs, no glucose, sediment: abundant erythrocytes and white blood cells and fine leukocytic and granular casts.

Serum C3 15 mg/dl, ,C4 6.1mg/dl, ANA, Anti-DNA, viral markers were all normal.

Renal USG revealed minimal increase in parenchymal echogenicity . Urine culture was negative.

**Renal biopsy diagnosis**: Acute postinfectious glomerulonephritis(APIGN) (Figs.21-22)

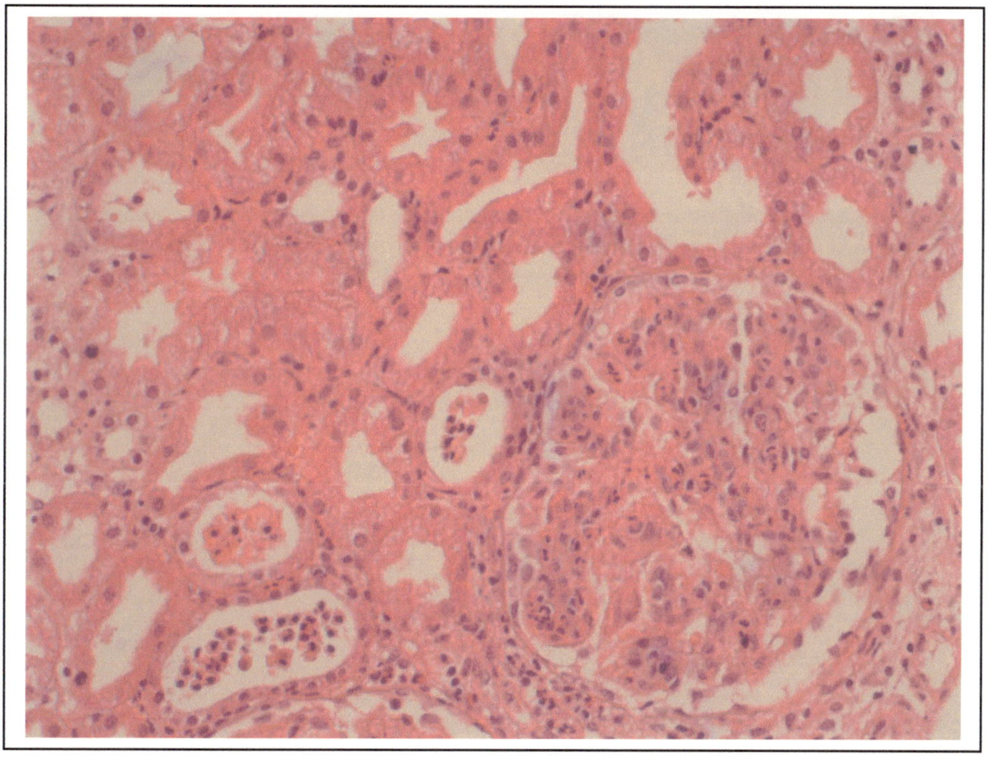

Fig. 21. Acute postinfectious glomerulonephritis. Light micrograph shows endocapillary proliferation with numerous neutrophils. There are also several neutrophils in tubular lumina.HEx200.

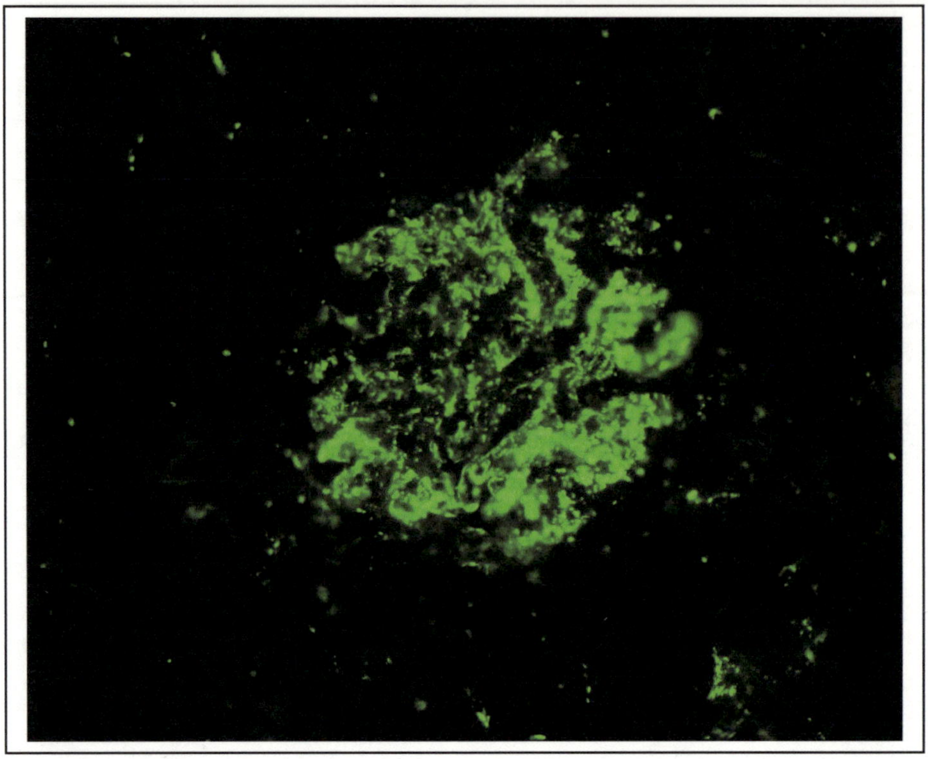

Fig. 22. Acute postinfectious GN. Immunofluorescence microphoto shows a starry sky pattern. There is a diffuse fine or coarse granular deposits of C3 in the GBM and mesangium. Immunofluorescence microscopyx200.

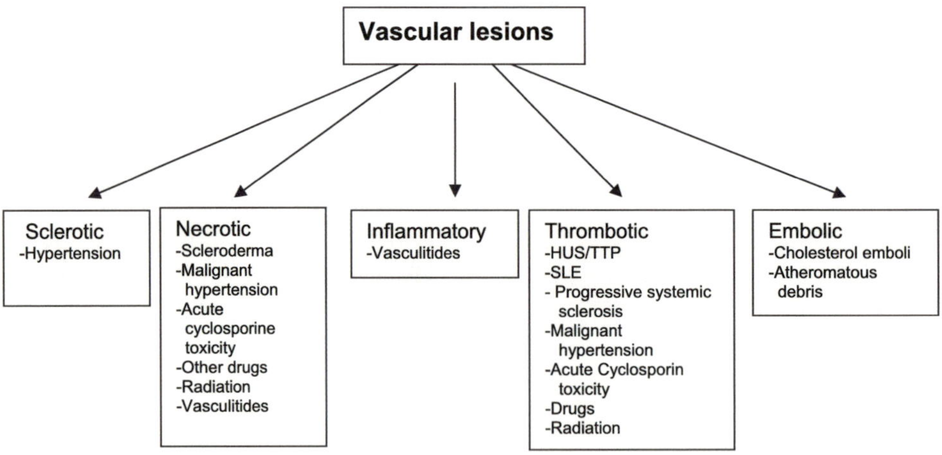


Fig. 23. An algorithm for interpretation of vascular lesions.(HUS: Hemolytic uremic syndrome, TTP: Thrombotic Thrombocytopenic purpura, SLE: Systemic lupus erythematosus)

### 2.1.2 Vascular lesions

Vascular lesions can be divided into five broad groups. Intimal fibrosis/medial fibrosis is associated with hypertension whereas necrosis may be a sign of progressive systemic sclerosis, vasculitis, drug hypersensitivity or radiation. Thrombotic lesions can be due to thrombotic microangiopathy/ hemolytic uremic syndrome, lupus nephritis + antiphospholipid syndrome, malignant hypertension and progressive systemic sclerosis. (Silvarin, 2011; Lindsay, 2011; Benz,2010) (Figures 24,25)

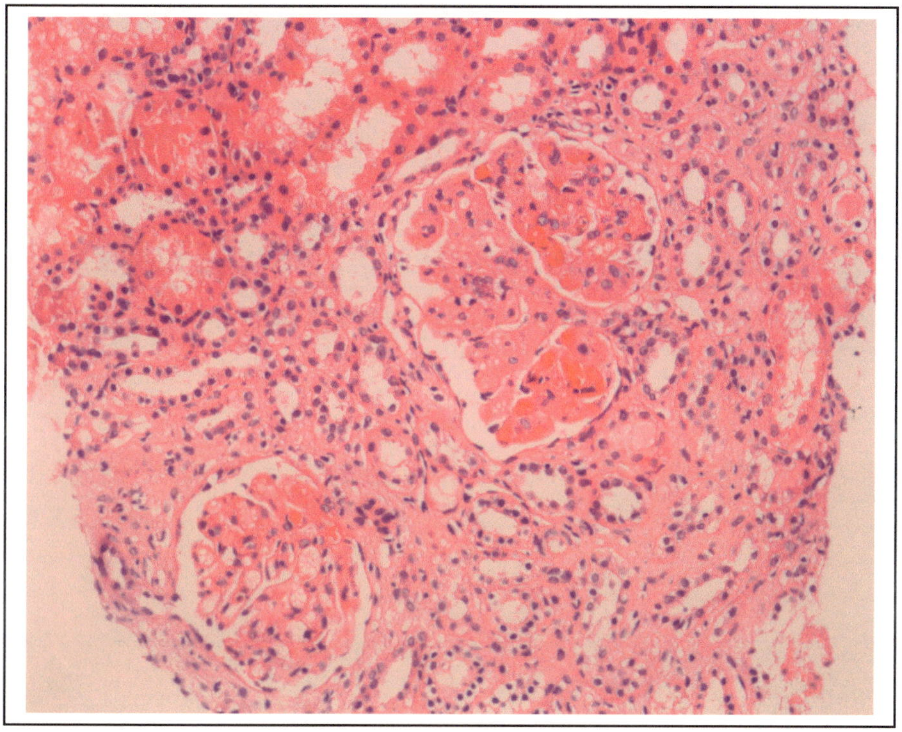

Fig. 24. Lupus nephritis+ thrombotic microangiopathy. Note 'wire-loops(down left) and fibrin thrombi obliterating glomerular capillary lumina. HEx100

### 2.1.3 Tubulointerstitial lesions

Tubulointerstitial lesions can be divided into five main categories including interstitial cellular infiltrates, necrosis, edema, tubular atrophy/fibrosis and tubular casts/deposits. If there is a significant infiltration in the tubulointerstitial area it is crucial to determine whether it is benign or malignant.(Figure 26). If benign, then the predominant cell type in the infiltration should be assessed or if there is no significant inflammation, necrosis, edema, tubular atrophy /fibrosis, tubular casts and deposits are investigated according to the main tubular abnormalities.(Figures 27,28) (Kowalewska,2011; Simms,2011; Wolf,2011; Midgley,2011;Chandra,2010)

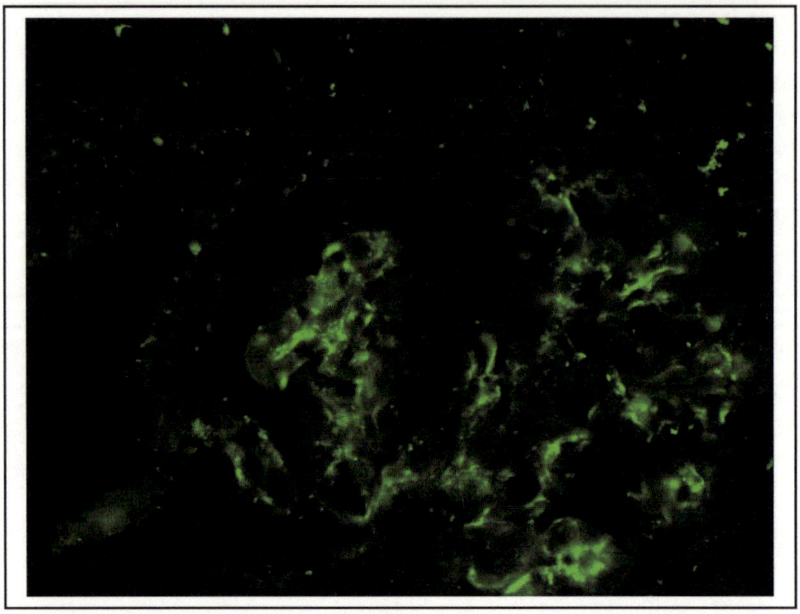

Fig. 25. Lupus nephritis+ thrombotic microangiopathy. IgG staining of glomerular basement membrane and mesangium. Immunofluorescence microscopyx400.

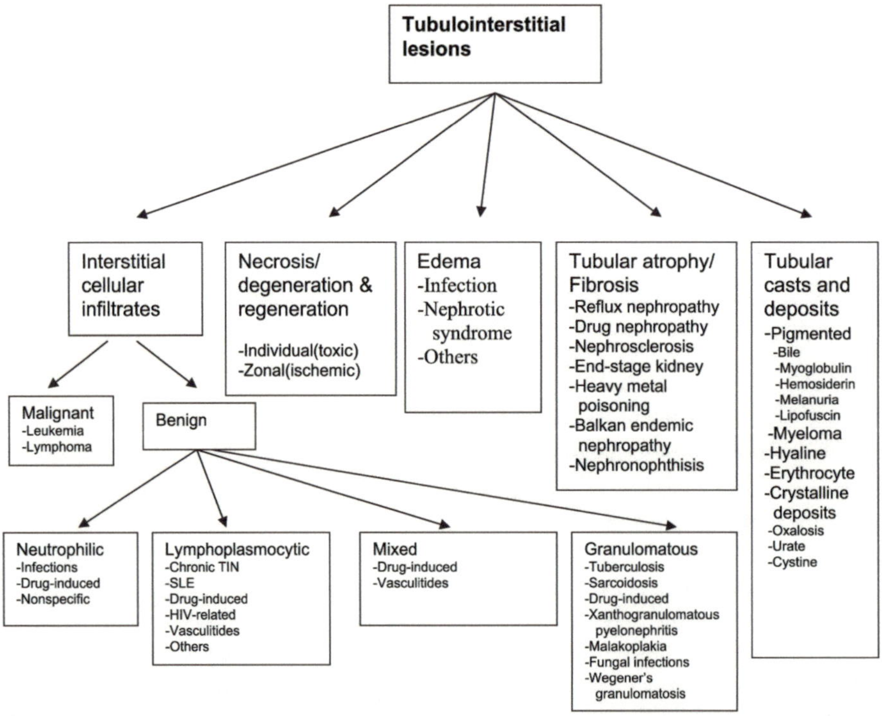


Fig. 26. An algorithm for interpretation of tubulointerstitial lesions. (TIN: Tubulointerstitial nephropathy, SLE:Systemic lupus erythematosus,HIV; Human immunodeficiency virus)

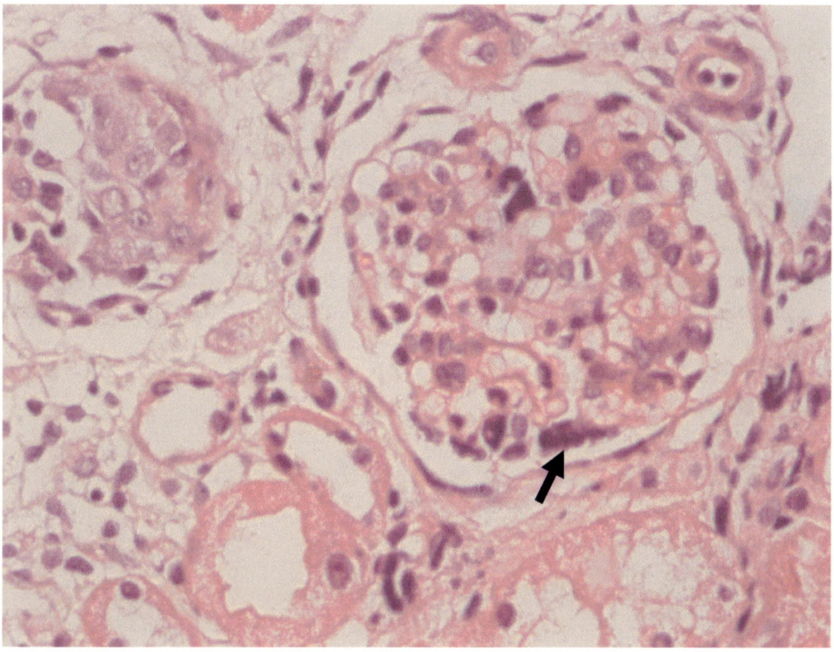

Fig. 27. Cystinosis. Multinuclear podocytes may be an early sign of cystinosis(arrow). HEx200.

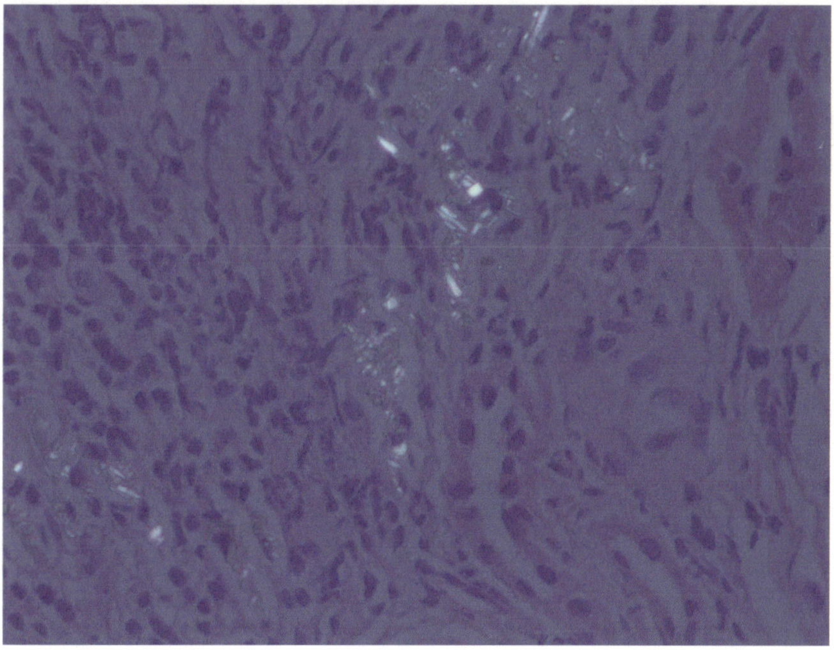

Fig. 28. Cystinosis. Cystine crystals in the interstitium under polarized light.HEx400.

**CASE 10.**

A 3 year-old-male presented with the complaints of polyuria, polydipsia and oliguria lasting eight months. No family history for kidney disease but 2nd degree consanguinity between parents.
Physical examination revealed a malnourished infant with failure to thrive.
Laboratory findings: Complete blood count and electrolytes were normal , Ca 9.8 mg/dl, P 3.97 mg/dl, BUN 30 mg/dl,Cr:0.7 mg/dl, Total protein/Albumin: 7.4/4.3 g/dl
Urinalysis: Density 1006, Proteinuria 200 mg/24hrs, glucose(+), sediment: 7-8 erythrocytes and 5-6 white blood cells. Serum C3 90 mg/dl, ,C20.1mg/dl, ANA, Anti-DNA, viral markers were all normal. Ultrasonography revealed increase in renal parenchymal echogenicity.
**Renal biopsy diagnosis**: Cystinosis (Figs.27-28)

### 2.2 Transplant kidney lesions

Renal allograft biopsy is still the gold standard for diagnosis of transplant rejection. A number of both immune complex( such as MPGN, IgA nephropathy etc.) or non-immune disease(FSGS,diabetic nephropathy etc.) can recur in transplanted kidneys. (Sun,2011; John,2010)(Figure 29)

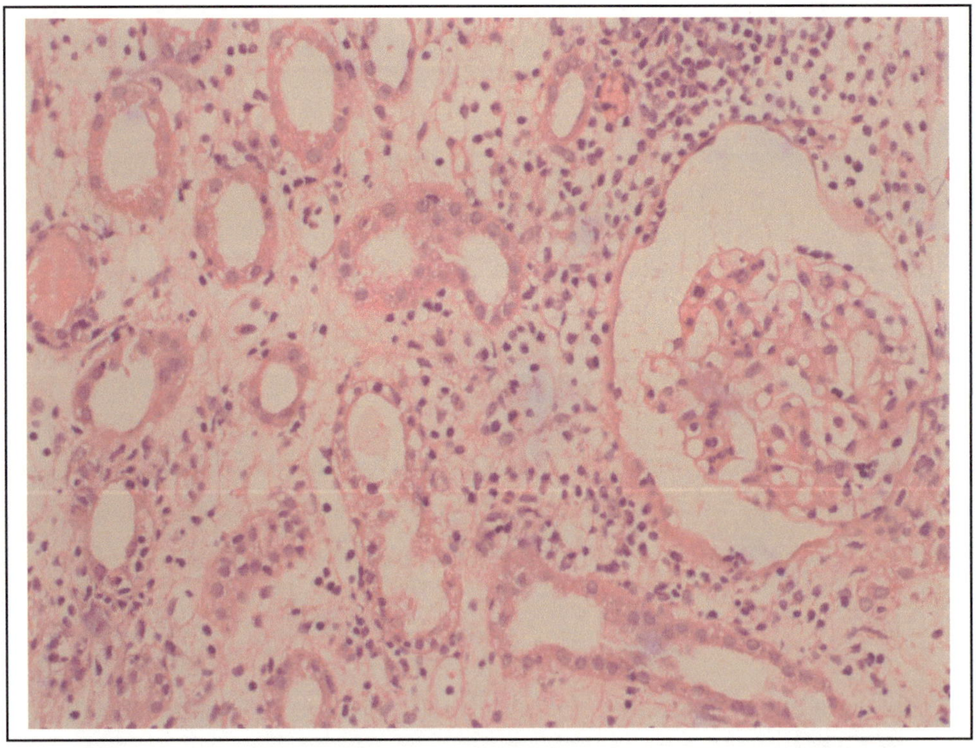

Fig. 29. Acute cellular rejection, Banff type 2. Light microscopic photo showing mild-moderate tubulitis along with tubulointerstitial inflammation. Note that the morphology of glomerulus is unremarkable.HEx100.

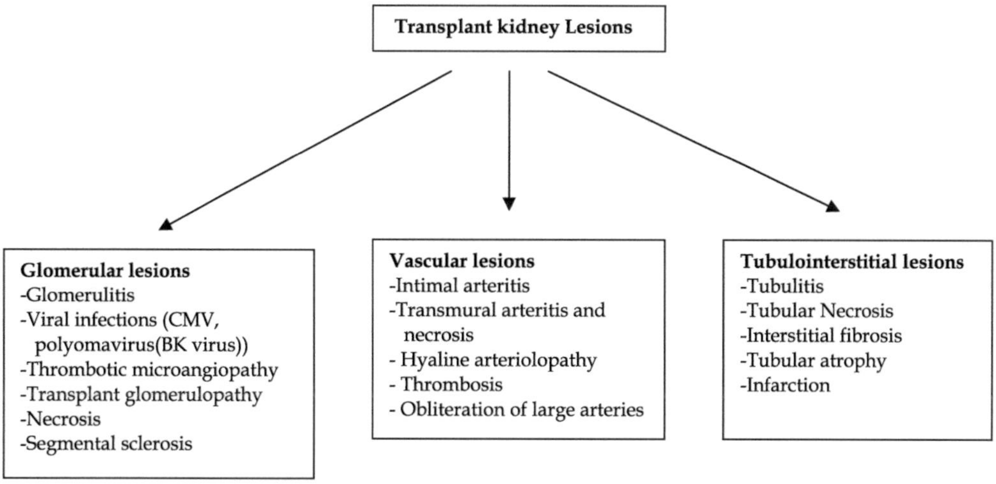


Fig. 30. Types of lesions commonly seen in transplanted kidneys. (CMV: Cytomegalovirus)

## 3. Conclusion

It should be remembered that these algorithms are designed for the diseases presenting with their classical patterns. Therefore, very rarely seen diseases or those without fully developed features are not included in the aforementioned algorithms. Since a number of disease may belong to more than one category because of diversity of the clinical and morphologic findings they may not clearly fall into any category. In addition, the best way to reach a correct diagnosis in a renal biopsy needs making a good correlation of morphological findings with appropriate clinical data.

In the future, a considerable amount of molecular genetic data are anticipated to be added. The aim is to use these data validated in large populations not only to create new algorithms providing the best approach to classify renal diseases but also to obtain complementary knowledge for appropriate prediction concerning diagnosis, therapy and prognosis of renal diseases.

## 4. References

Walker PD(2009). The renal biopsy. Archieves of Pathology & Laboratory Medicine, Vol. 133, No.2 ( February 2009), pp181-188, ISSN 0003-9985

Walker PD, Cavallo T& Bonsib SM, (2004).The Ad Hoc Committee on renal biopsy guidelines of the Renal Pathology Society. Practice Guidelines for the renal biopsy. Modern Pathology, Vol.17, No.12 ( December 2004), pp.1555-1563, ISSN 0893-3952

Kretzler M, Cohen CD, Doran P, Henger A, Madden S, Gröne EF, Nelson PJ, Schlöndorff D& Gröne HJ.(2002). Repuncturing the renal biopsy: strategies for molecular diagnosis in nephrology. Journal of the American Society of Nephrology, Vol.13 No.7, (July 2002), pp 1961-1972, ISSN 1555-9041

Fogo AB.(2003). Approach to Renal Biopsy. American Journal of Kidney Diseases, Vol.42, No.4, (October 2003), pp 826-836, ISSN 0272-6386

Furness PN.(2000). Acp. Best practice no 160. Renal biopsy specimens. Journal of Clinical Pathology, Vol.53, No.6, (June 2000), pp. 433-438, ISSN 0021-9746

Lajoie J & Silva FG. (1996). Appoach to the interpretation of Renal Biopsy. *Renal Biopsy Interpretation* Silva FG, D'agati VD, Nadasdy T(eds). pp 31-70.:Churchill Livingstone Inc.,0-443-07784-03, New York.

Mubarak M,. Kazi JI, Lanewala A, Hashmi S & Fazal Akhter .( 2011).Pathology of idiopathic nephrotic syndrome in children: are the adolescents different from young children? Nephrol. Dial. Transplant.;doi: 10.1093/ndt/gfr221

Zhang S, Audard V, Fan Q, Pawlak A, Lang P&Sahali D.(2011). Immunopathogenesis of idiopathic nephrotic syndrome. Contributions to Nephrology, Vol.169 No.1 (January 2011), pp. 94-106, ISSN 0302-5144

Kashtan CE.(2009). Familial hematuria. Pediatric Nephrology, Vol.24 No.10 (October 2009), pp 1951-1958, ISSN 0931-041X.

Savige J, Rana K, Tonna S, Buzza M, Dagher H&Wang YY.(2003). Thin basement membrane nephropathy. Kidney International, Vol.64, No.4 (October 2003), pp 1169-1178, ISSN 0085-2538

Haas M.(2009). Alport syndrome and thin glomerular basement membrane nephropathy: a practical approach to diagnosis. Archives of Pathology & Laboratory Medicine, Vol.133, No.2 (February 2009), pp 224-232, ISSN 0003-9985

Thomas DB.(2009). Focal segmental glomerulosclerosis: a morphologic diagnosis in evolution. Archives of Pathology & Laboratory Medicine, Vol.133, No.2 (February 2009), pp 217-223, ISSN 0003-9985

Gbadegesin R, Lavin P, Foreman J& Winn M.(2011). Pathogenesis and therapy of focal segmental glomerulosclerosis: an update. Pediatric Nephrology, Vol.26 No.7 (July 2011), pp 1001-1015, ISSN 0931-041X

Baskin E, Selda Bayrakci U, Alehan F, Ozdemir H, Oner A, Horvath R, Vega-Warner V, Hildebrandt F& Ozaltin F. Respiratory-chain deficiency presenting as diffuse mesangial sclerosis with NPHS3 mutation. Pediatric Nephrology, Vol.26 No.7 (July 2011), pp 1157-1161, ISSN 0931-041X

Emma F, Bertini E, Salviati Montini G.(2011) Renal involvement in mitochondrial cytopathies. Pediatr Nephrol. 10.1007/s00467-011-1926-6

Güçer S, Talim B, Aşan E, Korkusuz P, Ozen S, Unal S, Kalkanoğlu SH, Kale G&Cağlar M.(2005). Focal segmental glomerulosclerosis associated with mitochondrial cytopathy: report of two cases with special emphasis on podocytes. Pediatric and Developmental Pathology, Vol.8, No.6 (November-December 2005), pp 710-717 ISSN 1093-5266

Cybulsky AV. (2011).Membranous Nephropathy. Review.Contrib Nephrol.Vol.169, No.1 (January 2011), pp. ;107-25 , ISSN 0302-5144

Beck LH Jr.(2010). Membranous nephropathy and malignancy. Seminars in Nephrology, Vol.30, No.6 (November 2010), pp. 635-644, ISSN 0270-9295

Sen S, Sarsik B.(2010). A proposed histopathologic classification, scoring, and grading system for renal amyloidosis: standardization of renal amyloid biopsy report. Archives of Pathology & Laboratory Medicine, Vol.134, No.4 (April 2010), pp 532-544, ISSN 0003-9985

Hopfer H, Wiech T& Mihatsch J(2011). Renal amyloidosis revisited: amyloid distribution, dynamics and biochemical type. Nephrol Dial Transplant .doi: 10.1093/ndt/gfq831

Cattran DC, Coppo R, Cook HT, Feehally J, Roberts IS, Troyanov S, Alpers CE, Amore A, Barratt J, Berthoux F, Bonsib S, Bruijn JA, D'Agati V, D'Amico G, Emancipator S, Emma F, Ferrario F, Fervenza FC, Florquin S, Fogo A, Geddes CC, Groene HJ, Haas M, Herzenberg AM, Hill PA, Hogg RJ, Hsu SI, Jennette JC, Joh K, Julian BA, Kawamura T, Lai FM, Leung CB, Li LS, Li PK, Liu ZH, Mackinnon B, Mezzano S, Schena FP, Tomino Y, Walker PD, Wang H, Weening JJ, Yoshikawa N&Zhang H.(2009). Working Group of the International IgA Nephropathy Network and the Renal Pathology Society, The Oxford classification of IgA nephropathy: rationale, clinicopathological correlations, and classification. Kidney International, Vol.76, No.5 (September 2009), pp. 534-545, ISSN 0085-2538

Bellu SS, Troyanov, S, Hook T, Roberts ISD, on behalf of a Working Group of the International IgA Nephropathy Network and the Renal Pathology Society(2011). Immunostaining findings in IgA nephropathy: correlation with histology and clinical outcome in the Oxford classification patient cohort Nephrol Dial Transplant. doi: 10.1093/ndt/gfq812

Alchi B, Jayne D.(2010). Membranoproliferative glomerulonephritis. Pediatric Nephrology, Vol.25 No.8 (August 2010), pp 1409-1418, ISSN 0931-041X

Colucci G, Manno C, Grandaliano G, Schena FP. (2011). Cryoglobulinemic membranoproliferative glomerulonephritis: beyond conventional therapy. Clinical Nephrology, Vol. 74, No.4 (April 2010), pp. 374-379, ISSN 0301-0430

Nasr SH, Markowitz GS, Stokes MB, Said SM, Valeri AM, D'Agati VD.(2008). Acute postinfectious glomerulonephritis in the modern era: experience with 86 adults and review of the literature. Medicine (Baltimore), Vol.87, No.1 (January 2008), pp. 21-32 ISSN 1048-9614

Wen YK, Chen ML.(2010). The significance of atypical morphology in the changes of spectrum of postinfectious glomerulonephritis. Clinical Nephrology, Vol. 73, No.3 (March 2010), pp. 173-179, ISSN 0301-0430

Silvariño R, Sant F, Espinosa G, Pons-Estel G, Solé M, Cervera R, Arrizabalaga P.(2011). Nephropathy associated with antiphospholipid antibodies in patients with systemic lupus erythematosus. Lupus, Vol.20, No.7 (2011), pp. 721-729, ISSN 0961-2033

Keir L, Coward RJ.(2011). Advances in our understanding of the pathogenesis of glomerular thrombotic microangiopathy. Pediatric Nephrology, Vol.26 No.4 (April 2011), pp 523-533, ISSN 0931-041X

Benz K, Amann K.(2010). Thrombotic microangiopathy: new insights. Current Opinion in Nephrology and Hypertension, Vol.19, No.3 (May 2010), pp. 242-247, ISSN 1062-4821

Kowalewska J, Nicosia RF, Smith KD, Kats A, Alpers CE.(2011). Patterns of glomerular injury in kidneys infiltrated by lymphoplasmacytic neoplasms. Human Pathology, Vol.42, No.6 (June 2011), pp. 896-903, ISSN 0046-8177

Simms RJ, Hynes AM, Eley L, Sayer JA.(2011). Nephronophthisis: a genetically diverse ciliopathy. International Journal of Nephrology, Vol. No. (2011), pp. ISSN

Wolf MT, Hildebrandt F.(2011). Nephronophthisis. Pediatric Nephrology, Vol.26 No.2 (February 2011), pp 181-194, ISSN 0931-041X

Midgley JP, El-Kares R, Mathieu F, Goodyer P.(2011). Natural history of adolescent-onset cystinosis. Pediatric Nephrology, Vol.26 No.8 (August 2011), pp 1335-1337, ISSN 0931-041X

Chandra M, Stokes MB, Kaskel F.(2010). Multinucleated podocytes: a diagnostic clue to cystinosis. Kidney International, Vol.78, No.10 (November 2010), pp 1052, ISSN 0085-2538

Sun HJ, Zhou T, Wang Y, Fu YW, Jiang YP, Zhang LH, Zhang CB, Zhou HL, Gao BS, Shi YA, Wu S.(2011). Macrophages and T lymphocytes are the predominant cells in intimal arteritis of resected renal allografts undergoing acute rejection. Transplant Immunology, Vol.25, No.1 (July 2011), pp. 42-48, ISSN 0966-3274

John R, Herzenberg AM.(2010). Our approach to a renal transplant biopsy. Journal of Clinical Pathology, Vol.63, No.1, (January 2010), pp. 26-37, ISSN 0021-9746

# Part 3

## Glomerular Diseases

# 6

# The Many Faces of Thin Basement Membrane Nephropathy; A Population Based Study

Kyriacos Kyriacou et al.*
*Department of Electron Microscopy; Molecular Pathology*
*The Cyprus Institute of Neurology and Genetics, Nicosia*
*Cyprus*

## 1. Introduction

Thin basement membrane nephropathy (TBMN) or benign familial hematuria, is one of the commonest kidney disorders, characterized by recurrent benign hematuria, which is often associated with a family history (Gregory, 2005). It is generally considered to be a non-progressive, life long disorder with a rather benign course (Tryggvason & Patrakka, 2006), although data from some studies show that a proportion of patients manifest more severe symptoms, than originally described and eventually develop endstage renal disease (ESRD) (Dische, Weston, & Parsons, 1985; Frasca et al., 2005; Pierides et al., 2009; Tiebosch et al., 1989). TBMN was first described in 1926 (Baer, 1926) and at presentation is usually characterized by microscopic painless hematuria, by little or negligible proteinuria and normal renal function. TBMN is an autosomal dominant disorder and more than 50% of the cases have a family history of hematuria. In about 40% of families with a confirmed diagnosis of TBMN the condition co-segregates with heterozygous COL4A3/COL4A4 mutations (Lemmink et al., 1996). Mutations in the type IV collagen gene family which also includes the COL4A5 gene, also cause Alport syndrome (Hostikka et al., 1990). It is believed that these disorders are the result of defective, synthesis and/or assembly, of the critical glycoprotein components, that form the glomerular basement membranes (GBMs), among which type IV collagen, is the major constituent.

Clinically TBMN must be differentially diagnosed, between IgA nephropathy and Alport syndrome which are the other two main causes of hematuria, particularly in children. The need for differential diagnosis, often necessitates the examination of a kidney biopsy at the electron microscopical level, which also enables measurement of the thickness of the GBMs. Indeed Rogers et al (Rogers, Kurtzman, Bunn, & White, 1973) were the first to associate recurrent benign hematuria with the presence of thin GBMs. Currently the most widely

*Marianna Nearchou[1], Ioanna Zouvani[2], Christina Flouri[1], Maria Loizidou[1], Michael Hadjigavriel[3], Andreas Hadjisavvas[1] and Kyriacos Ioannou[4]
[1]*Department of Electron Microscopy/Molecular Pathology, The Cyprus Institute of Neurology and Genetics, Nicosia,*
[2]*Department of Histopathology, Nicosia General Hospital, Nicosia*
[3]*Department of Nephrology, Larnaca General Hospital, Larnaca*
[4]*Department of Nephrology, Nicosia General Hospital, Nicosia*
*Cyprus*

accepted pathognomonic hallmark for diagnosing TBMN is the presence of diffuse thinning of the GBM, in at least 50% of glomeruli examined. Accurate evaluation of the thickness of the GBM is best performed with the use of morphometry and requires the prior establishment of a normal range of GBM thickness, at each diagnostic centre.

It is well documented that the thickness of the normal GBM varies with age, gender and method of tissue preparation; thickness is also influenced by the method of measurement. According to general agreement, the GBM thickness is determined from samples fixed in glutaraldehyde. Recently it has been shown that even the choice of intermediate solvent and type of embedding resin are variables that also affect the thickness of the GBM (Edwards, Griffiths, Morgan, Pitman, & von Ruhland, 2009). Normal GBM thickness has been estimated in several reports (Coleman, Haynes, Dimopoulos, Barratt, & Jarvis, 1986; Das, Pickett, & Tungekar, 1996; Dische et al., 1985; Haas, 2009; Jovanovic GB, 1990). Since there is a lack of a general consensus on diagnostic criteria, it is recommended that a GBM normal range should be established for each laboratory (Dische et al., 1985; Tiebosch et al., 1989). This normal range is a necessary pre-requisite that facilitates the subsequent accurate diagnosis of TBMN. In our department we developed initially a detailed morphometric technique (Marquez et al., 1999) which was subsequently simplified to a more direct method, for measuring GBM thickness in kidney biopsies (Marquez et al., 2003). In this context we are one of a few electron microscopy departments which have been applying a standardized "in house" morphometric method, to diagnose TBMN cases, prospectively for more than 15 years. This method involves surveying the glomerulus and selecting the thinnest 4-5 peripheral glomerular capillary loops. Then the thickness of the GBM is measured in at least 4 different points per loop. If the average (arithmetic mean) of the measurements is less than 300nm, then the case is diagnosed as TBMN. We believe that this approach and practice have contributed to a more accurate estimate of the incidence of TBMN in our population (Zouvani et al., 2008).

In terms of histopathology, TBMN cases have normal glomeruli but some cases are often associated with mild and often premature glomerular changes. In some reports, the co-existence of thin GBMs with lesions compatible with focal segmental glomerulosclerosis (FSGS), affecting a variable number of glomeruli (up to 25%) was noted (Nieuwhof, de Heer, de Leeuw, & van Breda Vriesman, 1997; van Paassen, van Breda Vriesman, van Rie, & Tervaert, 2004). However, in our experience the occurrence of FSGS lesions in TBMN cases is more frequent and most of the glomeruli in TBMN cases show focal glomerulosclerosis. At the same time the importance of applying ultrastructural morphometry will be highlighted, as this is an essential component of accurate diagnosis. Our department operates as a referral diagnostic centre for the whole of Cyprus so the results are based on 1200 renal biopsies, from an unselected population sample, which is considered to be representative of our population. In this cohort of patients, a total of 75 renal biopsies showed thinning of GBMs, average thickness being less than 300nm and these cases were diagnosed as TBMN. The majority of glomeruli in these patients showed FSGS of different stages (different phases as described in the title), ranging from a mild segmental phenotype to more advance lesions of glomerulosclerosis. Another important aspect of TBMN is its association with other glomerulopathies, as shown by the histological examination of renal biopsy. This simultaneous presentation of TBMN with other glomerulopathies was present in seven of the 75 cases included in our study and gave rise to the selection of the title for this chapter. Consequently this title was chosen to reflect the progressive lesions of FSGS that are associated with TBMN, as well as the simultaneous occurrence of other glomerulopathies in the background of thin GBMs. In this review, the spectrum of histopathological and ultrastructural phenotypes detected in TBMN patients in our population will be described. We also illustrate the value of the direct GBM measurement method in detecting thin GBMs, in cases of TBMN presenting with more advanced glomerulosclerosis. In such cases the presence of thin GBMs may be overlooked, a factor which contributes to an underdiagnosis of this, rather common genetic disorder.

## 2. Aims

The main aims of the chapter are:

a. To present the histopathological features of TBMN in a population based study.
b. To highlight the fact that TBMN nephropathy is a more frequent disease and has a much higher incidence, than the 1-2% that is usually quoted in the literature.
c. To emphasize the need to use a standardized direct morphometric method for the accurate and systematic diagnosis of TBMN.
d. To highlight the observation that TBMN as a disease entity, may have different faces (phases), as histologically it is usually associated with different stages of glomerulosclerosis. Another factor that contributes to the different histological faces of TBMN is the phenomenon that TBMN is often associated with other glomerulopathies.

## 3. Materials and methods

### 3.1 Patients

In the last eighteen years, 1200 renal biopsies from Cypriot patients were investigated in the department of electron microscopy and 75 of these were diagnosed as TBMN. The TBMN group included 35 males and 40 females who at the time of biopsy had microscopic hematuria. Twenty-two patients had hematuria with proteinuria and of these eight had proteinuria in the nephrotic range. The majority of patients had normal renal function (Table 1). Detailed clinical data for some of these patients were described previously (Marquez et al., 2003; Zouvani et al., 2008). In this group of 75 patients, seven patients were diagnosed with TBMN which was associated with other glomerulopathies (Table 2). All patients included in the study were adults, above 18 years old.

### 3.2 Renal biopsies

Renal biopsies were obtained using a standard percutaneous technique under local anesthesia. The biopsies were examined and sectioned under an ordinary light microscope to select tissue containing glomeruli for light microscopy, immunofluorescence, and electron microscopy. All biopsies containing at least one glomerulus in the tissue submitted for electron microscopy were included.

### 3.3 Light microscopy

Tissue was fixed in 10% phosphate-buffered formalin and embedded in paraffin wax. Paraffin sections were cut at 4μm and stained with hematoxylin and eosin, periodic acid-Schiff (PAS), silver methanamine, Masson's trichrome and Congo red according to standard protocols.

### 3.4 Immunofluorescence

A small piece from each biopsy was embedded in optimal cutting temperature (OCT) compound and frozen directly in liquid nitrogen. Cryostat sections were cut at 4μm and incubated with a series of flourescein isothiocyanate (FITC)-linked mouse antibodies against human immunoglobulin A (IgA), IgG, IgM, C1q, C3 and fibrin, for direct immunofluorescence.

### 3.5 Routine electron microscopy

Specimens were fixed for a minimum of 4 h in 2.5% glutaraldehyde in 0.1 M phosphate buffer, pH 7.2, postfixed for 1 h in 1 % osmium tetroxide, dehydrated in a series of graded ethanols, cleared in propylene oxide, and embedded in an Epon/Araldite mixture. Blocks were sectioned with a Recheirt Jung Ultracut, ultramicrotome (Vienna, Austria). Semithin sections, 1μm thick, were stained with toluidine blue to locate glomeruli. Ultrathin sections of gold interference color were mounted on 200-mesh copper grids and stained with uranyl acetate and lead citrate. Electron microscopy was carried out in a JEM -1010 (JEOL-Tokyo) transmission electron microscope.

### 3.6 Morphometry

For measuring the thickness of the GBMs two approaches were used as our electron microscope was recently fitted with a digital camera. Consequently for the years spanning 1991-2008 the following methodology was used.

Each available block from a biopsy was serially sectioned to obtain the maximum number of glomeruli. In each glomerulus, each patent peripheral loop was photographed and this sometimes required a maximum of three separate micrographs per loop. Micrographs were taken at a magnification of x4,000 on 6.5 x 9cm Kodak electron microscope film. A grating replica with 2160 cross lines/mm was used for calibration (Electron Microscope Sciences, Washington, PA 19034). Prints were made to a final magnification of x12,000 and morphometric measurements were taken as described previously, using the simplified method (Marquez et al., 2003).

Since 2008 the software tool of the MEGAVIEM, Olympus Soft Imaging, system is being used to measure GBM thickness. In each biopsy every available glomerulus is scanned and at least four thin glomerular loops that are situated peripherally, are measured at a magnification of ×8000. For measurement, a square grid, size 2000x2000 nm, is superimposed over the glomerular capillaries and point measurements are taken at regions where the grid intersects the capillary loops exactly at right angles. Each point measures the distance from the cell membrane of the epithelial cell, as it attaches on the lamina rara externa, to the inner aspect of the endothelial cell membrane. In this manner a minimum of 16-20 separate points were measured in each peripheral glomerulus which represented 4-5 points per individual loop (Figs. 8 and 9b). In each patient the arithmetic mean of the GBM thickness was calculated, averaging measurements at 16 points, which is the minimum number of points measured per glomerulus. This approach was very similar to the direct method that was used previously (Marquez et al., 2003).

## 4. Results

### 4.1 Inclusion criteria

The selection criteria of biopsies for this study included:

a. Normal histology or minimal to moderate histological glomerular abnormalities.

b. Presence of thin GBMs having an arithmetic mean of less than 300 nm, or having more than 50% of the points measured below 300 nm upon direct measurement.
c. Presence of diffuse GBM thinning in a minimum number of four peripheral capillaries per glomerulus.
d. Absence of splitting or lamellation of the GBM.
e. Absence of diffuse fusion of podocytes in order to exclude primary FSGS.

### 4.2 Light microscopy

Seventy-five renal biopsies were selected for the present morphometric analysis based on the light microscopical observations and inclusion criteria outlined above (Table 1). On histology, 14 cases exhibited normal glomeruli. In 26 cases, up to 10% of glomeruli were affected by glomerulosclerosis (Figs. 1a and 1b) and in 27 cases glomerular sclerosis was present in between 10-50% of glomeruli (Figs. 2a and 2b). Focal glomerulosclerosis was characterized most often by an increase in mesangial matrix and very rarely this also included an increase in mesangial cells. In the remaining eight cases, glomerulosclerosis was evident in more than 50% of the total glomeruli identified in each biopsy (Fig. 3 and Table 1). These 75 patients included seven cases with the diagnosis of incidental TBMN which was associated with other glomerulopathies (Table 2).

### 4.3 Immunofluorescence

In all cases the immunofluorescence results were essentially negative except in the three cases that had a diagnosis of IgA nephropathy (IgAN), where moderate mesangial staining for IgA was present. In ten cases, there was mild and focal mesangial staining for IgM and two cases showed staining for C3.

### 4.4 Electron microscopy

All biopsy specimens, especially the ones obtained from patients with proteinuria showed a variable degree of epithelial cell foot process fusion. In all 75 cases foot process effacement was segmental and never global. In the selection process, renal biopsies showing global foot process fusion were excluded from the TBMN group, in order to eliminate inclusion of cases with primary FSGS. In terms of GBM thickness, 14 out of 75 patients who exhibited histologically normal glomeruli showed widespread thinning of the GBM. In the remaining patients, that showed glomerulosclerosis affecting between 10-50% of glomeruli, thinning of the GBM was more obvious in the glomerular segments that were unaffected by increased mesangial matrix and glomerulosclerosis. In all patients examined attenuation of GBM was the predominant finding. Thin GBMs were present in normal-looking capillary loops (Fig. 4) as well as in areas showing mild expansion of the mesangial matrix (Fig. 5). In some biopsies that exhibited a more marked increase in mesangial matrix, thin GBMs could still be distinguished even in severely affected areas, especially in peripheral glomerular capillaries (Fig. 6). In some patients, the thickness of the GBM was not uniform, and this was not related to orientation or differences in sectioning (Fig. 7). In such cases morphometry (see below) provided more accurate estimates of the GBM thickness.

### 4.5 Morphometry

For classifying our own patients, the normal adult mean GBM thickness range of 300–400nm was adopted. This is our "in-house" range of normal adult GBM thickness that was

| Number of patients | Total = 75 | TBMN = 68 | TBMN + associated GN=7 |
|---|---|---|---|
| Male/Female | 35/40 | 32/36 | 3/4 |
| Age-mean | 46 | 44 | 50 |
| Age range | 20-71 | 20-71 | 24-67 |
| Family history | 20 | 20 | 0 |
| Hematuria | 75 | 68 | 7 |
| Proteinuria | 22 | 15 | 7 |
| Normal renal function (serum creatinine <1.0 mg/dL) | 46 | 46 | 0 |
| Normal glomeruli | 14 | 14 | 0 |
| Glomerular sclerosis in <10% of glomeruli | 26 | 26 | 0 |
| Glomerular sclerosis in >10% - <50% of glomeruli | 27 | 20 | 7 |
| Glomerular sclerosis in >50% of glomeruli | 8 | 8 | 0 |
| Mean GBM thickness <200nm | 17 | 17 | 0 |
| Mean GBM thickness >200nm - <300nm | 58 | 51 | 7 |

Table 1. Demographic and clinicopathological findings in TBMN patients.

| Number of cases | 7 |
|---|---|
| IgA nephropathy (IgAN) | 3 |
| Mesangial proliferative GN (MesPGN) | 1 |
| Minimal change disease (MCD) | 2 |
| Transplant glomerulopathy (TG) | 1 |

Table 2. TBMN cases associated with other glomerulopathies.

established previously (Marquez et al., 1999). For the morphometric measurements of the thickness of GBM, the simplified method was used for biopsies obtained between 1991-2008; details of which were previously published (Marquez et al., 2003). For the renal biopsies investigated after 2008, the morphometric method using the iTEM software of the MEGAVIEW digital camera was applied as described in section 3.6 (Figs. 8 and 9b). Out of the 75 patients investigated 58 had an average GBM thickness between 200 and 300 nm, whereas for the remaining 17 patients the mean GBM thickness was below 200 nm. None of the 75 patients had a mean GBM thickness below 100nm.

In some cases showing progressive glomerulosclerosis, some glomerular capillaries exhibited uniformly thin GBMs (Fig. 10a), but other capillaries in adjacent areas, within the same glomerulus, required morphometry as there was a big variation in the thickness of the GBM (Fig. 10b). In many biopsies RBCs were frequently seen in the Bowman's space, as evidenced by the hematuria observed in this cohort of patients. Seven patients had TBMN associated with other glomerulopathies among which the commonest was IgA nephropathy. In these patients electron microscopy revealed the presence of isolated mesangial and subendothelial, electron dense deposits as well as thin GBMs (Figs. 11a and 11b).

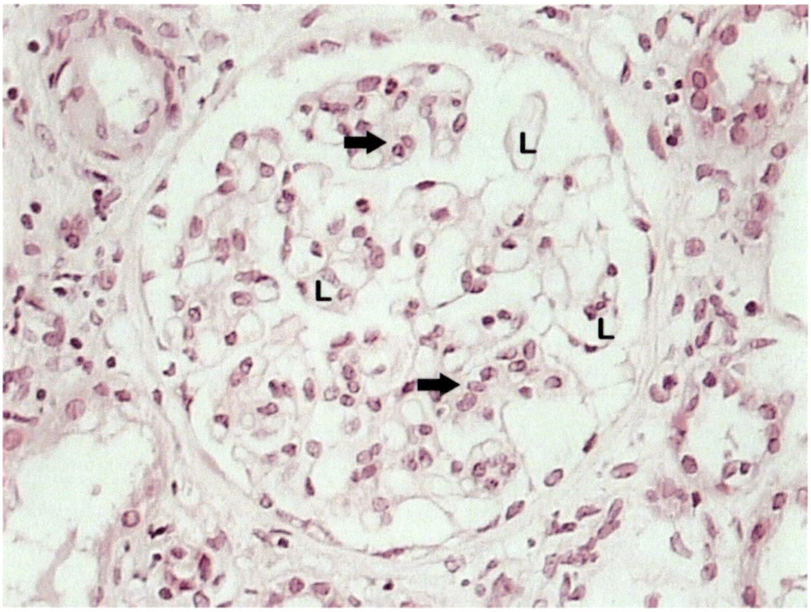


Fig. 1. a. Renal biopsy from a 35 year old male patient with hematuria. Light microscopy of renal biopsy stained with hematoxylin and eosin showing glomerulus with an almost normal histology. Early lesions of focal segmental glomerulosclerosis are shown (arrows) but most capillary loops are patent (L) (magnification x400).

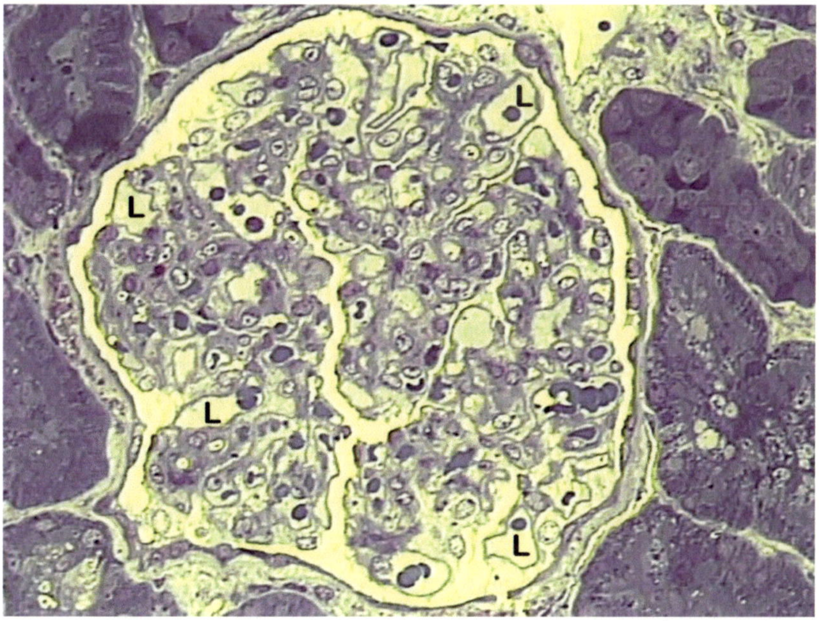


Fig. 1. b. Semithin araldite section stained with toluidine blue showing a glomerulus from the same patient as fig. 1a with patent peripheral capillary loops (L) (x400).

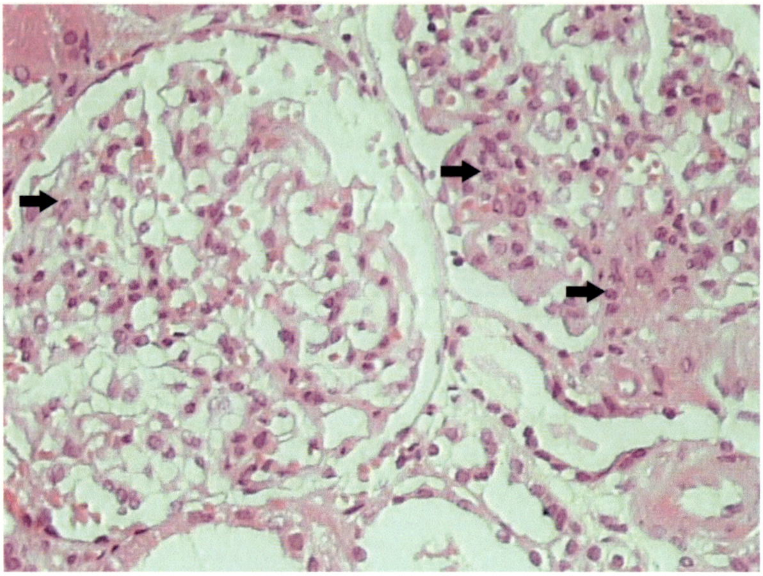

Fig. 2. a. Renal biopsy from a 45 year old male patient with hematuria. Light microscopy showing two adjacent glomeruli, with different stages of FSGS. On the left a mild lesion is present, whereas on the glomerulus on the right the lesions are more advanced (arrows). In this patient the GBM measured 230nm (Hematoxylin and eosin stained section) (x400).

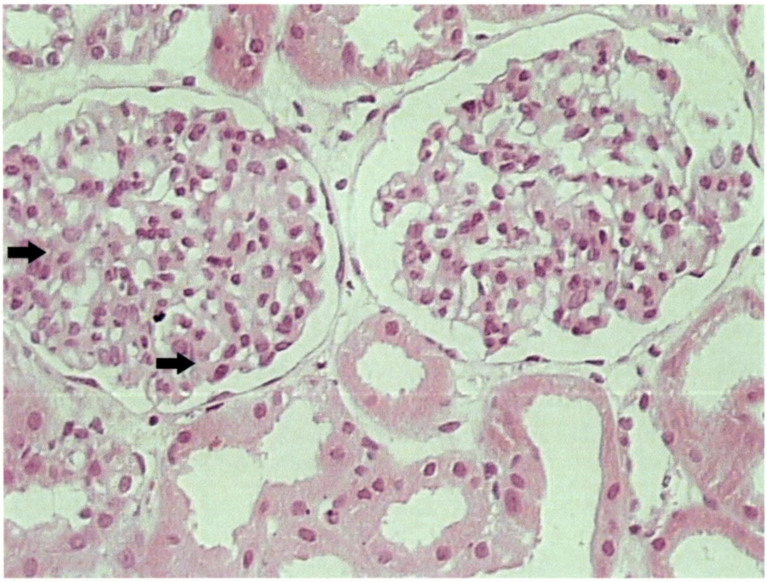

Fig. 2. b. Renal biopsy from a 50 year old female patient with hematuria and mild proteinuria. Light microscopy showing two adjacent glomeruli, with a different degree of glomerulosclerosis. Left glomerulus shows more advanced sclerosis (arrows) compared to the right. This patient had a mean GBM thickness, in unaffected glomeruli of 200 nm (Hematoxylin and eosin stained section) (x400).

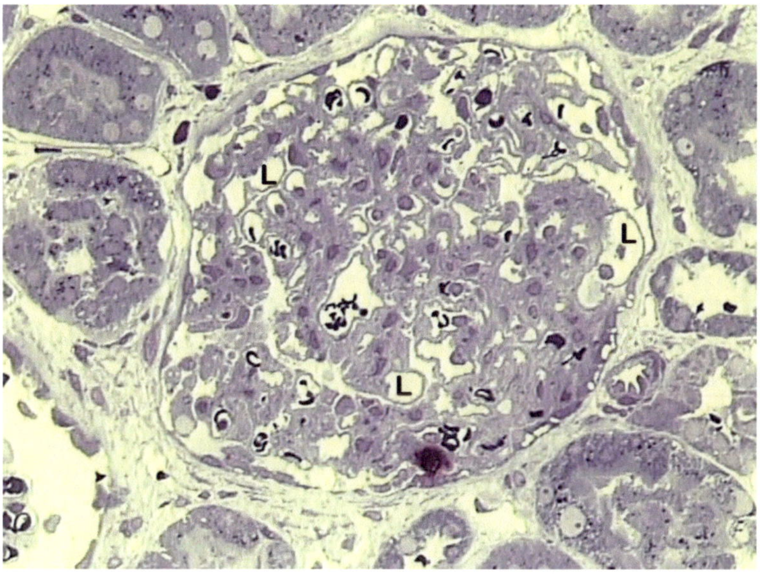


Fig. 3. Semithin araldite section stained with toluidine blue showing a glomerulus with more than 50% sclerosis. Patent capillary loops (L) are seen in the periphery of the glomerulus (x400).

## 5. Discussion

In the discussion that follows, the main aims of this chapter as outlined in section 2 will be discussed.

### 5.1 Histopathological features of TBMN

In this study we present the ultrastructural and histopathological features of a large series of TBMN cases diagnosed in the Cypriot population. TBMN is generally characterized by attenuation of GBMs, a finding that can be documented only by ultrastructural examination of kidney biopsies. This key ultrastructural feature was initially described by Rogers et al., in 1973; they were the first to associate the clinical symptoms of hematuria with the presence of thin GBMs. The above observations provided the basic criteria for distinguishing the more severe, Alport-type progressive nephritis, which ultrastructurally is characterized by thinning, thickening, and GBM lamellation from the more benign form of TBMN. It is well established that electron microscopy is absolutely essential for the accurate diagnosis of TBMN since the light microscopic alterations are usually nonspecific and include a spectrum of findings. Histology may show the presence of normal glomeruli or a range of pathological lesions such as focal glomerular sclerosis and mesangial matrix expansion. Direct immunofluorescence staining is usually negative, but sometimes traces of segmental mesangial staining for IgM and C3 may be present in some TBMN cases, as was observed in this study. In some renal biopsies, GBM attenuation can be observed histologically in Jones methenamine silver or PAS stains, but these findings are only suggestive of TBMN. Consequently, electron microscopy remains the only modality that can confirm the presence of thin GBMs. Our results show that the majority of TBMN cases on renal biopsy show early glomerular changes such as mesangial matrix increase that are compatible with FSGS. The association of TBMN with FSGS has been previously noted in other studies (Foster, Markowitz, & D'Agati, 2005; van Paassen et al., 2004). The presence of glomerular changes that inadvertently lead to increased mesangial matrix and thickening of GBMs, should be taken into consideration as this will affect the accurate diagnosis of TBMN. Indeed in our study, eight cases contained more than 50% glomerulosclerosis but on morphometry had GBM thickness of less than 300 nm. These eight cases, as well as the seven cases of TBMN associated with other glomerulopathies were included in our study as they had clinicopathological features resembling TBMN and fulfilled the inclusion criteria defined. In recent years it has become increasingly evident that within the TBMN group, the degree of thinning is quite variable, not only between patients but also within individual glomeruli from the same patient. Indeed, in some of our cases, we observed variations in the thickness of adjacent GBMs and even within the same capillary loop, GBM thinning was not uniform. Therefore, ultrastructural examination of renal biopsies has to include a detailed morphometric analysis in order to clearly define such cases accurately, and for confirming that the GBM attenuation is the major lesion.

### 5.2 Incidence of TBMN

TBMN is the commonest cause of recurrent glomerular hematuria that affects both children and adults (Tryggvason & Patrakka, 2006). Although a common nephropathy, the incidence of TBMN is poorly defined and estimates vary widely in the literature from 1% to 9% (Tryggvason & Patrakka, 2006), (Dische et al., 1990). Using electron microscopy in conjunction with a direct quantitative technique for measuring GBM thickness we recently estimated the incidence of TBMN to be 5.4% in the Cypriot population (Zouvani et al., 2008). These results are in agreement with those obtained by other studies (Cosio, Falkenhain, & Sedmak, 1994), where it was estimated that persistent hematuria occurs consistently in as much as 6% of both children and adults (Wang & Savige, 2005). Since some cases of Alport syndrome particularly the autosomal recessive type, can resemble TBMN ultrastructurally, children were excluded from this study as well as cases showing splitting or lamellation of the lamina densa (Haas, 2006).

The exact incidence of TBMN is difficult to assess, since the diagnosis is mostly made on the basis of persistent hematuria combined with minimal proteinuria. Indeed, the prevalence of hematuria in adults is not well known (Gregory, 2005). In addition, when estimating the prevalence of TBMN by analyzing the incidence of hematuria it should be remembered that not all patients who have TBMN have hematuria. Some patients with persistent hematuria, have other signs of renal dysfunction that exclude presence of TBMN, and most importantly, hematuria is not always of glomerular origin (Nieuwhof et al., 1997). In our case, the incidence was estimated on the basis of electron microscopic diagnosis and the presence of thin GBMs, having an arithmetic mean of less than 300 nm. However, the number of electron microscopic analyses of renal biopsies showing thin GBMs are few (Marquez et al., 1999), so many cases remain undiagnosed. It is likely that our figure of 5.4% is accurate, since it is based on the presence of thin GBMs as documented by electron microscopical examination, in a large series of consecutive kidney biopsies. These biopsies were unselected for a family history of hematuria or other familial renal disorder, so they represent an unbiased pool of samples on which our estimate is based. Therefore, it is not surprising that the incidence rate for TBMN in our population was estimated to 5.4%, (Zouvani et al., 2008) since our results are based on the actual presence of thin GBMs, which

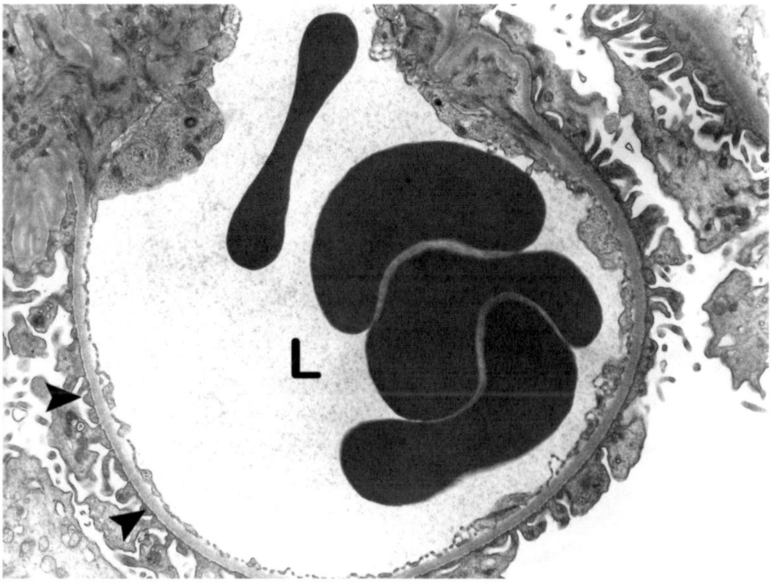


Fig. 4. Electron micrograph from the kidney biopsy of a 48-year old male patient presenting with hematuria showing uniform thinning of GBM of a peripheral glomerular capillary loop. The average thickness of the GBM was 220 nm. Note a widely patent capillary lumen (L) containing several RBCs. The foot processes are well preserved (arrowheads) (x15,000).

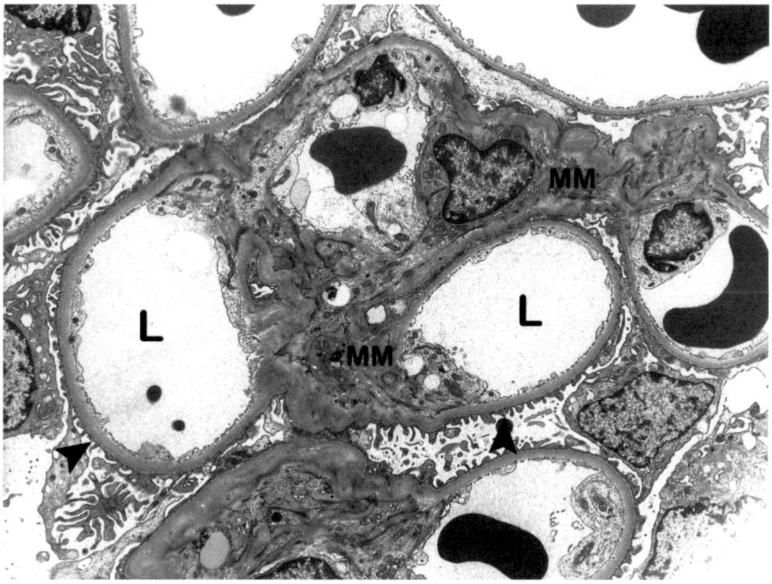


Fig. 5. Electron micrograph from the kidney biopsy of a 37-year old female patient presenting with hematuria showing variability in the thickness of the GBMs. The capillary lumina (L) are widely patent but areas of mesangial matrix increase are evident (MM). The foot processes (arrowheads) are well preserved. This patient had a mean GBM diameter of 250 nm (x9,000).

is the gold standard for diagnosing this disorder. Application of such morphometric methods at the ultrastructural level, are bound to increase the sensitivity and accuracy of the diagnosis, so it is not surprising that our incidence rate is much higher than the 1%, that is usually quoted. The accurate diagnosis of these TBMN cases by electron microscopy provided the basis and impetus for the subsequent molecular genetic studies that were recently published in this cohort of patients (Pierides et al., 2009; Voskarides, Patsias, Pierides, & Deltas, 2008). Another factor that could contribute to an increased incidence of TBMN in the Cypriot population is the recent characterization of founder mutations in our population (Voskarides et al., 2008).

### 5.3 Use of morphometry

It should be noted that the thickness of the GBM varies with age, gender, and method of tissue preservation. Considering the different results obtained by the various studies and the fact that there is no gold standard, as regards the method or cut off values for distinguishing between normal and thin GBMs, we established our "in house" normal range of GBM thickness as recommended (Dische et al., 1985).

In this context, previous morphometric work in our department at the ultrastructural level resulted in establishing the normal adult GBM thickness in our kidney biopsies to be between 300 and 400 nm (Marquez et al., 1999; Marquez et al., 2003). Using the above "in-house" GBM normal range values, our results show that the incidence of TBMN in Cyprus is 5.4%, which is much higher than the 1% usually quoted in the literature (Tryggvason & Patrakka, 2006). However, recent estimates put the incidence of TBMN to be not less than 1% and not greater than 10%. Indeed, our results agree with those of Wang and Savige (2005) who estimated that persistent hematuria occurs consistently in as much as 6% of both children and adults.

Indeed in such cases, if one applies the gold standard technique for estimating GBM thickness, from orthogonal intercepts recommended by others (McLay, Jackson, Meyboom, & Jones, 1992; Ramage et al., 2002), the presence of thin GBMs will almost certainly be missed. For this reason we recommend the use of a much simpler and direct measurement technique (Das et al., 1996 Marquez et al., 2003), which is performed in the thinnest GBM loops after surveying the glomeruli to be examined in each case. This approach contributed to the correct diagnosis of eight of the 75 cases presented in this report in which the presence of thin GBMs would have been overlooked. It is important to note that some of the cases show a progressive glomerulosclerosis and at the time of diagnosis, present with only isolated segments showing capillary loops with thin GBMs. These segments could be easily overlooked during the examination of the renal biopsy in the electron microscope and this could be another contributing factor to the wide variation that exists in the literature, regarding estimates of the incidence of TBMN.

### 5.4 TBMN, a disease with many faces (phases)

In our study, the majority of TBMN cases showed signs of FSGS, ranging from early lesions characterized by a mesangial matrix increase to the appearance of more progressive sclerosis, affecting more than 50% of the glomeruli in some cases.

In this context, when we first started to perform quantitative morphometric measurements for estimating GBM width in the mid 1990's we carefully selected cases that on histology showed a maximum of 10% sclerosed glomeruli (Das et al., 1996). However it is evident from our results and those of other studies (Foster et al., 2005; van Paassen et al., 2004) that

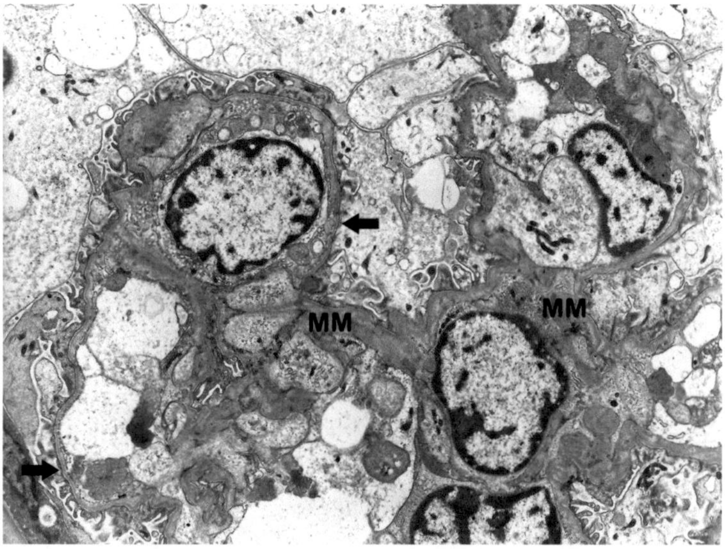


Fig. 6. Electron micrograph from the kidney biopsy of a 45-year old female patient showing increased mesangial matrix (MM) and very thin GBMs (arrows). The average GBM thickness was less than 200 nm (x10,000).

the most frequent morphologic entity associated with TBMN is FSGS. The extent and severity of glomerulosclerosis seen in each TBMN case is variable and ranges from mild, premature glomerular sclerotic changes, to more advanced stages presenting with glomerulosclerotic lesions that may affect up to 50% of the glomeruli. Although as a diagnostic entity TBMN may contain a heterogeneous group of conditions with different aetiologies, molecular genetic studies show that more than 40% of cases are known to be associated with heterozygous mutations in COL4A3 and COL4A4 genes (Tryggvason & Patrakka, 2006) (Lemmink et al., 1996). Recent genetic studies in Cyprus have revealed the presence of founder mutations in the COL4A3 gene in some Cypriot kindrends manifesting TBMN and FSGS (Voskarides et al., 2008). It is noted that the Cypriot population presents an interesting and rather isolated genetic pool, as novel founder mutations have also been characterized in other susceptibility genes, by our group such as the BRCA2 gene, that predisposes to the breast ovarian cancer syndrome (Hadjisavvas et al., 2004).

Patients with TBMN, or benign familial hematuria as the name implies, are believed to have a non-progressive, stable outcome, although some studies report that 30-40% of patients progress to ESRD (Dische et al., 1985; Frasca et al., 2005; Pierides et al., 2009; Tiebosch et al., 1989). At present very little is known about the mechanisms or the involvement of other genes in influencing the severity of the TBMN phenotype. As observed in the present as well as in other studies the extent of FSGS seen in patients, even from the same families is variable and does not depend on age of diagnosis (Voskarides et al., 2008). In some studies TBMN was divided into diffuse and segmental types (Ivanyi, Pap, & Ondrik, 2006), but it is possible that what was observed is different stages of FSGS. How mild or how severe, the glomerular sclerosis lesions are in each renal biopsy, depends on the interplay of other factors, genetic or not, of which little is known at present. Consequently the diagnosis of TBMN has clinical implications for the prognosis of patients, as now it is believed that it may not be as benign a lesion as was originally thought of. In addition, TBMN poses scientific challenges as there is a need to understand how mutations in GBM proteins, including the collagen type IV genes, produce thinning which alters glomerular physiology and leads to glomerulosclerosis in some patients. In the study by Voskarides et al. (2007) nearly 20% of patients, with adequate follow-up information, developed ESRD. Consequently the mechanisms that determine the outcome of TBMN need to be elucidated and research is in progress in our department towards achieving this aim. In this context, there is also increasing evidence that TBMN predisposes to the development of other nephropathies (Berthoux, Laurent, Alamartine, & Diab, 1996; Cosio et al., 1994).

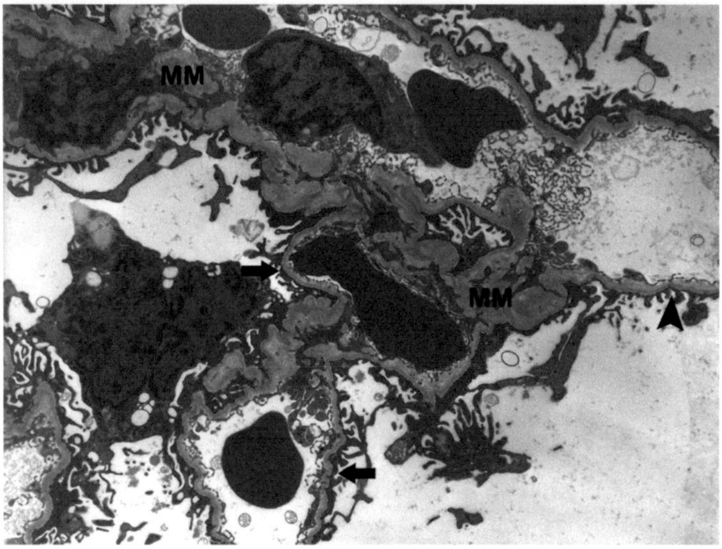


Fig. 7. Electron micrograph from the kidney biopsy of a 45-year old female patient, showing a marked increase in mesangial matrix (MM) and very thin GBMs (arrows), with an average GBM thickness of less than 200 nm. Note well preserved foot processes (arrowhead) (x10,000).

TBMN may occur in a familial setting and up to 50% of cases have a family history or it may be sporadic. The molecular defects underlying TBMN were characterized in the early 1990s, with the identification of type IV collagen genes, found to be mutated in Alport syndrome (Barker et al., 1990; Hostikka et al., 1990). Subsequently Lemmink et al (1996) noted that some carriers of the autosomal forms of Alport syndrome had thin GBMs, so they analyzed the COL4A3 and COL4A4 genes in patients with TBMN. They were the first to associate the presence of heterozygous mutations in these two genes with TBMN and thus provided the underlying genetic defect that explains about 40% of cases. The remaining cases may be sporadic and caused by de novo mutations or by defects in other genes that are as yet to be identified. It should be noted that such genetic tests are not widely available, because the presently known candidate genes COL4A3 and COL4A4 are quite large, consist of about 50 exons each, making genetic analysis expensive and rather insensitive. Furthermore, the occurrence of frequent polymorphisms in the COL4A3 and COL4A4 genes makes it difficult to confirm the pathogenicity of sequence variants with certainty. In addition, recent genetic studies in TBMN patients in Cyprus (Pierides et al., 2009; Voskarides et al., 2007; Voskarides et al., 2008), show that heterozygous carriers of mutations in the COL4A3 and COL4A4 manifest TBMN with many different clinical and histological features. Indeed, very little is known at present about the pathophysiologic mechanisms involved in the manifestation of thin GBMs, the development of which may lead to FSGS under the influence of as yet unknown modifier genes. In this context, the examination of a renal biopsy in the electron microscope and use of ultrastructural morphometry, remains the most accurate modality for correct diagnosis and prognosis of patients presenting with recurrent hematuria and proteinuria. An additional reason for the wider application of electron microscopy is the fact that several cases of TBMN are associated with other glomerulopathies, see section 5.5 below, which further necessitates the examination of a renal biopsy for correct diagnosis.

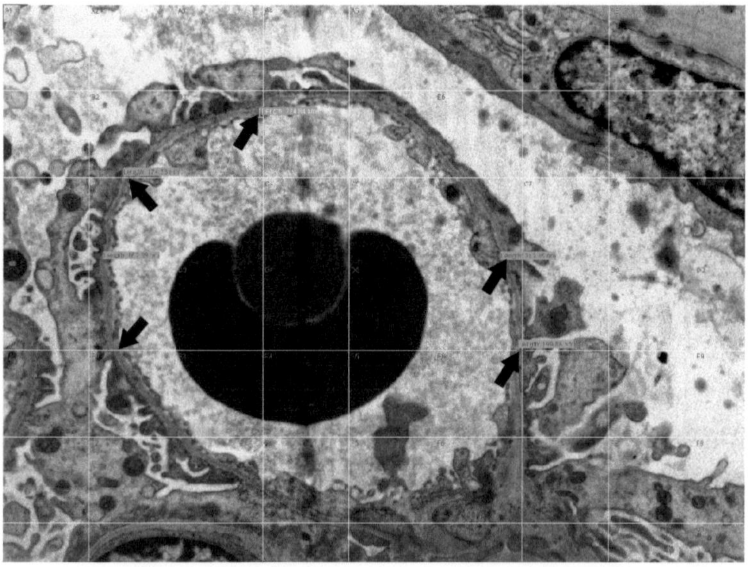

Fig. 8. Electron micrograph from a 48-year old male patient showing application of the morphometric method used for measuring the thickness of the GBM. The iTEM software of the MEGAVIEW digital camera was used to overlay a grid on top of the glomerular capillary. As shown 4-5 measurements were taken at points of the GBM, where the grid intersected the GBM exactly at right angles (arrows) (x15,000).

### 5.5 Association of TBMN with other diseases

TBMN is inherited as an autosomal dominant disease and is caused by the presence of heterozygous mutations in the COL4A3 and COL4A4 genes. Carriers of such pathogenic mutations, therefore have a pre-existing genetic condition, which predisposes them to the development of TBMN and thin GBMs. It is not unreasonable to expect that other glomerulopathies will develop in this setting as noted by other investigators (Cosio et al., 1994; Lanteri, Wilson, & Savige, 1996; Matsumae, et al., 1994). In our series of 1200 kidney biopsies and based on the selection criteria employed in our study, seventy-five biopsies were diagnosed as TBMN. Seven of these biopsies had additional glomerular changes that were characteristic of other glomerulopathies. As shown in table 2, three patients had IgAN, one had MesPGN, one had a TG, and two had MCD. The existence of TBMN with other glomerulonephropathies has been previously described (Cosio et al., 1994) and it was suggested that this disease entity may predispose to other glomerulopathies. In our study the concurrence of TBMN with other glomerulopathies was nearly 10%.

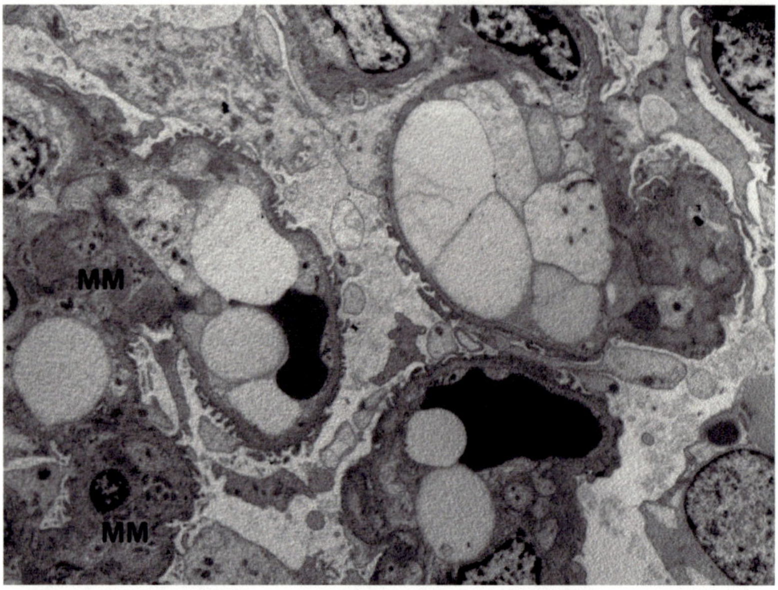


Fig. 9. a. Electron micrograph from the kidney biopsy of a 39 year old female presenting with hematuria showing a mild increase in mesangial matrix (MM) and patent capillary loops (x12,000).

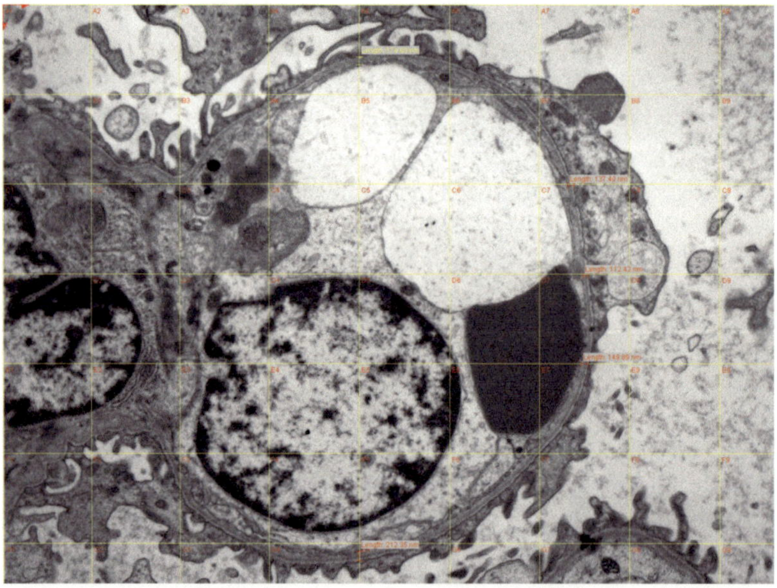

Fig. 9. b. Higher power electron micrograph from the kidney biopsy of the same patient showing application of the morphometric method used as described in the text and fig. 8, for measuring the thickness of the BM. The GBM measured 100nm (x15,000).

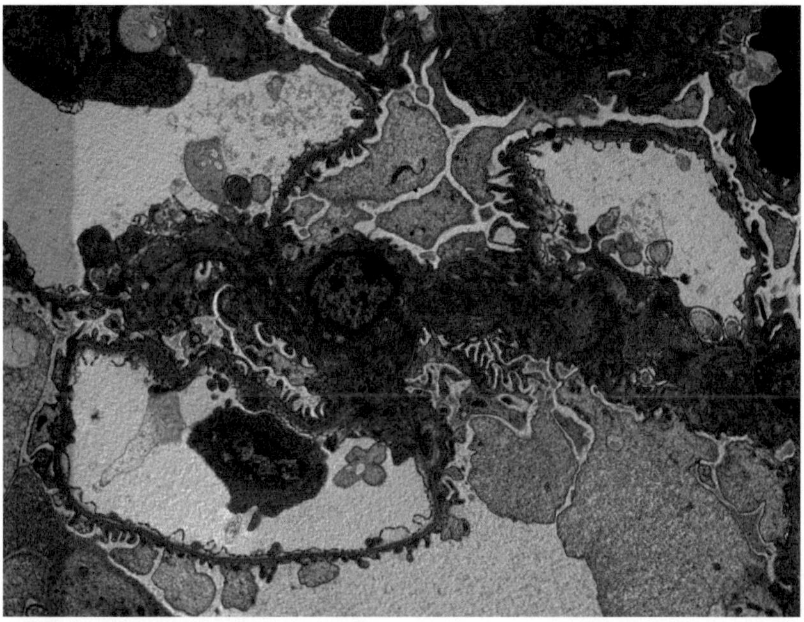

Fig. 10. a. Electron micrograph from the kidney biopsy of a 41 year old male presenting with hematuria, showing patent capillary loops with uniformly thin GBMs measuring 230nm (x12,000).

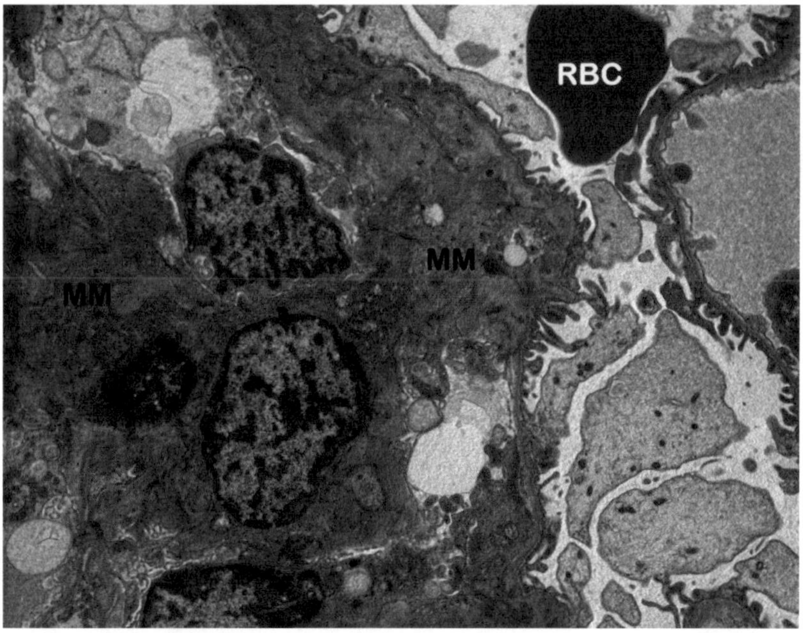


Fig. 10. b. Higher power electron micrograph from the same patient, showing increased mesangial matrix (MM) in the capillary on the left and thin GBM in the capillary on the right. An RBC is seen in the Bowman's space (x20,000).

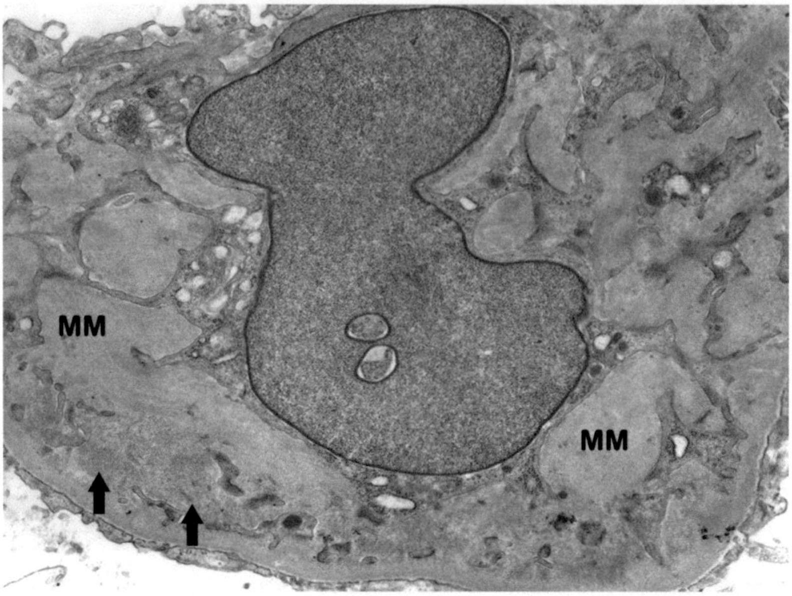


Fig. 11. a. Electron micrograph from the kidney biopsy of a 46 year old female patient presenting with hematuria showing the presence of subendothelial deposits (arrows) and increased mesangial matrix (MM). The patient had positive immunofluorescence of IgA and a mean GBM diameter of 200nm (x25,000).

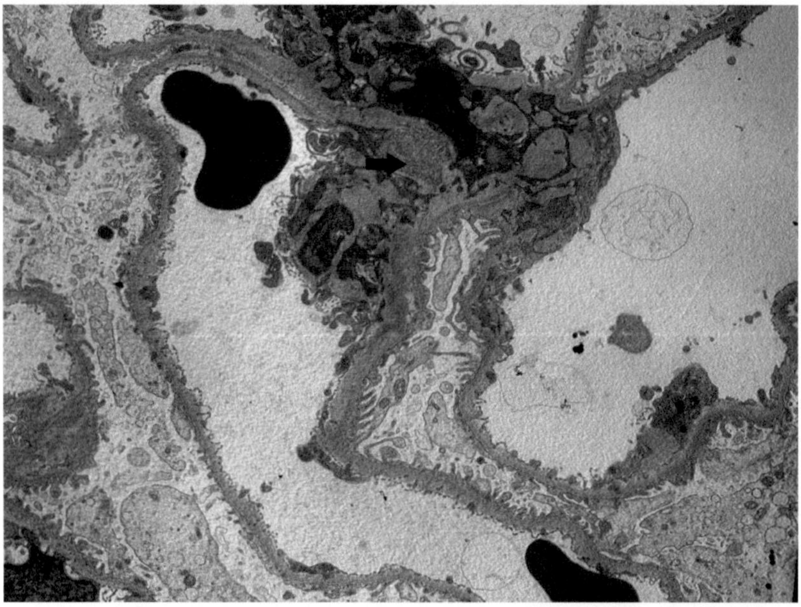

Fig. 11. b. Electron micrograph from the kidney biopsy of the same patient showing patent glomerular capillary loops with mesangial deposits (arrow) (x15,000).

## 6. Conclusion

When Rogers et al., (1973) first recognized and described TBMN, there was little expectation that he was actually describing one of the commonest genetic disorders, affecting glomerular structure and function. Generally, TBMN is characterized by recurrent hematuria and a non-progressive course; although recent data alert to the development of more progressive renal symptoms in 20-30% of patients. Accurate diagnosis relies on rigorous ultrastructural morphometric measurements and on the presence of thin GBMs even in cases that show glomerulosclerosis in more than 50% of glomeruli, as alluded to in this study. Our results demonstrate that the majority of TBMN cases are associated with glomerular histopathology that resembles FSGS; this finding should be taken into consideration when morphometry is applied for accurate diagnosis. Recent advances in genetics, particularly in relation to the collagen IV family of genes have greatly improved our understanding of the underlying genetic causes that lead to TBMN.

However, our knowledge of the pathophysiologic mechanisms involved in the manifestation of TBMN is limited. There is a pressing need to identify markers that can aid in the better diagnosis and prognosis of patients diagnosed with this heterogeneous disease, in order to provide more effective patient management strategies and prevent progression to ESRD.

## 7. Acknowledgement

This study was supported by the Cyprus Institute of Neurology and Genetics, the Cyprus Ministry of Health and the Cyprus Research Promotion Foundation Grant (KY/ROM/0609/08).

## 8. References

Baer, G. (1926). Benign and curable form of hemorrhagic nephritis. *JAMA,* Vol. 86, pp. 1001-1004.

Barker, D. F., Hostikka, S. L., Zhou, J., Chow, L. T., Oliphant, A. R., Gerken, S. C., et al. (1990). Identification of mutations in the COL4A5 collagen gene in Alport syndrome. *Science,* Vol. 248, No.4960, pp. 1224-1227.

Berthoux, F. C., Laurent, B., Alamartine, E., & Diab, N. (1996). New subgroup of primary IgA nephritis with thin glomerular basement membrane (GBM): syndrome or association. *Nephrology, dialysis, transplantation : official publication of the European Dialysis and Transplant Association - European Renal Association,* Vol. 11, No.3, pp. 558-559.

Coleman, M., Haynes, W. D., Dimopoulos, P., Barratt, L. J., & Jarvis, L. R. (1986). Glomerular basement membrane abnormalities associated with apparently idiopathic hematuria: ultrastructural morphometric analysis. *Hum Pathol,* Vol. 17, No.10, pp. 1022-1030.

Cosio, F. G., Falkenhain, M. E., & Sedmak, D. D. (1994). Association of thin glomerular basement membrane with other glomerulopathies. *Kidney Int,* Vol. 46, No.2, pp. 471-474.

Das, A. K., Pickett, T. M., & Tungekar, M. F. (1996). Glomerular basement membrane thickness - a comparison of two methods of measurement in patients with unexplained haematuria. *Nephrol Dial Transplant,* Vol. 11, No.7, pp. 1256-1260.

Dische, F. E., Anderson, V. E., Keane, S. J., Taube, D., Bewick, M., & Parsons, V. (1990). Incidence of thin membrane nephropathy: morphometric investigation of a population sample. *J Clin Pathol,* Vol. 43, No.6, pp. 457-460.

Dische, F. E., Weston, M. J., & Parsons, V. (1985). Abnormally thin glomerular basement membranes associated with hematuria, proteinuria or renal failure in adults. *Am J Nephrol,* Vol. 5, No.2, pp. 103-109.

Edwards, K., Griffiths, D., Morgan, J., Pitman, R., & von Ruhland, C. (2009). Can the choice of intermediate solvent or resin affect glomerular basement membrane thickness? *Nephrol Dial Transplant,* Vol. 24, No.2, pp. 400-403.

Foster, K., Markowitz, G. S., & D'Agati, V. D. (2005). Pathology of thin basement membrane nephropathy. *Seminars in nephrology,* Vol. 25, No.3, pp. 149-158.

Frasca, G. M., Onetti-Muda, A., Mari, F., Longo, I., Scala, E., Pescucci, C., et al. (2005). Thin glomerular basement membrane disease: clinical significance of a morphological diagnosis--a collaborative study of the Italian Renal Immunopathology Group. *Nephrol Dial Transplant,* Vol. 20, No.3, pp. 545-551.

Gregory, M. C. (2005). The clinical features of thin basement membrane nephropathy. *Semin Nephrol,* Vol. 25, No.3, pp. 140-145.

Haas, M. (2006). Thin glomerular basement membrane nephropathy: incidence in 3471 consecutive renal biopsies examined by electron microscopy. *Archives of pathology & laboratory medicine,* Vol. 130, No.5, pp. 699-706.

Haas, M. (2009). Alport syndrome and thin glomerular basement membrane nephropathy: a practical approach to diagnosis. *Arch Pathol Lab Med,* Vol. 133, No.2, pp. 224-232.

Hadjisavvas, A., Charalambous, E., Adamou, A., Neuhausen, S. L., Christodoulou, C. G., & Kyriacou, K. (2004). Hereditary breast and ovarian cancer in Cyprus: identification of a founder BRCA2 mutation. *Cancer Genet Cytogenet,* Vol. 151, No.2, pp. 152-156.

Hostikka, S. L., Eddy, R. L., Byers, M. G., Hoyhtya, M., Shows, T. B., & Tryggvason, K. (1990). Identification of a distinct type IV collagen alpha chain with restricted kidney distribution and assignment of its gene to the locus of X chromosome-linked Alport syndrome. *Proc Natl Acad Sci U S A,* Vol. 87, No.4, pp. 1606-1610.

Ivanyi, B., Pap, R., & Ondrik, Z. (2006). Thin basement membrane nephropathy: diffuse and segmental types. *Arch Pathol Lab Med,* Vol. 130, No.10, pp. 1533-1537.

Jovanovic GB, V. V., Gil J, Kim DU, Dikman SH, Cheurg J:. (1990). Morphometric analysis of glomerular basement membranes (GBM) in thin basement membrane disease (TBMD). *Clin Nephrol,* Vol. 33, pp. 110-114.

Lanteri, M., Wilson, D., & Savige, J. (1996). Clinical features in two patients with IgA glomerulonephritis and thin-basement-membrane disease. *Nephrology, dialysis, transplantation : official publication of the European Dialysis and Transplant Association - European Renal Association,* Vol. 11, No.5, pp. 791-793.

Lemmink, H. H., Nillesen, W. N., Mochizuki, T., Schroder, C. H., Brunner, H. G., van Oost, B. A., et al. (1996). Benign familial hematuria due to mutation of the type IV collagen alpha4 gene. *J Clin Invest,* Vol. 98, No.5, pp. 1114-1118.

Marquez, B., Stavrou, F., Zouvani, I., Anastasiades, E., Patsias, C., Pierides, A., et al. (1999). Thin glomerular basement membranes in patients with hematuria and minimal change disease. *Ultrastruct Pathol,* Vol. 23, No.3, pp. 149-156.

Marquez, B., Zouvani, I., Karagrigoriou, A., Anastasiades, E., Pierides, A., & Kyriacou, K. (2003). A simplified method for measuring the thickness of glomerular basement membranes. *Ultrastruct Pathol,* Vol. 27, No.6, pp. 409-416.

Matsumae, T., Fukusaki, M., Sakata, N., Takebayashi, S., & Naito, S. (1994). Thin glomerular basement membrane in diabetic patients with urinary abnormalities. *Clinical nephrology,* Vol. 42, No.4, pp. 221-226.

McLay, A. L., Jackson, R., Meyboom, F., & Jones, J. M. (1992). Glomerular basement membrane thinning in adults: clinicopathological correlations of a new diagnostic approach. *Nephrol Dial Transplant,* Vol. 7, No.3, pp. 191-199.

Nieuwhof, C. M., de Heer, F., de Leeuw, P., & van Breda Vriesman, P. J. (1997). Thin GBM nephropathy: premature glomerular obsolescence is associated with hypertension and late onset renal failure. *Kidney international,* Vol. 51, No.5, pp. 1596-1601.

Pierides, A., Voskarides, K., Athanasiou, Y., Ioannou, K., Damianou, L., Arsali, M., et al. (2009). Clinico-pathological correlations in 127 patients in 11 large pedigrees, segregating one of three heterozygous mutations in the COL4A3/ COL4A4 genes associated with familial haematuria and significant late progression to proteinuria and chronic kidney disease from focal segmental glomerulosclerosis. *Nephrology, dialysis, transplantation : official publication of the European Dialysis and Transplant Association - European Renal Association,* Vol. 24, No.9, pp. 2721-2729.

Ramage, I. J., Howatson, A. G., McColl, J. H., Maxwell, H., Murphy, A. V., & Beattie, T. J. (2002). Glomerular basement membrane thickness in children: a stereologic assessment. *Kidney Int,* Vol. 62, No.3, pp. 895-900.

Rogers, P. W., Kurtzman, N. A., Bunn, S. M., Jr., & White, M. G. (1973). Familial benign essential hematuria. *Arch Intern Med,* Vol. 131, No.2, pp. 257-262.

Tiebosch, A. T., Frederik, P. M., van Breda Vriesman, P. J., Mooy, J. M., van Rie, H., van de Wiel, T. W., et al. (1989). Thin-basement-membrane nephropathy in adults with persistent hematuria. *N Engl J Med,* Vol. 320, No.1, pp. 14-18.

Tryggvason, K., & Patrakka, J. (2006). Thin basement membrane nephropathy. *J Am Soc Nephrol,* Vol. 17, No.3, pp. 813-822.

van Paassen, P., van Breda Vriesman, P. J., van Rie, H., & Tervaert, J. W. (2004). Signs and symptoms of thin basement membrane nephropathy: a prospective regional study on primary glomerular disease-The Limburg Renal Registry. *Kidney Int,* Vol. 66, No.3, pp. 909-913.

Voskarides, K., Damianou, L., Neocleous, V., Zouvani, I., Christodoulidou, S., Hadjiconstantinou, V., et al. (2007). COL4A3/COL4A4 mutations producing focal segmental glomerulosclerosis and renal failure in thin basement membrane nephropathy. *Journal of the American Society of Nephrology : JASN,* Vol. 18, No.11, pp. 3004-3016.

Voskarides, K., Patsias, C., Pierides, A., & Deltas, C. (2008). COL4A3 founder mutations in Greek-Cypriot families with thin basement membrane nephropathy and focal segmental glomerulosclerosis dating from around 18th century. *Genet Test,* Vol. 12, No.2, pp. 273-278.

Wang, Y. Y., & Savige, J. (2005). The epidemiology of thin basement membrane nephropathy. *Semin Nephrol,* Vol. 25, No.3, pp. 136-139.

Zouvani, I., Aristodemou, S., Hadjisavvas, A., Michael, T., Vassiliou, M., Patsias, C., et al. (2008). Incidence of thin basement membrane nephropathy in 990 consecutive renal biopsies examined with electron microscopy. *Ultrastruct Pathol,* Vol. 32, No.6, pp. 221-226.

# 7

# Update on IgM Nephropathy

Javed I. Kazi and Muhammed Mubarak
*Sindh Institute of Urology and Transplantation, Karachi*
*Pakistan*

## 1. Introduction

IgM nephropathy (IgMN) is a relatively recently described, and still a controversial clinico-immunopathologic entity which presents mainly as idiopathic nephrotic syndrome (INS) in both children and adults (Al-Eisa et al., 1996). The disease, like IgA nephropathy (IgAN), is defined by its immunohistologic features: the presence of immunoglobulin M (IgM) as the sole or dominant immunoglobulin in the mesangium of the glomeruli in a diffuse (all glomeruli) and global (whole glomerulus) distribution (Bhasin et al., 1978; Cohen et al., 1978). Similar to IgAN, the light microscopic (LM) features on renal biopsy are very heterogeneous, ranging from minimal change lesion to variable degree of mesangial proliferation to focal segmental glomerulosclerosis (FSGS) (Mubarak et al., 2010). Electron-dense deposits in the mesangium are a variable ultrastructural feature. Its epidemiology is interesting; the disease is reported mostly from South East Asia and Eastern Europe, but sparse studies have also appeared from USA, Canada, and parts of Western Europe. Its etiology and pathogenesis are still not well understood (Myllimaki et al., 2003). Owing chiefly to controversy over its distinct nature, it has attracted little interest in the scientific community. There are very few studies on the prognostic factors (Jungthirapanich et al., 1997; Myllimaki et al., 2003). Currently, IgMN is treated along the similar lines as minimal change disease (MCD) or FSGS, but the response to steroids is less favorable than that of MCD. Its prognosis is relatively guarded as compared with MCD. Upto one third of individuals with IgMN develop renal insufficiency or one fourth, the end-stage renal disease (ESRD) over 15 years of follow-up (Myllimaki et al., 2003). In this chapter, we briefly discuss the historical background, etiology, pathogenesis, pathology, clinical manifestations, treatment, and prognosis of this relatively young and still largely controversial primary glomerulopathy. Further long term longitudinal studies are needed to clarify the status of the disease among the primary glomerulopathies.

## 2. Historical background

Although, it is widely believed that this lesion was described for the first time in 1978 by two independent research groups led by Cohen (1978), and Bhasin (1978) in patients presenting with heavy proteinuria, the deposits of predominant IgM in the glomeruli, in fact, were first described in renal biopsies in 1974 by Putte et al. (1974) in patients presenting with persistent or recurrent hematuria. Soon after the formal recognition of the disease as a distinct entity in 1978, many series were reported on the disease mostly from USA, UK, other countries of Europe, and South East Asia (Al-Eisa et al., 1996; Cavalo & Johnson, 1981;

Kobayashi et al., 1982; Hamed 2003; Helin et al., 1982; Hsu et al., 1984; Jungthirapanich et al., 1997; Lawler et al., 1980; Mampaso et al., 1981; Myllimaki et al., 2003; Pardo et al., 1984; Saha et al., 1989). Among these, the large series of patients with this disease from Finland are of note (Helin et al., 1982; Myllimaki et al., 2003; Saha et al., 1989). However, the interest in the disease soon faded, and many investigators, especially in the western world, were reluctant to accept the disease as a distinct clinicopathologic entity. The disease is however still being reported from different parts of the world (Mubarak et al., 2011).

## 3. Epidemiology

Few studies have been reported on the population based incidence and prevalence, mode of presentation, immunopathologic features, pattern of steroid response and the long term prognosis of IgMN in either children or adults (Myllymaki et al., 1993). Most of the studies have reported the prevalence of the disease as frequency or percentage of renal biopsies with a diagnosis of IgMN. The frequency of IgMN reported in literature has varied considerably from 2% to 18.5% (Al-Eisa et al., 1996; Cavalo et al., 1981; Kazi et al., 2010; Kopolovic et al., 1987; Lawler et al., 1980; Mampaso et al., 1981; Cavalo & Johnson, 1981; Chan et al., 2000; Donia et al., 2000; Hsu et al., 1984; Jungthirapanich et al., 1997; Kobayashi et al., 1982; Mubarak et al., 2011; Singhai et al., 2011; Tejani & Nicastri, 1983). The first two pioneering studies found frequencies of 2 and 6.1% respectively in their biopsy series (Cohen et al., 1978; Bhasin et al., 1978). Soon thereafter, a frequency of 11.7% of IgMN was reported in a study by Lawler et al. from UK (1980). Hsu et al. (1984) found a frequency of 10% of IgMN in all biopsies with primary glomerular disease. One of the largest and long-term longitudinal series on IgMN has come from Finland, comprising of 110 patients, including both adults and children (Myllimaki et al., 2003). More recently, we have published our experience in the largest study ever carried out on 135 children with INS and IgMN as the biopsy diagnosis (Mubarak et al., 2011). The exact cause for this wide variation in the prevalence of IgMN is unclear but may be partly due to varying biopsy indications, varying criteria for the diagnosis of this lesion used in different studies, and partly to genetic or environmental factors. Most of the studies have been undertaken on native renal biopsies; however, occasional cases of its occurrence in renal transplant recipients have also been reported (Salmon AH et al., 2004).

## 4. Etiology

As with IgAN, the etiology of this common form of primary GN is still largely unknown. IgM deposits in the glomeruli may be seen in a variety of systemic diseases, such as systemic lupus erythematosus (SLE), rheumatoid arthritis, diabetes mellitus, Alport's syndrome, and paraproteinemia. For a diagnosis of primary IgMN, the above conditions must be excluded.

## 5. Pathogenesis

As with the etiology, the pathogenesis of this disease is also still elusive. Very few studies have been undertaken on the pathogenesis of this condition, mainly because this disease is not accepted widely as a distinct entity in most of the western countries (Border, 1988). Some investigators have suggested classical immune complex mediated activation of complement system leading to mesangial injury and reaction (Hsu et al., 1984). They cite as evidence the presence of C1q and C4 deposits along with IgM in glomerular mesangium in majority of cases, while properdin and factor B were not found (Hsu et al., 1984). Others have found C3 in majority of cases and C1q only infrequently (Mubarak et al., 2011). The source of antigens triggering immune complex formation is not known, but it is hypothesized that certain antigens in the food or environment which preferentially elicit IgM response may be responsible. Abnormalities of T-lymphocyte function or a disturbance in immune complex clearance by mesangial cells have also been suggested (Hsu et al., 1984). Many studies have found increased serum IgM or IgM immune complex concentrations in patients with IgMN (Disciullo et al., 1988; Hsu et al., 1984). No abnormalities of IgM molecule, as are observed in IgA, have been detected or reported as yet. Similarly, no animal studies have been conducted on this disease till now.

## 6. Pathology

The diagnosis of IgMN requires, like IgAN, examination of renal biopsy by at least LM and IF methods. EM is not essential but optional and often confirms the findings seen on LM and IF. The pathologic findings are correlated with clinical and serological studies to diagnose the primary form of the disease.

### 6.1 Light microscopy

The LM findings in IgMN are heterogeneous, as in IgAN. The spectrum of changes is however not as wide as in IgAN and includes minor changes, variable degree of mesangial proliferation, usually of mild to moderate degree, and FSGS (Mubarak et al., 2011; Myllimaki et al., 2003) (Fig. 1, 2). Many biopsies also display small cellular crescents (Lawler et al., 1980; Kishimoto & Arakawa, 1999). The most common morphologic change reported consists of mesangial proliferation of the glomeruli, mostly of mild to moderate degree (Hsu et al., 1984). In a minority of cases, severe mesangial proliferation with interpositioning of the expanded mesangium into the peripheral capillary walls with consequent splitting and tram-track appearance have also been noted (Kishimoto & Arakawa, 1999). Minor changes on LM are reported in about one third of cases (Hsu et al., 1984; Mubarak et al., 2011; Myllimaki et al., 2003). FSGS morphology is also commonly reported in IgMN. These cases show diffuse mesangial positivity of IgM in contrast to nonspecific, segmental trapping of IgM in idiopathic FSGS. The previously reported prevalence of this morphologic pattern in biopsies of IgMN shows wide variation (Lawler et al., 1980; Mubarak et al., 2011; Myllimaki et al., 2003). Some investigators have entirely excluded this lesion in their study patients; others have included those cases of FSGS showing diffuse mesangial positivity of IgM in the category of IgMN, as in our study (Mubarak et al., 2011). The reported rates of this lesion have varied from 9 to 65.2% (Mubarak et al., 2011; Myllimaki et al., 2003). This pattern was also noted in one third of the cases in our study (Mubarak et al., 2011). Still other investigators have reported progression of IgMN cases with minor changes or mesangial proliferation into FSGS on repeat biopsies (Myllimaki et al., 2003; Zeis et al., 2001). We have observed one case each of florid crescentic GN and a case of collapsing FSGS as a morphologic expression of IgMN (unpublished data). Tubular atrophy and interstitial scarring are also commonly observed on renal biopsies of IgMN at the time of diagnosis and are usually mild (Mubarak et al., 2011; Myllimaki et al., 2003). Moderate and severe tubular atrophy have been rarely reported. Mild fibrointimal thickening of arteries has also been reported in a minority of cases (Mubarak et al., 2011).

### 6.2 Immunoflourescence

Like IgAN, IgMN is a diagnosis of IF microscopy. Characteristic of the disease is a diffuse and global mesangial positivity of IgM (either as sole immunogloblulin or predominant) of at least 1+ intensity on a scale of 0-3+ (where 0 is absent, 1+ is mild, 2+ is moderate, and 3+ is marked) (Mubarak et al., 2011; Myllimaki et al., 2003) (Fig. 3). Some studies have included trace positivity of IgM on IF as IgMN. Concomitant but not dominant deposits of IgA and IgG are found in a small percentage of cases (Mubarak et al., 2011; Myllimaki et al., 2003). Complement fragments of C3 and C1q are found in majority of cases co-localized with IgM deposits (Mubarak et al., 2011; Myllimaki et al., 2003; Zeis et al., 2001).

### 6.3 Electron microscopy

There are very few studies on the ultrastructural features of IgMN. In majority of cases, no EM was done and the diagnosis was made solely on IF microscopy. The few studies that have carried out EM examination have noted small, granular to short linear, electron-dense deposits in the mesangium and paramesangium, along with variable degrees of mesangial cell proliferation and mesangial matrix expansion. Variable degrees of fusion of foot processes commensurate with the degree of proteinuria have also been observed. The electron-dense deposits have typically been of low volume and low density, and in many cases, rather ill-defined (Al-Eisa et al., 1996; Hsu et al., 1984; Myllimaki et al., 2003).

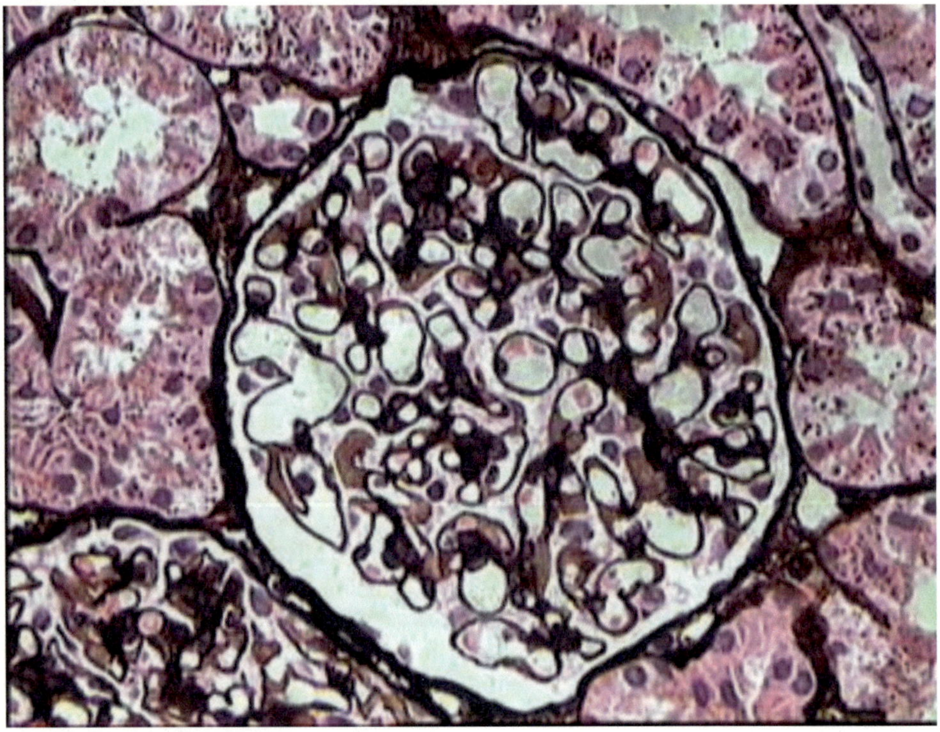

Fig. 1. Medium-power view showing a glomerulus with minor changes on light microscopy. There is no significant mesangial proliferation. Capillary lumena are intact. This morphological pattern is observed in about one third of cases of IgM nephropathy. (Jone's methenamine silver, ×200).

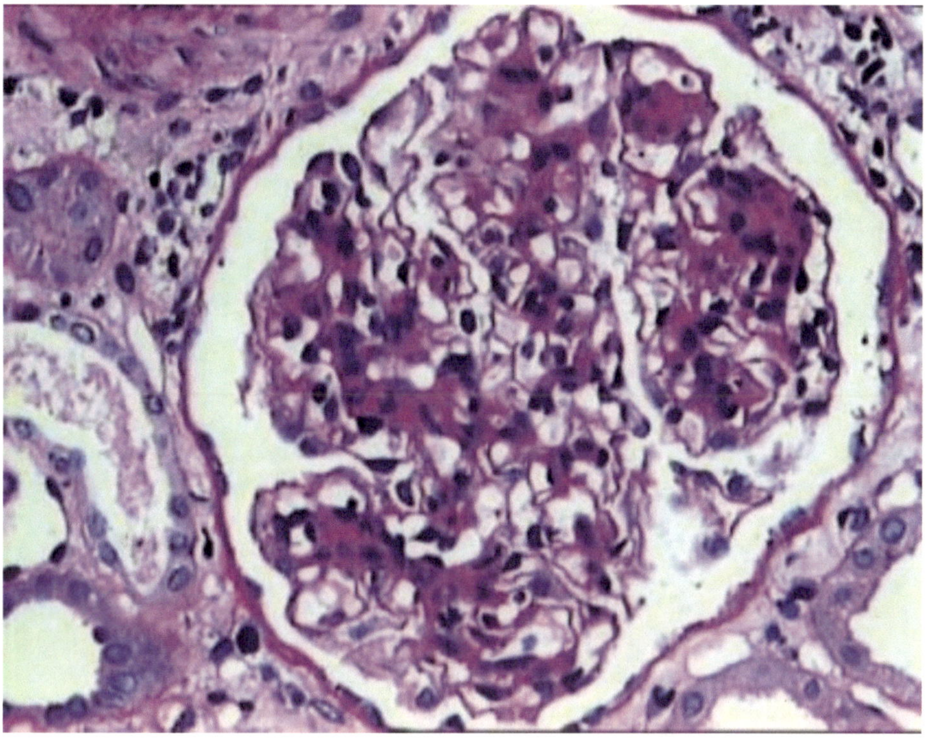

Fig. 2. High-power view showing a glomerulus with mild mesangial cell proliferation and moderate mesangial matrix expansion. Peripheral capillary walls are thin. This is the most common morphological pattern observed in cases of IgM nephropathy. (PAS, ×400).

## 7. Clinical manifestations

Clinically, the disease most commonly presents with INS in both children and adults. The disease also frequently presents with hematuria (HU) or asymptomatic urinary abnormalities (AUA). However, in many centers of the world, patients with the later manifestations are not subjected to renal biopsy, which accounts for the low number of patients presenting with these manifestations. It is believed that patients with HU, especially adult females, have a good prognosis, as compared with patients with NS or proteinuria (PU) (Myllimaki et al., 2003). Hypertension is frequent at presentation or biopsy, being found in roughly one third of cases. Its prevalence increases with increasing duration of the disease approaching 50% at 15 years of follow-up (Myllimaki et al., 2003).

The disease predominantly affects males as compared with females. Some studies have found a female preponderance, especially in those patients presenting with HU. Isolated HU or proteinuria-hematuria (PU-HU) have constituted almost half of biopsy indications in some previous reports (Myllimaki et al., 2003). This may have implications for the severity of the pathological lesions observed on renal biopsy and the long term outcome of disease. It has been observed, however, that IgMN in children mostly presents as INS rather than as HU or PU, as shown in the study by Myllimaki et al. (2003), in which 32 of 36 children with IgMN presented as NS and only four children presented with non nephrotic proteinuria and none presented with PU-HU or HU.

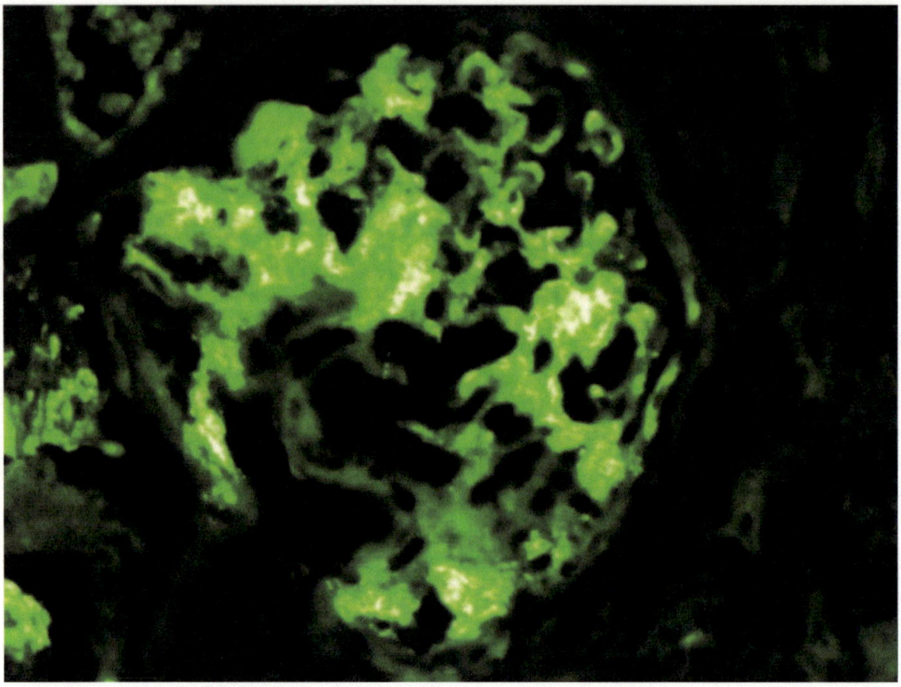

Fig. 3. Medium-power view showing a glomerulus with bright (3+ on a scale of 0 to 3+), granular, and global positivity of IgM mainly in the mesangium of the glomerulus on immunoflourescence. (Immunoflourescence for IgM, ×200).

## 8. Treatment

IgMN is treated in the same manner as MCD or FSGS. Corticosteroids form the mainstay of treatment. Similar to its prevalence, the steroid response pattern in IgMN varies considerably; steroid resistance reported varies from 0 to 52% (Border, 1988). We found a steroid resistance pattern in about one third of our children presenting with INS. Border (1988). also found a mean of 28% steroid resistance on a review of nine published studies of IgMN (Border, 1988). It follows from these studies that IgMN responds less well to steroids compared to typical minimal change disease (MCD), and favors the hypothesis that IgMN is distinct from MCD (Mubarak et al., 2011; Myllimaki et al., 2003). Other researchers have not found any significant differences in clinical, pathological or steroid response pattern among these diseases (Al-Eisa et al., 1996; Ji-Yun et al., 1984).

## 9. Clinical course and prognosis

The clinical course and prognosis of IgMN are also very variable. Part of the variation in the studies is due to variable length of follow-up of the patients and variable case definitions. In the largest and longest follow-up study from Finland, renal insufficiency was observed in 35% of cases at 15 years after biopsy, and ESRD was found in 23% of cases (Myllimaki et al., 2003). They also looked for clinical and pathological prognostic factors leading to renal insufficiency or ESRD. In multivariate analysis, hypertension was the only factor that predicted renal insufficiency; on the other hand, none of the multiple factors analyzed was

predictive of ESRD. They proposed that this may be due to small number of patients reaching ESRD in their study (Myllimaki et al., 2003). Another study identified microscopic HU, extent of mesangial proliferation, and global glomerulosclerosis as independent prognostic markers on multivariate analysis (O'Donoghue et al., 1991).
One important complication of IgMN is the transition of the usual mesangial proliferative lesion into the morphologic expression of FSGS. The later is diagnosed only in re-biopsies (Myllimaki et al., 2003; Zeis et al., 2001).

## 10. Conclusion

In conclusion, IgMN is an important cause of renal morbidity in both children and adults in many parts of the world. It shows a spectrum of morphologic changes ranging from minor changes to FSGS. Immunoflourescence is necessary for its diagnosis. Clinically, a poor response to steroid therapy distinguishes this disease from MCD. Further long term longitudinal studies are needed to clarify the status of the disease among the primary glomerulopathies. More studies are also needed to elucidate the etiology and pathogenesis of this disease and develop effective therapeutic regimens.

## 11. References

Al Eisa A, Carner JE, Lirenman DS, & Magil AB. (1996). Childhood IgM nephropathy: comparison with minimal change disease. *Nephron*, Vol. 72, No. 1, pp. 37-43.

Bhasin HK, Abeulo JG, Nayak R, & Esparza AR. (1978). Mesangial proliferative glomerulonephritis. *Lab Invest*, Vol. 39, No. 1, pp. 21-9.

Border WA. (1988). Distinguishing minimal change disease from mesangial disorders. *Kidney Int*, Vol. 34, No. 3, pp. 419-24.

Cavalo T, Johnson MP. (1981). Immunopathologic study of minimal change glomerular disease with mesangial IgM deposits. *Nephron*, Vol. 27, No. 6, pp. 281-4.

Chan YH, Wong KM, Choi KS, Chak WL, Cheung CY. (2000). Clinical manifestation and progression of IgM mesangial nephropathy: a single center perspective. *Hong Kong J Nephrol*, Vo. 2, No. 1, pp. 23-6.

Cohen AH, Border WA, Glassock RJ. (1978). Nephrotic syndrome with glomerular mesangial IgM deposits. *Lab Invest*, Vol. 38, No. pp. 610-9.

Disciullo SO, Abeulo JG, Moalli K, & Pezzullo JC. (1988). Circulating heavy IgM in IgM nephropathy. *Clin Exp Immunol*, Vol. 73, No. 3, pp. 395-400.

Donia AF, Sobh MA, Moustafa FE, Bakr MA, Foda MA. (2000). Clinical significance and long term evolution of minimal change histopathologic variants and of IgM nephropathy among Egyptians. *J Nephrol*, Vol. 13, No. 4, pp. 275-81.

Habib R, Girardin E, Gagnadoux M-F, Hinglais N, Levy M, Broyer M. (1988). Immunopathological findings in idiopathic nephrosis:clinical significance of glomerular "immune deposits". *Pediatr Nephrol*, Vol. 2, No. pp. 402-8.

Hamed RM. (2003). Clinical significance and long term evolution of mesangial proliferative IgM nephropathy among Jordanian children. *Ann Saudi Med*, Vol. 23, No. 5, pp. 323-7.

Helin H, Mustonen J, Pasternack A, Antonen J. (1982). IgM associated glomerulonephritis. *Nephron*, Vol. 31, No. 1, pp.11-6.

Hsu HC, Chen WY, Lin GJ, Chen L, Kao S-L, Huang C-C, et al. (1984). Clinical and immunopathologic study of mesangial IgM nephropathy: report of 41 cases. *Histopathology*, Vol. 8, No. 3, pp. 435-46.

Ji-Yun Y, Melvin T, Sibley R, Michael AF. (1984). No evidence for a specific role of IgM in mesangial proliferation of idiopathic nephrotic syndrome. *Kidney Int,* Vol 25, No. 1, pp. 100-6.

Jungthirapanich J, Singkhwa V, Watana D, Futrakul P, Sensirivatana R, Yenrudi S. (1997). Significance of tubulointerstitial fibrosis in paediatric IgM nephropathy. *Nephrology,* Vol. 3, No. pp. 509-14.

Kazi JI, Mubarak M, Mallick S. Clinicopathologic characteristics of IgM nephropathy in pediatric nephrotic population from Pakistan. Letter to the editor. J Pak Med Assoc 2010;76:878.

Kishimoto H, Arakawa M. (1999). Clinico-pathological characterization of mesangial proliferative glomerulonephritis with predominant deposition of IgM. *Clin Exp Nephrol,* Vol. 3, No. 2, pp. 110-5.

Kopolovic J, Shvil Y, Pomeranz A, Ron N, Rubinger D, Oren R. (1987). IgM nephropathy: morphological study related to clinical findings. *Am J Nephrol,* Vol. 7, No. 4, pp. 275-80.

Lawler W, Williams G, Tarpey P, Mallick NP. (1980). IgM associated primary diffuse mesangial proliferative glomerulonephritis. *J Clin Pathol,* Vol. 33, No. 11, pp. 1029-38.

Mampaso F, Gonzalo A, Teruel J, Losada M, Gallego N, Ortuno J, & Bellas C. (1981). Mesangial deposits of IgM in patients with the nephrotic syndrome. *Clin Nephrol,* Vol. 16, No. 5, pp. 230-4.

Mubarak M, Kazi JI, Malik S, Lanewala A, Hashmi S. (2011). Clinicopathologic characteristics and steroid response of IgM nephropathy in children presenting with idiopathic nephrotic syndrome. *APMIS,* Vol. 119, No. pp. 180-6.

Mubarak M, Lanewala A, Kazi JI, Akhter F, Sher A, Fayyaz A, et al. (2009). Histopathological spectrum of childhood nephrotic syndrome in children in Pakistan. *Clin Exp Nephrol,* Vol. 13, No. 6, pp. 589-93.

Myllymaki J, Saha H, Mustonen J, Helin H, Pasternack A. (2003). IgM nephropathy: clinical picture and long term prognosis. *Am J Kidney Dis,* Vol. 41, No. 2, pp. 343-50.

O'Donoghue DJ, Lawler W, Hunt LP, Acheson EJ, & Mallick NP (1991). IgM associated primary diffuse mesangial proliferative glomerulonephritis: natural history and prognostic indicators. *Q Med J,* Vol. 79, No. 1, pp. 333-50.

Pardo V, Riesgo I, Zilleruelo G, Strauss J. (1984). The clinical significance of mesangial IgM deposits and mesangial hypercellularity in minimal change nephrotic syndrome. *Am J Kidney Dis,* Vol. 3, No. 4, pp. 264-9.

Saha H, Mustonen J, Pasternack A, Helin H. (1989). Clinical follow up of 54 patients with IgM nephropathy. *Am J Nephrol,* Vol. 9, No. 2, pp. 124-8.

Salmon AH, Kamel D, & Mathieson PW. (2004). Recurrence of IgM nephropathy in a renal allograft. *Nephrol Dial Transplant,* Vol. 19, No. 10, pp. 2650-2.

Singhai AM, Vanikar AV, Goplani KR, Kanodia KV, Patel RD, Suthar KS, Patel HV, Gumber MR, Shah PR, & Trivedi HL. (2011) Immunoglobulin M nephropathy in adults and adolescents in India: a single center study of natural history. *Indian J Pathol Microbiol,* Vol. 54, No. 1, pp. 3-6

Tejani A, Nicastri AD. (1983). Mesangial IgM nephropathy. *Nephron,* Vol. 35, No. 1, pp. 1-5.

Van de Putte LBA, DeLa Riviere GB, Van Breda Vriesman PJC. (1974). Recurrent or persistent hematuria, sign of mesangial immune-complex deposition. *N Engl J Med,* Vol. 290, No. 21, pp. 1165–70.

Zeis PS, Kavazarakis E, Nakopoulou L, Moustaki M, Messaritaki A, Zeis MP, & Nicolaidou P. (2001). Glomerulopathy with mesangial IgM deposits: long-term follow up of 64 children. *Pediatr Int,* Vol. 43, No. 3, pp. 287-92.

8

# Recent Developments in the Pathogenesis and the Pathological Classification of IgA Nephropathy

Muhammed Mubarak and Javed I. Kazi
*Histopathology Department, Sindh Institute of Urology and Transplantation, Karachi Pakistan*

## 1. Introduction

IgA nephropathy (IgAN), also known as Berger's disease, is the most common primary glomerular disease world wide and a significant cause of end-stage renal disease (ESRD) in many parts of the world (Floege & Feehally, 2000; Geddes et al., 2003; Julian et al., 1988). It was first described in 1968 in Paris, France (Berger & Hingalis, 1968), but now the disease is known to have a cosmopolitan distribution (Ballardie et al., 1987; Chandrika, 2009; D'Amico, 1985; Koyama et al., 1997; Lai et al., 1999; Mubarak, 2009; Power et al., 185; Rivera et al., 2004; Schena, 1997; Seedat et al., 1988; Sinniah, 1980; Strata P, et al., 1995; Yahya et al., 1997). Significant advancements have been made during last four decades in understanding the etiology, pathogenesis, classification, and treatment of this enigmatic disease. In this chapter, we discuss briefly about the historical background, epidemiology, etiology, pathogenesis, pathology, treatment, and recent developments in the diagnosis and prognosis of IgAN with particular emphasis on a recent clinicopathological classification developed through international collaboration by the members of International IgAN network in conjunction with renal pathology society (RPS). This classification is simple, easy to apply, fairly reproducible, and clinically pre-validated, and provides a role model for classifying other renal diseases in similar manner.

## 2. Historical background

IgAN was first described by Berger and Hingalis in France in 1968 as a renal glomerular disease characterized by the predominant or co-dominant IgA containing immune complex deposits in the mesangium of the glomeruli (Berger & Hingalis, 1968). Thus, its diagnosis required, and still so, the histopathologic and immunoflourescence (IF) evaluation of the invasive procedure of renal biopsy. No blood or urinary test has been developed yet to replace the renal biopsy for its accurate diagnosis. Traditionally, the disease was considered to be a benign disease, due mainly to its very slow rate of progression, as is apparent from its earlier synonym of "benign familial hematuria" and to be confined to France. However, soon it was realized, as evidence accumulated from subsequent long term follow-up studies from different parts of the world, that both the above assumptions about IgAN were wrong, as will be discussed below in the epidemiology and the prognosis of the disease.

## 3. Epidemiology and magnitude of the problem

The epidemiology of IgAN is both interesting and intriguing in that, although cosmopolitan in distribution, there is a significant variability in the reported incidence and prevalence of the disease in different countries. Very few population based incidence studies on IgAN have been reported in the literature. The reported incidence in different parts of Western Europe has varied from 15 to 40 new cases per million population per year (Rivera et al., 2004; Schena, 1997; Strata P, et al., 1995). Majority of the studies have calculated the frequency of IgAN as a percent of all native renal biopsies performed for a variety of clinical indications. The highest prevalence (upto 60%) has been reported in native renal biopsy series from Japan, Korea, China, Singapore, Western Europe, and Australia (Ballardie et al., 1987; D'Amico, 1985; Kazi et al., 2009; Koyama et al., 1997; Lai et al., 1999; Power et al., 185; Rivera et al., 2004; Schena, 1997; 1988; Sinniah, 1980; Strata P, et al., 1995). In contrast, studies from United States have reported very low rates at 2 to 10 percent, with the exception of a 38 percent incidence in the Navajo Indians in New Mexico (Julian et al., 1988). Nearly similar rates have been reported from Africa, Middle East, and some parts of Asia, including India, and Pakistan (Chandrika, 2009; D'Amico, 1985; Mubarak, 2009; Narasimhan et al., 2006; Seedat et al., 1988; Yahya et al., 1997). The exact cause for this marked variability in the epidemiology of the disease is not known, but it most probably is related to the differences in biopsy indications and the extent of pathologic evaluation of the renal biopsies.

## 4. Etiology

The vast majority of cases of IgAN are primary or idiopathic, and as their name suggests, their etiology is still not known (Barratt et al., 2004; Donadio & Grande, 2002; Floege & Feehally, 2000; Galla, 1995). The disease is, in most cases, a sporadic disorder. However, cases of familial and secondary IgAN are well documented and these have proved very useful for the insight they have provided for a better understanding of the pathogenetic mechanisms underlying the disease (Barratt et al., 2004; Donadio & Grande, 2002; Galla, 1995). A list of these secondary causes is shown in table 1.

| |
|---|
| **Diseases of the liver:** alcoholic, primary biliary, or cryptogenic cirrhosis; hepatitis B; chronic schistosomiasis |
| **Diseases of the gastrointestinal tract:** celiac disease; chronic ulcerative colitis; Crohn's disease |
| **Dermatologic diseases:** dermatitis herpetiformis; psoriasis |
| **Pulmonary diseases:** sarcoidosis, idiopathic pulmonary hemosiderosis; cystic fibrosis; bronchiolitis obliterans |
| **Malignant neoplasms:** carcinoma of the lung, larynx, and pancreas; mycosis fungoides |
| **Infective agents:** human immunodeficiency virus; leprosy |
| **Immunologic disorders:** systemic lupus erythematosus; rheumatoid arthritis; cryoimmunoglobulinemia; psoriatic arthritis; ankylosing spondylitis; Sjögren's syndrome; Behçet's syndrome; Reiter's syndrome; familial immune thrombocytopenia; Goodpasture's syndrome |

Table 1. List of diseases/conditions associated with IgA deposits in the kidney.

## 5. The pathogenetic mechanisms

The mechanism of development of IgAN is still largely unresolved. However, many advances have been made, especially during the last decade in unraveling some of the steps involved in the pathogenetic pathway of the disease. This has been made possible by the numerous experimental studies conducted on animal models and clinical studies in humans on the sporadic as well as rare genetic forms of the disease (Barratt et al., 2004; Donadio & Grande, 2002; Floege & Feehally, 2000; Galla, 1995). The postulated mechanisms of pathogenesis are shown in Fig. 1.

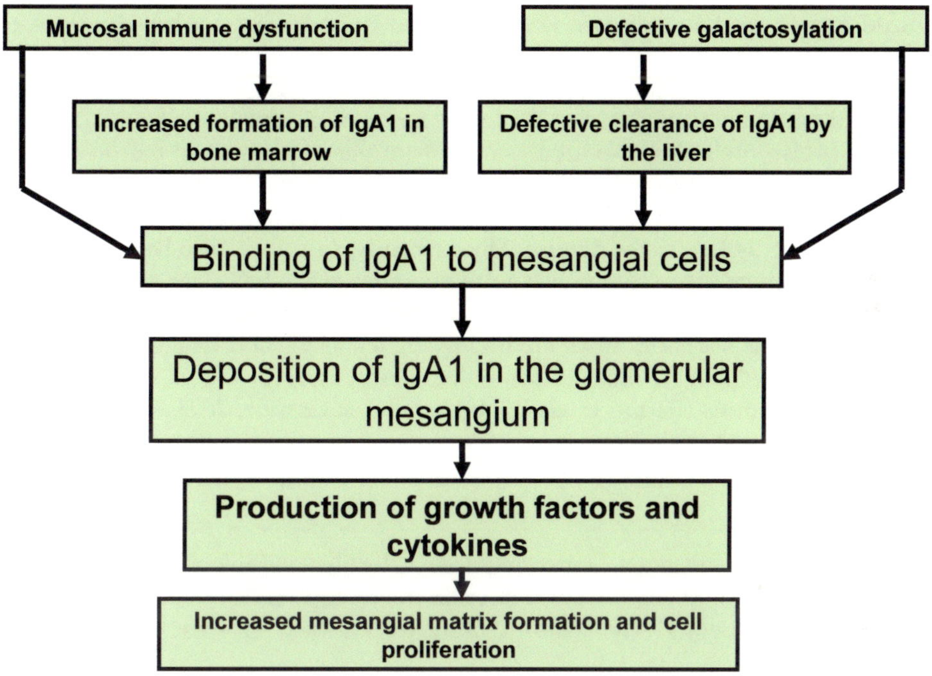


Fig. 1. Schematic diagram showing the main steps involved in the pathogenesis of IgA nephropathy. The final common step consists of deposition of polymers of IgA1 molecules or their complexes in the mesangium. These, then induce injury and stimulate mesangial cells and recruited inflammatory cells to release mediators which result in the morphological expression of glomerular abnormaliteis.

As is apparent from this figure, the final common pathway in the process consists of an accumulation of an abnormally galactosylated polymers of IgA1 (pIgA1) molecules and/or complexes in the mesangial regions of the glomeruli. It is plausible that numerous pathogenetic pathways are involved and converge on this central and unifying stage in the pathway (Barratt et al., 2004). The likely events of pathogenesis implicated in different studies run the whole span of IgA immune system abnormalities from increased production of aberrantly galactosylated pIgA1 molecules by a putative abnormal subclone of B lymphocytes, to decreased clearance by the liver, to host immune response to abnormal pIgA1 molecules, to physicochemical mechanisms leading to abnormal accumulation of pIgA1 in the mesangium (Coppo & Amore, 2004). These bind to and interact with mesangial cells leading to their activation and proliferation. Activated mesangial cells as well as infiltrating inflammatory cells, not only proliferate but also produce pro-inflammatory cytokines, chemokines, and growth factors, which initiate tissue injury. A number of cytokines have been studied in detail including platelet derived growth factor (PDGF) β- chain and transforming growth factor-β (TGF- β) for their roles in the ultimate expression of the disease (Barratt et al., 2004; Donadio & Grande, 2002; Floege & Feehally, 2000; Galla, 1995). There is also evidence of local complement activation induced by alternative pathway triggered by pIgA1 molecules in the mesangium. There are species differences in the molecular structure of IgA and unique features of human IgA1 have prevented development of satisfactory animal models for the early stages of IgAN. A fully humanized mouse model of disease is still awaited to better extrapolate the steps of the pathogenesis to clinical disease in humans. It is probable that events downstream of pIgA1 deposition, which result in glomerular inflammation and scarring, are not specific to IgAN but generic to many immune complex mediated forms of glomerulonephritis (Barrat et al., 2004). There is also preliminary evidence in favor of genetic factors in the predisposition, development, and progression of the disease (Hsu et al., 2000). However, there is no single "IgA gene" involved, and it is likely that multiple interacting genes will eventually be discovered that predispose to the disease. More recently, IgAN has also been categorized as a form of auto-immune disease, in which autoantibodies of the IgG class are formed against aberrantly galactosylated IgA1 molecules. A complete understanding of the pathogenesis along with etiology is necessary if we are to develop a specific and targeted therapy for the disease. Future molecular biologic studies will certainly help in this discovery of missing steps in the pathogenesis (Barratt et al., 2004; Donadio & Grande, 2002; Floege & Feehally, 2000; Galla, 1995; Novak et al., 2001).

## 6. Pathology

The diagnosis of IgAN on renal biopsy requires a detailed pathological evaluation of the biopsy by light microscopy (LM), IF, and electron microscopy (EM). In particular, IgAN is a diagnosis of IF microscopy. The features of IgAN on each of these investigations are described below:

### 6.1 Light microscopy

IgAN is primarily an immune-complex mediated GN, and like lupus nephritis manifests a wide range of morphological appearances on LM. Thus, on LM, IgAN is quite heterogenous. The range of morphologic alterations seen on renal biopsy under the LM spans the whole spectrum from minor changes in the glomeruli and the surrounding parenchyma to full blown crescentic GN (CresGN), except for pure membranous pattern. The list of morphological patterns seen in IgAN is shown in table 2 and in figures 2 to 6. All the above patterns of glomerular injury in IgAN are unified by the presence of predominant or co-dominant IgA deposits in the glomerular mesangium on IF microscopy (Galla, 1995). The reason for this varying phenotypic expression of the disease in different patients is not completely known, but may be related to both the abnormalities of IgA molecule and the host factors. This phenotypic variability of IgAN on LM is expressed as clinical heterogeneity of the disease, but the clinical histologic correlation is not perfect. This variability in morphology of the disease has led to efforts to classify the disease into prognostic groups.

**Light microscopy**

**Glomeruli**
Minor changes
Varying degrees of mesangial proliferation
Mesangiocapillary pattern
Focal segmental glomerular sclerosis
Crescentic GN
Diffuse proliferative and exudative GN
Chronic sclerosing GN

**Tubulo-interstitial component**
Varying degrees of tubular atrophy and interstitial scarring, usually commensurate with glomerular changes

**Vascular changes**
Usually mild fibro-intimal thickening of arteries, commensurate with the degree and duration of hypertension
Thrombotic microangiopathy

**Immunoflourescence**
IgA-dominant or co-dominant, is sine qua non for the diagnosis of IgA nephropathy
Other immunoglobulins and complement components- variably present
Lambda chain predominant

**Electron microscopy**
Variable degree of mesangial proliferation and glomerular inflammation
Large electron dense deposits in the mesangium, paramesangium and occasionally, in other locations

Table 2. Pathologic features of IgA nephropathy on light microscopy, immunoflourescence and electron microscopy.

Many pathological classifications have been proposed over time, but none has achieved international acceptance (Hass, 1997; Manno et al., 2007). More recently, a new pathological classification of IgAN, termed "The Oxford classification of IgAN" has been formulated and published (Cattran et al., 2009; Roberts et al., 2009). It is unique and unprecedented type of classification that was validated before it was formulated and published, in contrast to the traditional approach to disease classifications.

It is very simple and based on only four pathological features on renal biopsy and is easy to apply in routine practice. This classification is pre-validated, evidence based, and of good interobserver reproducibility and most important of all, proves independent prognostic value of pathological features on renal biopsy. Although, pre-validated, the scheme does require more validation studies in routine practice in prospective cohorts and in different study populations. The reasons are; although the sample size in the original study cohort was large, it was limited in scope, the retrospective design of the study, the use of only LM assessment for the classification, and most important of all, the unaddressed issue of treatment strategies. LM features are of independent prognostic value in IgAN and have been investigated by many researchers for classification purpose.

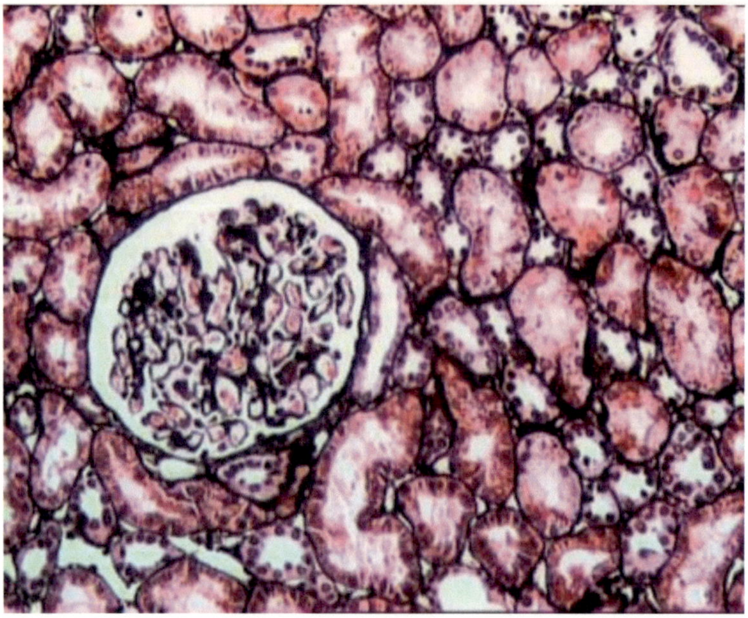

Fig. 2. Medium-power view showing a glomerulus with minor changes on light microscopy. Although rare, this pattern can be seen in IgA nephropathy. The surrounding tubules and interstitium show no significant pathology. (Jones' methenamine silver, ×200).

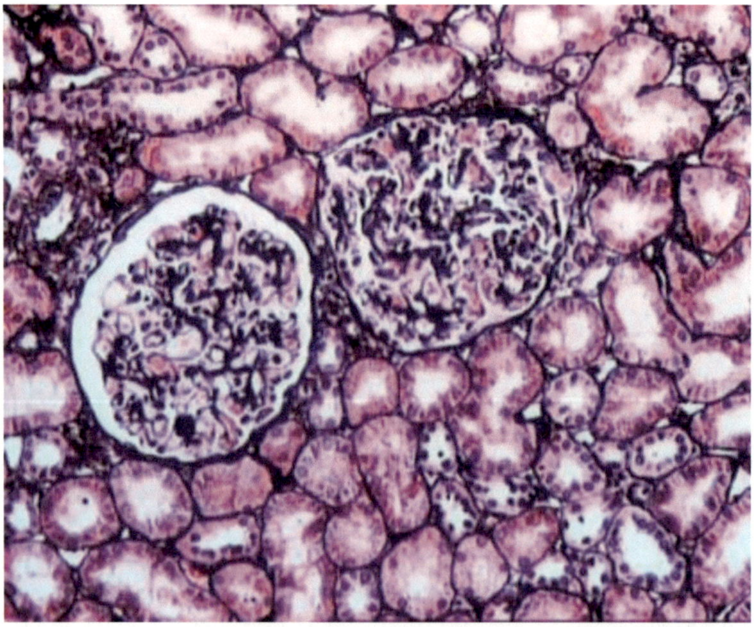

Fig. 3. Medium-power view showing two glomeruli showing mild prominence of the mesangium, but there is no significant increase in the mesangial cellularity in another case of IgA nephropathy. Surrounding parenchyma is unremarkable. (Jones' methenamine silver, ×200).

### 6.2 Immunoflourescence microscopy

The sine qua non for the diagnosis of IgAN is the presence of dominant or co-dominant deposits of IgA in the mesangial area of the glomeruli on IF microscopy. The intensity of staining can vary from 1+ to 3+ on a semiquantitative scale of 0 to 3+ (Fig. 7). A trace positivity of IgA is not sufficient for the definitive diagnosis of IgAN. The distribution of IgA is predominantly mesangial, with extension of the deposits into peripheral capillary walls in approximately one third of cases. The deposited IgA consists mainly of IgA1 rather than IgA2, and is accompanied by other immunoglobulins and complement components in many cases. IgG and IgM are frequently present, but their intensity is generally lower than that of IgA. In contrast, C3 deposits are almost universal and bright in intensity, whereas C1q is found only rarely and usually is of low intensity. The presence of dominant C1q with bright IgA should raise a differential diagnosis of lupus nephritis. Light chain typing of IgAN on IF shows a predominance of lambda light chains over kappa chains, a distinctive feature of IgAN. Fibrin may be found in severe forms of IgAN with crescent formation. Some IF features, such as peripheral capillary location of IgA and mesangial IgG, are supposedly of prognostic importance in IgAN (Bellur et al., 2011).

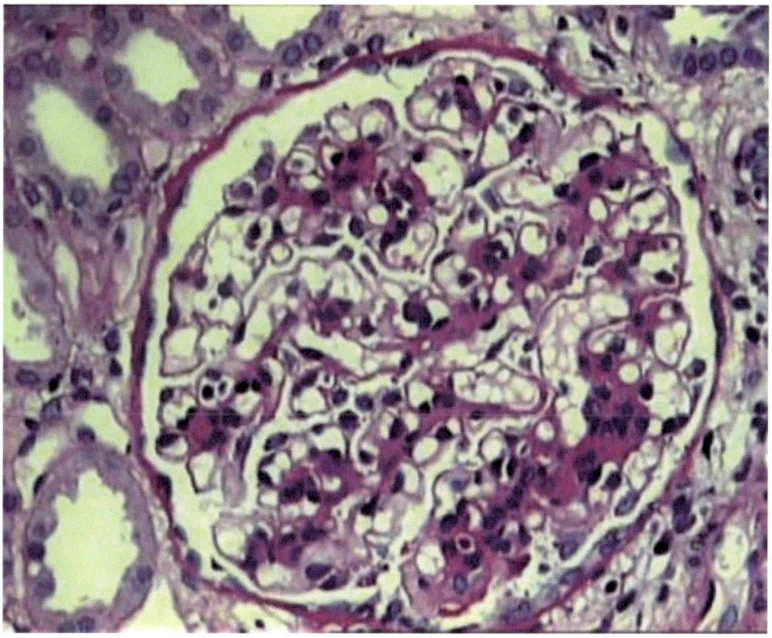

Fig. 4. High-power view showing a glomerulus with segmental and moderate degree mesangial hypercellularity. The patchy involvement of the glomeruli is characteristic of IgA nephropathy. Peripheral capillary walls are thin and capillary lumena patent. The later features distinguishes this pattern from mesangiocapillary pattern. This is the typical and the most common morphological pattern seen in IgA nephropathy. (PAS, ×400).

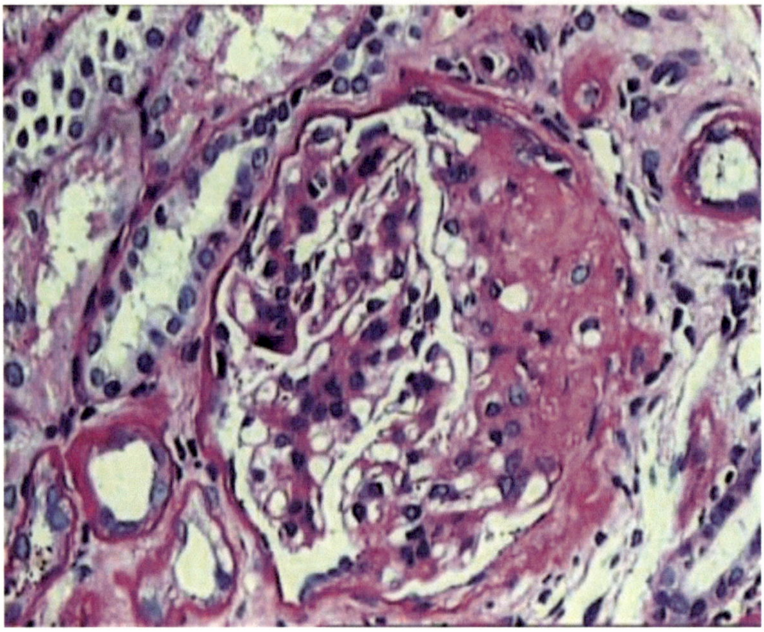

Fig. 5. High-power view showing a segmental scar with adhesion formation with Bowman's capsule. The unscarred portion of the glomerulus shows mild mesangial hypercellularity. This morphologic pattern is common in IgA nephropathy and is distinguished from idiopathic focal segmental glomerulosclerosis by the presence of IgA deposits on immunoflourescence and electron microscopy. (PAS, ×400).

### 6.3 Electron microscopy

Ultra-structurally, the main finding apart from the secondary changes of mesangial proliferation and other alterations, is the deposition of large, frequently triangular shaped, electron-dense deposits, most often, in the mesangium and para-mesangial area of the glomeruli (Fig. 8, 9). The deposits may on rare occasions be found in other locations within the glomeruli. The amount of deposits varies from case to case, and in some cases, massive deposits are found throughout the mesangium, extending into the sub-endothelial location. Peripheral capillary wall deposits in subepithelial, subendothelial, and intramembranous locations are found in approximately one fourth to one third of cases of IgAN. The deposits in these loci are more common in histologically severe forms of the disease, such as cresGN and rare in the mild forms of the disease. Electron-dense deposits may not occasionally be found in typical cases of IgAN diagnosed on IF microscopy. This does not rule out the diagnosis of IgAN, as the disease is a diagnosis of IF microscopy. Moreover, the deposits may be patchy and not included in the scanty material usually examined under the EM.

In addition to the electron-dense deposits, the glomeruli show expansion of the mesangium and mesangial cell proliferation. These alterations parallel those seen on LM. There is also focal to diffuse loss of foot processes of podocytes, especially in those cases presenting with nephrotic range proteinuria. Focal areas of irregular thinning of GBM are seen in many cases of IgAN; these are not synonymous with concurrent IgAN and thin basement membrane disease (TBMD), and may contribute to the hematuria. Occasionally, IgAN co-exists with other glomerulopathies, such as TBMD, minimal change disease (MCD), membranous GN

(MN), etc. In those cases, features of both diseases will be found on ultrastructural study. No prognostic importance is attached with the ultrastructural alterations in IgAN.

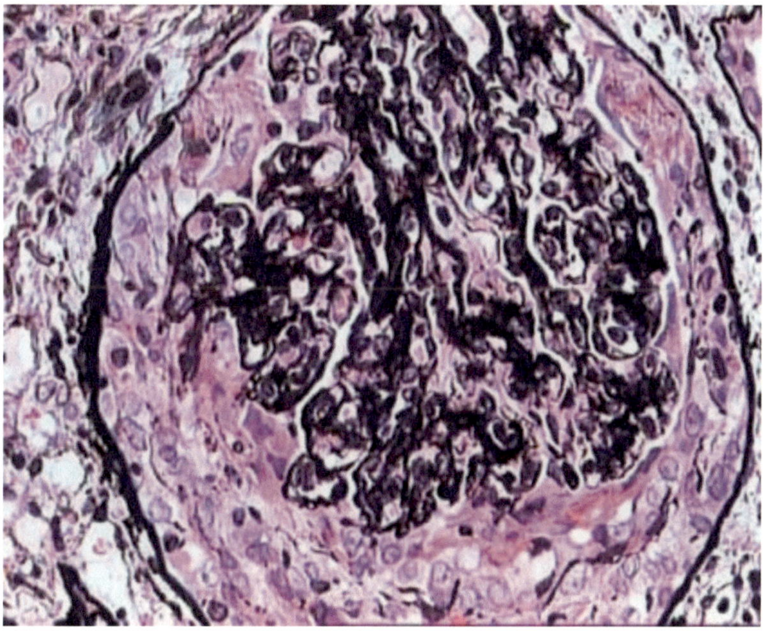

Fig. 6. High-power view showing a glomerulus with marked extracapillary cellular proliferation forming a crescent. The glomerular tufts are collapsed. This morphological pattern is rare in IgA nephropathy, but is well described, and leads rapidly to renal failure. (Jones' methenamine silver, ×400).

## 7. Clinical presentation

Similar to its pathology and clinical course, IgAN is also heterogeneous in clinical presentation. It presents in a variety of ways. It can occur at any age, but majority of cases are seen in adolescents and young adults. The disease is more common in males than females, the male to female varying from less than 2:1 in Japan and other oriental studies to more than 6:1 in the studies from northern Europe and United States. The classic presentation is with painless usually episodic gross or persistent microscopic hematuria, usually developing concurrently with upper respiratory tract infection (hence the use of synonym of synpharyngitic GN), gastroenteritis, or pneumonia. The presenting illness of episodic, grossly visible hematuria is more common in younger patients, whereas that of microscopic hematuria and proteinuria is more frequent in older individuals. Proteinuria is usually mild and usually associated with persistent microscopic hematuria. Occasional cases present with nephrotic range proteinuria. IgAN may rarely present with acute or chronic renal failure. Hypertension is rarely diagnosed at the time of presentation, but its frequency increases as the disease duration is increased or when patients develop ESRD (Barratt et al., 2004; Donadio & Grande, 2002; Floege & Feehally, 2000; Galla, 1995).

## 8. Differential diagnosis

A wide range of diseases are associated with the deposition of IgA in the glomeruli, and these come into the differential diagnosis of IgAN. The most common being Henoch-Schonlein purpura (HSP), believed to be a systemic form of the same disease process as IgAN, with similar histopathological and IF findings in the glomeruli. The presence of systemic symptoms, such as purpuric rash, arthralgias, and abdominal pain help in this differential diagnosis. Post-infectious GN (PIGN) may also present with microscopic hematuria and comes in the clinical differential of IgAN, but the onset of hematuria occurs 7 to 14 days after, and not at the time of infection as in IgAN. A large number of other diseases are characterized by renal pathology resembling IgAN. These are listed in table 1 and are distinguished from primary IgAN by their associated signs and symptoms.

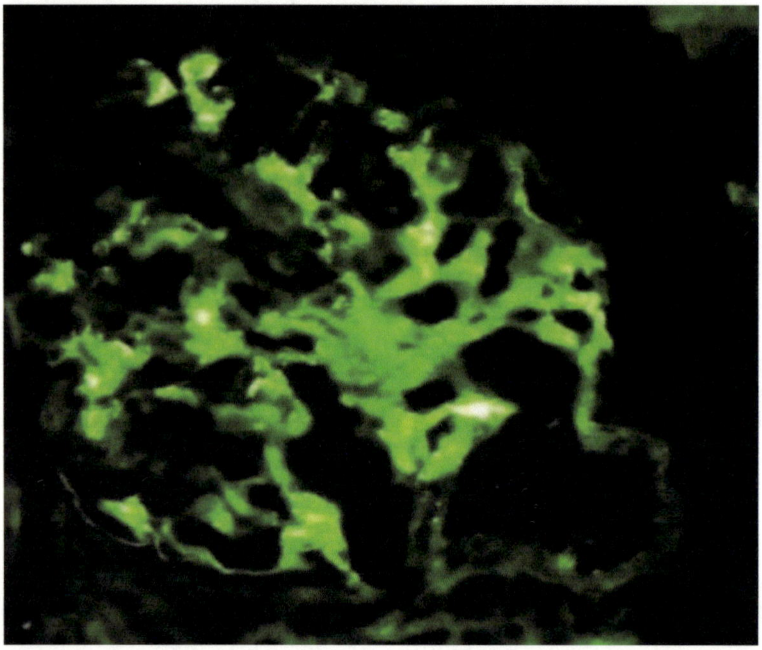

Fig. 7. High-power view showing a glomerulus with diffuse, granular, strong (3+ on a scale of 0 to 3+) deposits of IgA in the mesangial regions. Focally, the deposits are extending into the peripheral capillary walls. (FITC-conjugated IgA, ×400).

## 9. Risk of progression and classification systems

Just like its morphology, the disease is also heterogeneous in its clinical evolution. Although the disease was traditionally considered as benign process, it is now known to lead to a slowly progressive decline in renal function with ESRD developing in upto 30-40% of patients 20 years after initial presentation (Barratt et al., 2004; Donadio & Grande, 2002; Galla, 1995; Geddes et al., 2003).

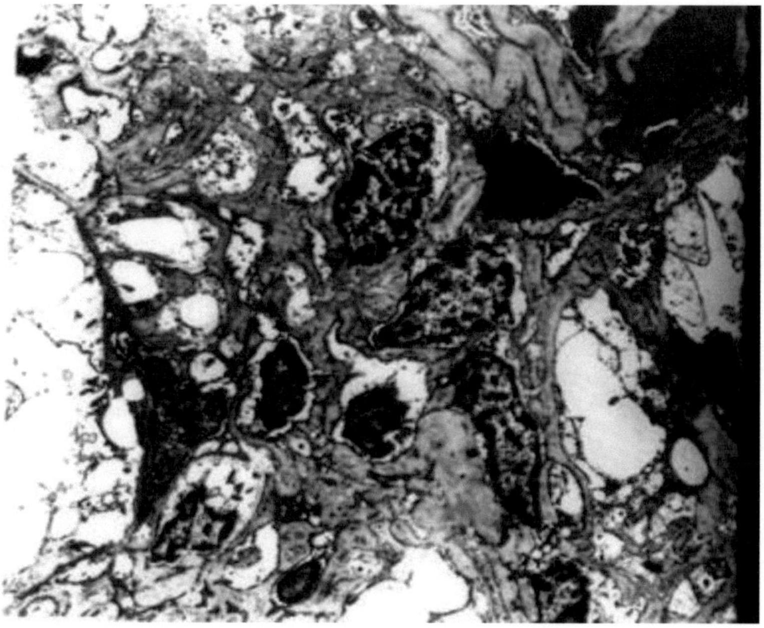

Fig. 8. Low-power electron photomicrograph showing mild mesangial proliferation associated with many large, triangular shaped, electron dense deposits in the mesangium. (Lead citrate & Uranyl acetate, ×5000).

The clinical course in other patients is non-progressive, while in a minority of individuals it leads to a rapidly progressive course to ESRD. Most of the research is focused on identifying the predictive factors for the subset of patients with slowly progressive forms of the disease. Long term follow up studies show variable rates of disease progression in different parts of the world (Geddes et al., 2003). Many attempts have been made in recent past in identifying clinical, familial, laboratory, immunological, genetic, and morphologic features on renal biopsies which can predict the outcome in individual patients. However, many of these parameters have been investigated by simple univariate analysis, and the independent prognostic value of these factors has not been established. Among these, the predictive value of serial estimations of clinical and laboratory parameters is proved beyond any doubt. But whether, pathological features on renal biopsy are of any significant and independent predictive value has remained controversial till very recently. This is because of the fact that almost all pathologic studies carried out by different investigators in different parts of the world have produced conflicting results. Some investigators tried to incorporate the various morphological features observed under LM into a pathologic classification of IgAN, but none succeeded in achieving international approval (Hass, 1997; Lee et al., 2005; Manno et al., 2007). More recently, an international working group of nephrologists and nephropathologists with keen interest and expertise in IgAN have promulgated a novel classification of IgAN, termed "The Oxford classification of IgAN" (Cattran et al., 2009; Roberts et al., 2009).

This scheme was developed by using a novel and unique approach to the pathological classification of IgAN, inasmuch as no arbitrary classes or grades are constructed, as in

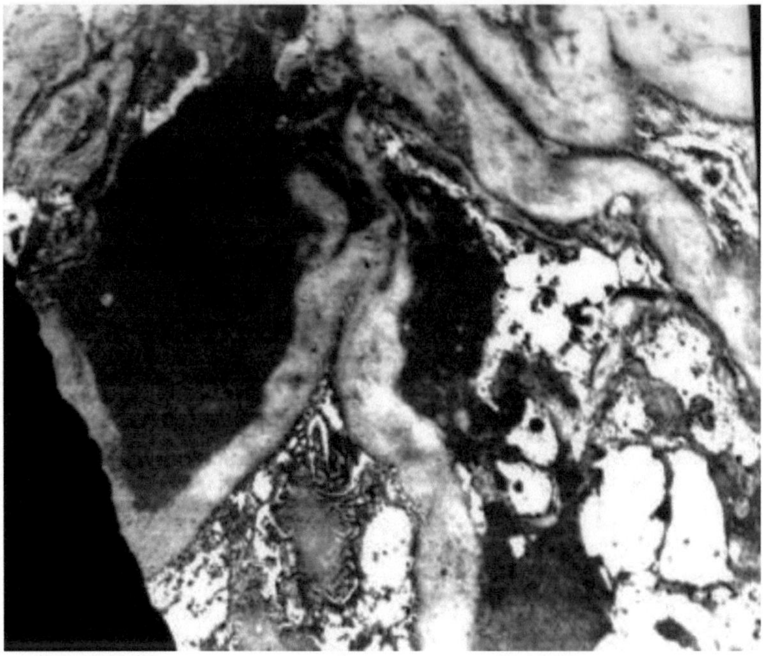

Fig. 9. High-power electron photomicrograph showing large, triangular shaped, uniformly electron dense deposits in the para-mesangial regions of the glomerulus. (Lead citrate & Uranyl acetate, ×25000).

previous classifications. Instead, specific pathological variables of prognostic importance independent of clinical data at the time of biopsy and follow up have been identified and scored by a rigorous iterative methodology of first defining the lesions and then testing for reproducibility and ease of scoring and finally testing them for their predictive power. This type of rigorous effort has never been employed previously in the classification of renal diseases (Cattran et al., 2009; Roberts et al., 2009). The study cohort for the final study validation project consisted of 265 adults and children with biopsy-proven IgAN from eight different countries from four continents, with a median follow-up period of 5 years. The study cohort can be considered as fairly but not completely representative of the entire clinicopathological spectrum of IgAN. It included both males and females, children and adults, nearly all racial groups, and nearly all grades of severity of the disease. However, there was a marked underrepresentation of some grades of disease, for example, very mild cases and very severe cases were very few. This classification is based on detailed analysis of retrospective clinical data obtained on these patients in concert with intense and detailed pathological review of their renal biopsy material for the identified prognostic pathological features. Thus, the classification was validated before its formulation. A set of six distinct pathology variables were identified, from around 24 original pathological features tested, on the basis of sufficient reproducibility among the nephropathologists, least propensity for sampling error, and the ease of scoring in routine practice while avoiding strong co-linearity (mesangial hypercellularity score, segmental glomerulosclerosis or adhesion, endocapillary hypercellularity, cellular or fibrocellular crescents, tubular atrophy/interstitial fibrosis, artery score). Four of them (mesangial hypercellularity score, endocapillary hypercellularity, segmental glomerulosclerosis or adhesion, and tubular atrophy/interstitial fibrosis) were shown in the final analysis to have independent predictive value for the final renal outcome even after taking into account all clinical and laboratory parameters available at the time of biopsy as well as during follow up. These pathological variables along with their proposed scoring (so called MEST score), which are recommended by the Oxford group, to be included in the pathology report of renal biopsy specimens from patients with IgAN, are shown in Table 3. These variables showed the independent prognostic value and a significant correlation with the clinical outcome in both univariate and multivariate analysis. The classification could not address the prognostic value of crescents due to their low prevalence in the enrolled cohort which did not include rapidly progressive cases. This classification is clinically pre-validated, evidence based with acceptable interobserver reproducibility, and most important of all, relatively simple to apply in routine practice (Cattran et al., 2009; Mubarak, 2009; Roberts et al., 2009). The case mix was fairly varied; the cases were collected from eight different centers from four main continents, to ensure international participation and consensus development. However, there are certain limitations of the classification scheme; the classification was developed by dedicated, research-oriented nephropathologists with special interest in IgAN and on a limited repertoire of cases. As discussed previously, both mild (non-progressive) and severe (rapidly-progressive) ends of IgA spectrum were not enrolled. It was retrospective by design and the impact of treatment was not explored in detail. There is definitely a scope for further refinement and validation of the scheme in other prospective cohorts of patients. It needs to be validated in routine practice among practicing pathologists throughout the world on a wide range of cases (Herzenberg et al., 2011). Moreover, the original classification is based purely on light microscopic assessment of pathological features on renal biopsies (Mubarak, 2009). No correlation with IF or EM variables was carried out during the development of this classification. More recently, the question of clinical value of immunohistologic findings in the context of the original study patients' cohort has been addressed by the core group of the researchers involved in the development of the original classification (Bellur et al., 2011). They conclude that the glomerular location of IgA and the presence of IgG correlate with mesangial and endocapillary cellularity. It is likely that the immunohistologic findings may be added to the classification in near future as more data accumulate.

| **Pathological features** | **Score** |
|---|---|
| 1. Mesangial hypercellularity | |
| Present in ≤50% of the glomeruli | M0 |
| Present in >50% of the glomeruli | M1 |
| 2. Endocapillary hypercellularity | |
| Absent | E0 |
| Present | E1 |
| 3. Segmental glomerulosclerosis | |
| Absent | S0 |
| Present | S1 |
| 4. Tubular atrophy/interstitial fibrosis | |
| ≤ 25% of the cortex | T0 |
| 26–50% of the cortex | T1 |
| >50% of the cortex | T2 |

Table 3. The four key pathological features that are recommended by the Oxford group to be included in the standardized pathology reports for patients with IgA nephropathy.

There is also need to investigate the effect of additional features which had enrollment bias in the original study ( rapidly progressive and non-progressive cases) and to investigate the combined prognostic value of adding clinical data to biological scores (e.g. proteinuria at the time of renal biopsy or during follow-up), and the last, but not the least, to detect for each lesion, the most effective treatment and the point of no return when no treatment is effective.

## 10. Future prospects

During recent past, a series of important advancements in the areas of molecular pathogenesis and experimental therapy have taken place, reflected in a molecular paradigm shift in the techniques and approaches applied to the study of IgAN (Novak et al., 2001). Ongoing and future investigations in this area will lead to the development of new non-invasive molecular tests for the diagnosis and prognosis, and the application of these discoveries to the rational design of tailored therapeutic agents.

## 11. References

Ballardie FW, O'Donoghue DJ, & Feehally J. (1987). Increasing frequency of adult IgA nephropathy in the UK? *Lancet*, Vol. 330, No. 8568, pp.1205.

Barratt J, Feehally J, & Smith AC. (2004). Pathogenesis of IgA nephropathy. *Semin Nephrol*, Vol. 24, No. 3, pp. 197–217.

Bartosik LP, Lajoie G, Sugar L, & Cattran DC. (2001). Predicting progression in IgA nephropathy. *Am J Kidney Dis*, Vol. 38, No. 4, pp. 728–35.

Bellur SS, Troyanov S, Cook HT, & Roberts ISD. (2011). Immunostaining findings in IgA nephropathy: correlation with histology and clinical outcome in the Oxford classification patient cohort. *Nephrol Dial Transplant*, Vol. 26, No. 8, pp. 2533-36.

Berger J, & Hinglais N. (1968). Les dépôts intercapillaires d'IgA-IgG. *J Urol Nephrol*, Vol. 74, pp. 694-5.

Floege J, & Feehally J. (2000). IgA nephropathy: recent developments. *J Am Soc Nephrol*, Vol. 11, No. 12, pp. 2395–2403.

Coppo R, & Amore A. (2004). Aberrant glycosylation in IgA nephropathy (IgAN). *Kidney Int*, Vol. 65, No. 5, pp. 1544–7.

Cattran DC, Coppo R, Cook T, Feehally J, Roberts ISD, Troyanov S, Alpers CE, Amore A, Barratt J, Berthoux F, Bonsib S, Bruijn JA, D'Agati V, D'Amico G, Emancipator S, Emma F, Ferrario F, Fervenza FC, Florquin S, Fogo A, Geddes CC, Groene HJ, Haas M, Herzenberg AM, Hill PA, Hogg RJ, Hsu SI, Jennette JC, Joh K, Julian BA, Kawamura T, Lai FM, Leung CB, Li LS, Li PK, Liu ZH, Mackinnon B, Mezzano S, Schena FP, Tomino Y, Walker PD, Wang H, Weening JJ, Yoshikawa N, & Zhang H. (2009). The Oxford classification of IgA nephropathy: rationale, clinicopathologic correlations, and classification. *Kidney Int*, Vol. 76, No. 5, pp. 534–45.

Chandrika BK. (2009). IgA nephropathy in Kerala, India: a retrospective study. *Indian J Pathol Microbiol*, Vol. 52, No. 1, pp.14-16.

D'Amico G. (2004). Natural history of idiopathic IgA nephropathy and factors predictive of disease outcome. *Semin Nephrol* Vol. 24, No. 3, pp. 179–96.

D'Amico G. (1985). The commonest glomerulonephritis in the world: IgA nephropathy. *Q J Med*, Vol. 64, No. 245, pp. 709-27.

Donadio JV, & Grande JP. IgA nephropathy. (2002). *New Engl J Med,* 347, No. 10, p. 738-48.

Galla JH. (1995). IgA nephropathy. *Kidney Int,* Vol. 47, No. 2, pp. 377-87.

Geddes CC, Rauta V, Gronhagen-Riska C, Bartosik LP, Jardine AG, Ibels LS, Pei Y, & Cattran DC. (2003). A tricontinental view of IgA nephropathy. *Nephrol Dial Transplant,* Vol. 18, No. 8, pp. 1541-8.

Hass M. (1997). Histologic sub-classification of IgA nephropathy: a clinicopathologic study of 244 cases. *Am J Kidney Dis,* Vol. 29, No. 6, pp. 829-42.

Herzenberg AM, Fogo AB, Reich HN, Troyanov S, Bavbek N, Massat AE, Hunley TE, Hladunewich MA, Julian BA, Fervenza FC, Cattran DC. (2011). Validation of the Oxford classification of IgA nephropathy. *Kidney Int,* Vol. 80, pp. 310-7.

Hsu SI, Ramirez SB, Winn MP, Bonventre JV, & Owen WF. (2000). Evidence for genetic factors in the development and progression of IgA nephropathy. *Kidney Int,* Vol. 57, No. 5, pp. 1818-35.

Julian BA, Waldo FB, Rifai A, & Mestecki J. (1988). IgA nephropathy, the most common glomerulonephritis worldwide. A neglected disease in the United States? *Am J Med,* Vol. 84, No. 1, pp. 129-32.

Kazi JI, Mubarak M, Ahmed E, Akhter F, Naqvi SAA, & Rizvi SAH. (2009). Spectrum of glomerulonephritides in adults with nephrotic syndrome in Pakistan. *ClinExp Nephrol,* Vol. 13, No. 1, pp. 38-43.

Koyama A, Igarashi M, & Kobayashi M. Members and coworkers of the Research group on progressive renal diseases. (1997). Natural history and risk factors for Immunoglobulin A nephropathy in Japan. *Am J Kidney Dis,* Vol. 29, No. 4, pp. 526-32.

Lai FMM, To KF, Choi PCL, & Li PKT. (1999). Primary immunoglobulin A nephropathy through the retrospectroscope. *Hong Kong Med J,* Vol. 5, No. 4, pp. 375-82.

Lee HS, Lee MS, Lee SM, Lee SY, Lee ES, Lee EY, et al. (2005). Histological grading of IgA nephropathy predicting renal outcome: Revisiting H.S. Lee's glomerular grading system. *Nephrol Dial Transplant,* Vol. 20, No. 2, pp. 342–8.

Manno C, Strippoli G, D'Altri C, Torres D, Rossini M, & Schena F. (2007). A novel simpler histological classification for renal survival in IgA Nephropathy: A retrospective study. *Am J Kidney Dis,,* Vol. 49, No. 6, pp. 763-75.

Mubarak M. (2009). The prevalence of IgA nephropathy in Pakistan: only a tip of the iceberg. *J Pak Med Assoc,* Vol. 59, No. 10, pp. 733.

Mubarak M, Lanewala A, Kazi JI, Akhter F, Sher A, Fayyaz A, & Bhatti S. (2009). Histopathological spectrum of childhood nephrotic syndrome in Pakistan. *Clin Exp Nephrol,* Vol. 13, No. 6, pp. 589-93.

Mubarak M. (2009). Nomenclature of the Oxford classification of IgA nephropathy: do we need to be careful? *Kidney Int,* Vol. 77, No. 1, pp. 74.

Narasimhan B, Chacko B, John GT, Korula A, Kirubakaran MG, & Jacob CK. (2006). Characterization of kidney lesions in Indian adults: towards a renal biopsy registry. *J Nephrol,* Vol. 19, No. 2, pp. 205-10.

Novak J, Julian BA, Tomana M, & Mestecky J. (2001). Progress in molecular and genetic studies of IgA nephropathy. *J Clin Immunol,* Vol. 21, No. 5, pp. 310-27.

Power DA, Murhead N, & Simpson JG. (1985). IgA nephropathy is not a rare disease in the United Kingdom. *Nephron* Vo. 40, No. 2, pp. 180-4.

Rivera F, Lopez-Gomez JM, & Perez Garcia R. (2004). Clinicopathologic correlations of renal pathology in Spain. *Kidney Int,* Vol. 66, No. 3, pp. 898-904.

Roberts ISD, Cook T, Troyanov S, Alpers CE, Amore A, Barratt J, Berthoux F, Bonsib S, Bruijn JA, Cattran DC, Coppo R, D'Agati V, D'Amico G, Emancipator S, Emma F, Feehally J, Ferrario F, Fervenza FC, Florquin S, Fogo A, Geddes CC, Groene HJ, Haas M, Herzenberg AM, Hill PA, Hogg RJ, Hsu SI, Jennette JC, Joh K, Julian BA, Kawamura T, Lai FM, Li LS, Li PK, Liu ZH, Mackinnon B, Mezzano S, Schena FP, Tomino Y, Walker PD, Wang H, Weening JJ, Yoshikawa N, & Zhang H. (2009). The Oxford classification of IgA nephropathy: pathology definitions, correlations and reproducibility. *Kidney Int,* Vol. 76, No. 5, pp. 546–56.

Schena FP and the Italian Group of Renal Immunopathology. Survey of the Italian Registry of renal biopsies. (1997). Frequency of the renal diseases for 7 consecutive years. *Nephrol Dial Transplant,* Vol. 12, No. pp. 3, pp. 418-26.

Seedat YK, Nathoo BC, Parag KB, Naiker IP, & Ramsaroop R. (1988). IgA nephropathy in Blacks and Indians of Natal. *Nephron,* Vol. 50, No. 2, pp. 37-41.

Sinniah R. (1980). Renal disease in Singapore with particular reference to glomerulonephritis in adults. *Singapore Med J,* Vol. 21, No. 3, pp. 583-91.

Stratta P, Segoloni GP, Canavese C, Sandri L, Mazzucco G, Roccatello D, Manganaro M, & Versellone A. (1996). Incidence of biopsy-proven primary glomerulonephritis in an Italian province. *Am J Kidney Dis,* Vol. 27, No. 5, pp. 631-9.

Yahya TM, Pingle A, Boobes Y, & Pingle S. (1997). Analysis of 490 kidney biopsies: data from the United Arab Emirates renal diseases registry. *J Nephrol,* Vol. 11, No. 3, pp. 148-50.

# 9

# Collapsing Glomerulopathy: The Expanding Etiologic Spectrum of a Shrinking Glomerular Lesion

Muhammed Mubarak and Javed I. Kazi
*Histopathology Department, Sindh Institute of Urology and Transplantation, Karachi Pakistan*

## 1. Introduction

Collapsing glomerulopathy (CG) is a relatively recently described pattern of renal parenchymal injury that is being increasingly recognized as a common cause of end-stage renal disease (ESRD) throughout the world (Albaqumi et al., 2006). Although, it is currently classified officially as one of the pathological variants of focal segmental glomerulosclerosis (FSGS), its defining morphological alterations are in marked contrast to those observed in other variants of FSGS. During the initial stages of the disease, the lesion is characterized morphologically by an implosive, segmental and/or global wrinkling and retraction of the glomerular capillary tufts, pronounced hypertrophy and proliferation of the visceral epithelial cells (VECs) or podocytes, and severe tubulointerstitial damage. With disease progression, segmental and/or global glomerulosclerosis is also observed in addition to the pathognomonic collapsing lesions. Often, both the active and chronic lesions (collapsing and sclerotic) co-exist at the time of pathologic diagnosis, hence its classification as a variant of FSGS (Albaqumi et al., 2006; Albaqumi & Barisoni, 2006). The exact cause of this mysterious lesion is still not known, but a growing list of both genetic and acquired diseases/conditions is being reported in association with this morphologic pattern of renal parenchymal injury (Albaqumi et al., 2006). The pathogenesis of CG is also still incompletely understood, but many advances have been made during the past two to three decades, especially in the development and study of animal models of the disease and the discovery of genetic abnormalities leading to CG. Various triggering agents typically cause discreet epithelial cell injury in different anatomical compartments of the renal parenchyma leading to cell cycle dysregulation and a proliferative cellular phenotype (Albaqumi et al., 2006; Albaqumi & Barisoni, 2006; Schwimmer et al., 2003). Clinically, CG is characterized by its black racial predilection, a high incidence and severity of nephrotic syndrome (NS), a poor response to the currently used empirical therapy, and a rapid downhill course to ESRD (Albaqumi & Barisoni, 2006; Schwimmer et al., 2003). Although most of the early studies were reported in the native kidneys, the disease has also been found more recently to afflict the transplanted kidneys, either as a recurrent or de novo disease, frequently leading to loss of the allograft (Schwimmer et al., 2003; Canaud et al., 2010; Gupta et al., 2011; Nadasday et al., 2002; Stokes et al., 1996; Swaminathan et al., 2006). Most of the cases have been reported from the western countries, but the lesion is also being increasingly recognized in the tropical regions

(Kazi & Mubarak, 2007; Mubarak & Kazi, 2010; Nada et al., 2009). The recent increase in the reporting of CG partly reflects a genuine increase in the incidence of the disease and partly a detection bias resulting from heightened recognition by the pathologists (Albaqumi et al., 2006). There is no specific treatment for the disorder at present. Newer insights into the pathogenesis may pave the pathway for the development of targeted and specific therapy in not too distant future (Albaqumi et al., 2006; Albaqumi & Barisoni, 2006). This chapter discusses the nomenclature and historical background, epidemiology, etiology, pathogenesis, pathology, clinical manifestations, treatment and the prognosis of the condition.

## 2. The changing nomenclature of the lesion and the historical background

The nomenclature of CG has undergone interesting metamorphosis over the time and is still controversial. Although, the lesion was first recognized as a distinct clinicopathological entity (with a question mark!) in 1986, cases with similar morphology and clinical course in the literature trace back to early 1970's, when they were described as "malignant FSGS" (Albaqumi & Barisoni, 2006). During late 1980s and early 1990s, the term CG, was popular for this lesion (Weis et al., 1986). However, during mid to late 1990s reports started appearing in the literature linking this lesion to the expanding spectrum of FSGS; the main reason for this was the clinical presentation and concurrence of sclerotic lesions along with collapsing lesions on renal biopsies at the time of pathologic diagnosis (Detwiler et al., 1994; Valeri et al., 1996). Indeed, it has been suggested that the morphological lesions of CG may represent an early stage in the evolution that eventually are converted into the discrete segmental scars typical of FSGS (Detwiler et al., 1994). Another term, "cellular lesion," was also used for this lesion in 1980s (Schwartz & Lewis, 1985). The Columbia classification of FSGS officially classified this lesion as a subtype of FSGS (D'Agati et al., 2004). The Columbia classification also suggests using "cellular lesion" for a variant of FSGS characterized by expansion of the glomerular capillaries by intracapillary hypercellularity, in contrast to the intracapillary hypocellularity and collapse of CG. More recent studies suggest that the lesion may be distinct from FSGS and merits classification as a separate nosologic entity (Meyrier, 1999). Indeed, Barisoni et al. in a recently proposed classification of the podocytopathies have categorized CG separately from FSGS and further subdivided it into three major subtypes: idiopathic, genetic, and secondary or reactive (Barisoni et al., 2007). Further studies are needed to clarify this nosologic puzzle.

## 3. The magnitude of the problem and the epidemiology

Although the first report of CG included only six patients, this was soon followed by a series of fairly large studies from different centers mostly from United States, and subsequently from Europe and more recently from the developing countries (Agarwal et al., 2008; Bariety et al., 1998; Deegans et al., 2008; Detwiler et al., 1994; Grcevska & Polenakovik, 1999; Kazi & Mubarak, 2007; Laurinavicious et al., 1999; Meyrier, 1999; Mubarak & Kazi, 2010; Nada et al., 2009; Valeri et al., 1996; Weis et al., 1986). However, a wide variation is noted in the reported frequency of the lesion among all cases of FSGS. The disease thus has a cosmopolitan distribution and the wide geographical disparity in the reporting of CG appears to be mostly due to detection bias rather than true difference in the prevalence of the disorder, as more recently, rates of its diagnosis in both the native and the transplanted kidneys approaching the western studies have been reported (Gupta et al., 2011; Mubarak, 2011). The increasing reporting of CG in the literature from both the western and the developing countries reflects both a true increase in the incidence of the lesion and the diagnostic bias (Albaqumi et al., 2006). The increase in the incidence of this lesion has been clearly shown in studies from United States and Europe. This lesion constituted 11% of all idiopathic FSGS at Columbia Presbyterian Medical Center from 1979 to 1985, 20% from 1986 to 1989, and 24% from 1990 to 1993 (Valeri et al., 1996). It is interesting to note their first case with the typical morphological features of CG was identified in 1979 on retrospective review of the renal biopsies, well before the formal recognition of this lesion, and represents the first documented case of idiopathic CG in the literature. Even more importantly, this lesion comprised 11% of all cases of idiopathic FSGS diagnosed on renal biopsies in pre-recognition era of CG in their report during the study period from 1979 to 1985 (Valeri et al., 1996). Another retrospective study by Haas et al. (1995), also from United States, from 1974 to 1993, identified their first case of CG after 1980, and during the time period of 1980 to 1993, CG represented 5.3% of cases of idiopathic FSGS in their series. A follow up study by the same authors from 1995 to 1997 identified CG in 9% of patients with idiopathic FSGS (Haas et al., 1997). Although less common than in the United States, Europe has also not lagged behind in the reporting of CG (Meyrier, 1999). The exact cause for the increase in the incidence of CG is not known, but may be due to a possible change in the exposure to certain infective organisms, chemical agents, or other environmental factors. Similarly, high rates of detection have been reported both in native and transplanted kidneys from developing countries, but no formal upward trend analysis of CG has been reported from developing countries till date (Gupta et al., 2011; Kazi & Mubarak, 2007; Mubarak & Kazi, 2010; Nada et al., 2009).

## 4. The etiology and the associated conditions

The most common form of CG is the primary or idiopathic one and the exact cause of this, as is evident from the name, is still not known. What is apparent from the increased reporting of CG is, however, that it is not a single disease but rather a unique pattern of renal parenchymal injury, which may result from a multitude of causes (Albaqumi et al., 2006; Amoura et al. 2006). Indeed, one outcome from the growing awareness of the lesion has been the exponential increase in reporting its association with disorders other than human immunodeficiency virus (HIV)-1 infection or idiopathic. There are many reports of secondary or reactive and genetic causes of this lesion and these provide an insight into the widening etiopathogenetic pathways of the condition (Table 1).

When broadly categorized, these associated disorders fall into seven classes: infections, drug toxicity, autoimmune diseases, malignant tumors, genetic diseases, ischemic causes, and during the posttransplant period. Among all the known causes/associations, HIV-1 infection is the most common cause and the disease caused by HIV-1 infection is called HIV associated nephropathy (HIVAN) (D'Agati & Appel, 1998). Other infectious agents and immunologic derangements are next common reported associations (Albaqumi et al., 2006). The list of the associated conditions/etiologic agents is growing day by day. As alluded to earlier, this wide heterogeneity of the underlying causes/associated conditions clearly shows that CG is not a single disease entity, but rather a common final pathway resulting from these various insults, all sharing the similar morphologic appearance on renal biopsy.

One peculiar scenario for the development of CG is the posttransplant period, where the disease can occur as recurrent, or more commonly, as de novo disease (Canaud et al., 2010; Gupta et al., 2011; Nadasday et al., 2002; Stokes et al., 1996; Swaminathan et al., 2006).

| |
|---|
| **Infections** |
| Human Immunodeficiency Virus-1 infection |
| Parvovirus B19 |
| Cytomegalovirus infection |
| Human T cell Lymphotropic Virus-1 |
| Hepatitis C Virus |
| Pulmonary tuberculosis |
| Leishmaniasis |
| Febrile illness |
| **Autoimmune diseases** |
| Systemic lupus erythematosus |
| Adult Still's disease |
| Mixed connective tissue disorder |
| Giant cell arteritis |
| Lupus-like syndrome |
| **Malignant tumors** |
| Multiple myeloma |
| Acute monoblastic leukemia |
| Hemophagocytic syndrome |
| **Genetic disorders** |
| Action myoclonus-renal failure syndrome |
| Mitochondrial cytopathy |
| Familial |
| Sickle cell anemia |
| **Drugs/chemotherapeutic agents** |
| Interferon-α |
| Pamidronate |
| Cyclosporin A |
| **Post renal and other solid organ transplantation** |
| Recurrent |
| De novo |
| Hyaline arteriolopathy |
| Acute vascular rejection |
| Thrombotic microangiopathy |

Table 1. List of known etiologic factors/clinical conditions associated with collapsing FSGS in humans.

However, the etiological and clinical associations of CG following kidney transplantation are still not fully known. Recent studies have implicated ischemia and drug toxicity as major predisposing factors in the development of posttransplant CG (Swaminathan et al., 2006). Recurrent CG provides a unique opportunity to study the evolution of the lesions of CG by sequential biopsies with no interference of the confounding secondary causes (Bariety et al., 2001).

## 5. Pathogenetic mechanisms

Given the wide range of etiologic associations, a variety of hypotheses for the pathogenesis of CG have been proposed over the years, but till date no one definable pathogenic trigger has emerged clearly from studying these disparate disorders as a group. However, significant advances have been made during past two to three decades in unraveling many of the pathways leading to the final common manifestation of the disease. As discussed previously in the etiology of the condition, the discovery of secondary and genetic causes of CG had been very instrumental in understanding the pathogenesis of the disorder. Similarly, the discovery of a number of susceptibility genes for CG in mice and humans, and the development of more than a dozen independent mouse models of the disease in different centers of the world, represent landmark achievements for studying the disease process both in vivo and in a wider perspective (Albaqumi et al., 2006). The mouse models can be broadly categorized in to four types based on the nature of the triggering agents. In marked contrast to human disease, the pathogenic triggers in each of the four types of mouse models of CG are known. These include; HIV-1 gene products, immunoglobulins (Ig), oxidative stress, and the disturbance of podocyte paracrine/autocrine regulatory loop (Albaqumi et al., 2006). How these different triggering agents lead to the stereotyped morphological appearance is still not known. However, a hypothetical "best-fit" model has been proposed to explain the final common expression of the disease caused by such seemingly divergent initiating stimuli. According to this model, the initiating event consists of discreet epithelial cell injury caused by either intrinsic or extrinsic agents involving different compartments of renal parenchyma, i.e., both the podocytes and the renal tubular epithelium. The injured epithelial cells undergo either apoptosis or necrosis, and relay signals to the surrounding un-injured epithelial cells and resident immune cells, principally the dendritic cells. Conditioned by the genetic and other environmental factors, the surrounding uninjured epithelial cells, subsequently respond to the injury, not by the normal repair or regeneration, but in a perverted manner, by the processes of dedifferentiation, proliferation and transdifferentiation of, for example, podocytes to the macrophage-like phenotype in the glomerular compartment (Albaqumi et al., 2006). These phenotypic changes are accompanied by changes in the behavior of these cells and their immunophenotypic profile. The immunophenotypic markers of maturity are lost, and the markers of immature phenotype, proliferation and macrophage lineage are expressed, the latter phenomenon being known as transdifferentiation (Bariety et al., 1998) (Table 2).

The podocytes become cuboidal to epithelioid cell like, lose primary foot processes, and detach from the glomerular basement membrane (GBM) and proliferate to form pseudo-crescents. Many of these detached podocytes are also passed into the tubules. These phenotypic changes result in marked alterations in the normal structure-function relationships of the different compartments of the nephron with consequent drastic changes in the function, so characteristic of this disease. The luminal factors and the preexisting disturbance in the immune system, coupled with genetic susceptibility, likely contribute to the above sequence of events (Albaqumi et al., 2006). Similar changes in tubular epithelium give rise to both acute and chronic damage of the tubules, with microcystic transformation of the tubules in many forms of CG, especially that induced by HIV-1 infection (Fig. 1). Although this hypothetical "best-fit" model has not been studied directly in humans, but preliminary studies to characterize the earliest changes in the development of CG in some mouse models have shown that necrosis or apoptosis of epithelial cells occurs before the aberrant proliferation of the surviving epithelium. This podocytopenia is transient, short-lived, and not often seen on renal biopsies in human CG, and is in contrast with the prominent and pathogenetic podocytopenia in non-collapsing FSGS. We have observed this phenomenon in some of our sequential renal allograft biopsies done for the investigation of posttransplant proteinuria (unpublished observations) (Fig. 1). Indeed, renal allograft represents one of the best models to study the evolution and natural history of CG in humans.

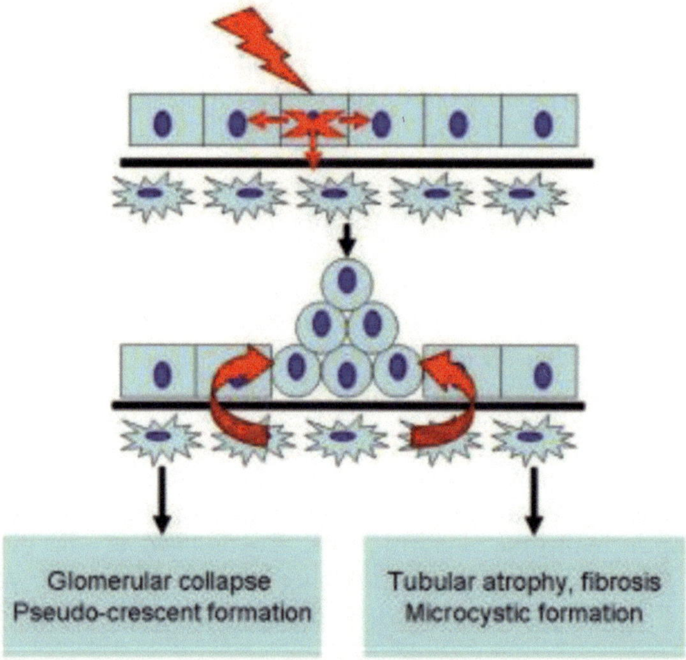


Fig. 1. Schematic diagram showing a hypothetical "best-fit" model for the pathogenesis of collapsing glomerulopathy. According to this model, an intrinsic or extrinsic injurious agent discreetly damages some epithelial cells. These cells undergo either apoptosis or necrosis and send signals to neighboring epithelial cells and dendritic and other innate immune cells. These cells, instead of inducing normal repair or cell cycle arrest upon contact with adjacent epithelial cells, cause aberrant hyperplasia of surrounding epithelial cells. These ultimately manifest in the form of glomerular collapse and pseudocrescent formation in the glomeruli, and in tubular atrophy, microcystic formation in the tubular compartment with interstitial inflammation and fibrosis. These structural alterations result in profound disturbances in the functions of respective elements of the renal parenchyma.

| Underexpressed markers | Overexpressed markers |
|---|---|
| CD10 | Cyclin D1 |
| Glomerular epithelial protein 1 | Cyclin E |
| Podocalyxin | Cyclin A |
| Synaptopodin | Ki-67 |
| Wilms' tumor-1 | Desmin |
| p27 | Cytokeratin |
| p57 | CD68 |

Table 2. The main immunohistochemical (IHC) markers of the aberrant podocyte phenotype observed in collapsing glomerulopathy.

Two major common pathways have been proposed to explain the stereotyped response of the renal parenchyma to a wide variety of conditions in CG: activation of the immune system and the dysregulation of the mitochondrial function ((Albaqumi et al., 2006)) (Fig. 2). Many of the diseases associated with CG involve a disturbance of immune homeostasis, suggesting at least some role for immune activation in the development of CG. The precise immunologic mechanisms are still not completely clear, but studies show that many involve T helper type 1 lymphocyte responses, an immune perturbation that already is known to aggravate and accelerate other proliferative parenchymal renal diseases, particularly crescentic glomerulonephritis (CresGN), the disease that CG mimics most closely on renal biopsies.

The second major common pathway involves some form of acute ischemic insult to the kidney such as that resulting from thrombotic microangiopathy (TMA), cyclosporine A (CsA) toxicity and severe hyaline arteriopathy ((Albaqumi et al., 2006)). This phenomenon has been particularly observed in transplanted kidneys. Recently, three cases of CG have been reported in renal allografts on allograft biopsies in association with areas of frank segmental infarction (Canaud et al., 2010). We have also observed similar phenomenon on renal biopsies from patients with acute cortical necrosis in native kidneys (Kazi & Mubarak, 2011). Thus, ischemic injury to the glomeruli does have a role in the development of CG. This may be mediated by dysregulation of the mitochondrial function and/or altered autocrine/paracrine interaction of podocytes, endothelial cells, and/or parietal epithelial cells ((Albaqumi et al., 2006)).

## 6. Diagnosis and histopathology

Although the diagnosis of CG may be suspected on clinical grounds, it can only be confirmed on the invasive test of renal biopsy. It is diagnosed pathologically by its characteristic morphological features in the glomeruli on light microscopy (LM) of renal biopsy (Albaqumi et al., 2006; Schwimmer et al., 2003). These consist of focal to diffuse, segmental to global, implosive collapse of the glomerular capillary tufts associated with marked proliferation and swelling of overlying podocytes (Fig. 3-7). These proliferating podocytes form a number of cell layers and fill the Bowman's space caused by collapsed tufts, resulting in the formation of pseudo-crescents, which differ from the true crescents of CresGN by their visceral location, the presence of a cleft like space between the pseudo-crescents and the parietal epithelium, the epithelioid appearance of the cells forming the pseudo-crescents, and the absence of fibrin in the pseudo-crescents (Fig. 5, 6). These extracapillary cells lack the spindle cell appearance or pericellular matrix with collagen fibers typically noted in true crescents. Another distinguishing feature is that Bowman's capsule itself is intact, without the ruptures typical of cellular crescents of the inflammatory type. The proliferating podocytes also exhibit marked cytoplasmic vacuolization and prominent, hyaline, protein resorption droplets (Figure 5). There is usually also concurrent segmental and/or global glomerulosclerosis at the time of pathologic diagnosis of CG (Fig. 7). The distribution of lesions may be segmental or global, focal or diffuse and may involve any number of the glomeruli (Fig. 4). Due primarily to its poor prognosis among all the other variants of FSGS, even a single glomerulus with the characteristic collapsing lesion is sufficient for the diagnosis of CG on the biopsy. Although, CG is defined on the basis of glomerular lesions, the tubulointerstitial disease is an equally important component of the condition and often appears out of proportion to the degree of glomerular sclerosis.

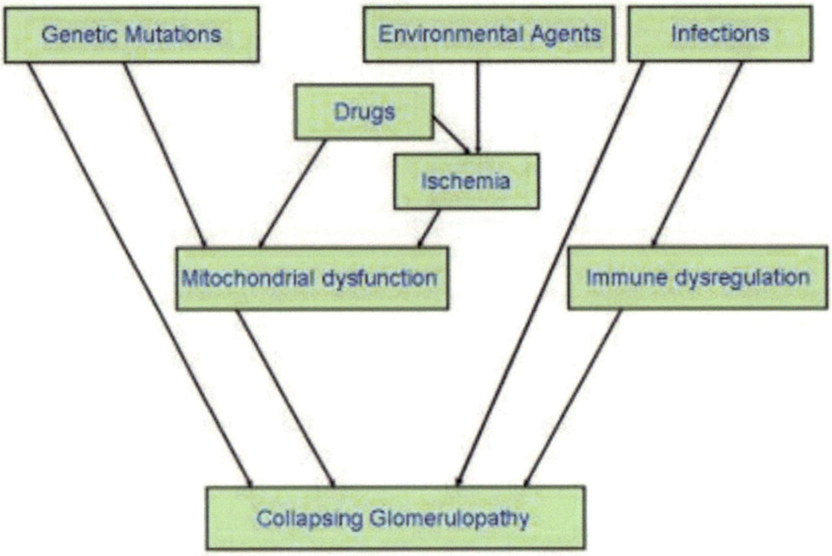


Fig. 2. Schematic diagram showing the pathogenesis of collapsing glomerulopathy. As is evident from this diagram, several mechanisms are involved in the pathogenesis of CG. A variety of triggering agents act through two major common pathways: dysregulation of the immune system and mitochondrial dysfunction. Some factors, eg. Infections, can directly lead to CG, while others produce lesions of CG by the disturbances in mitochondrial activity and immune function.

It has been suggested that the poor prognosis of the condition results from tubulointerstitial pathology rather than glomerular lesions (Meyrier, 1999). The tubulointerstitial component shows both acute and chronic changes. These include variable degrees of tubular atrophy, interstitial fibrosis, edema, and inflammation, associated with widespread degenerative and regenerative changes of the tubular epithelium, including microcyst formation, as shown in Fig. 8 and 9. The later are filled with hyaline casts with scalloped margins, as shown in Fig. 9. It has been proposed that the extent of tubulointerstitial involvement varies depending on the etiology of CG and may help in the differential diagnosis of different causes of CG (Albaqumi & Barisoni, 2006).

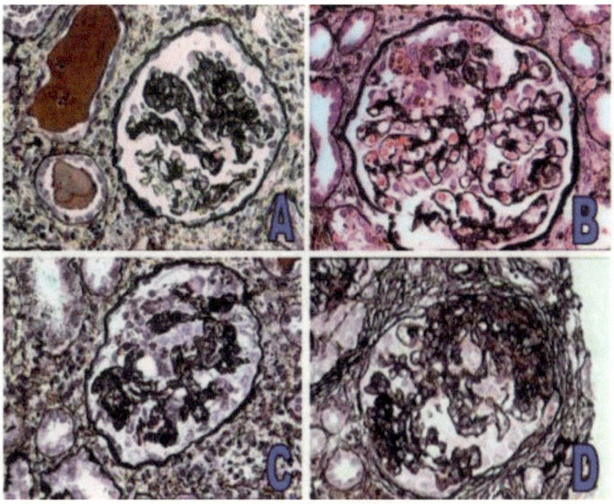


Fig. 3. The morphologic evolution of the lesions of collapsing glomerulopathy. A. Medium-power view showing segmental collapse of capillary tufts. The overlying podocytes have not yet markedly proliferated or hypertrophied. They are forming a cobblestone structure directly overlying the collapsed tufts. B. Medium-power view showing mild hypertrophy and hyperplasia of podocytes overlying the segment of capillary collapse. The hypertrophied podocytes are forming a focal crescent-like structure. Many hypertrophied podocytes contain protein resorption droplets in their cytoplasm. C. Medium-power view showing marked hypertrophy and hyperplasia of podocytes forming a cellular crescent-like structure, known as pseudo-crescent. An irregular cleft like space separates the viscerally located pseudo-crescent from the Bowman's capsule. D. Advanced stages of collapsing glomerulopathy showing the evolution of collapsed tufts to areas of segmental scar formation and adhesion with Bowman's capsule. Areas of capillary collapse and mild hypertrophy of podocytes are still visible.

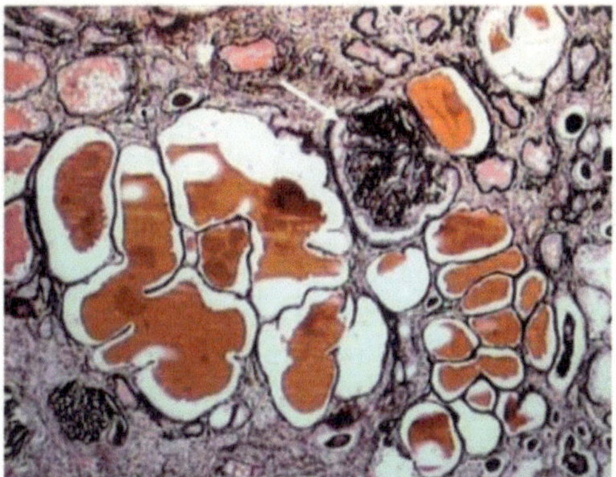

Fig. 4. Low-power photomicrograph showing one glomerulus with global retraction of the capillary tufts associated with prominent podocytes arranged as cobblestone-like collar on the surface of collapsed capillary tufts. These podocytes have not yet proliferated profusely. There is also marked tubulointerstitial involvement with tubular atrophy, microcystic dilatation and protein casts in dilated tubules. (Jones' methenamine silver, ×200)

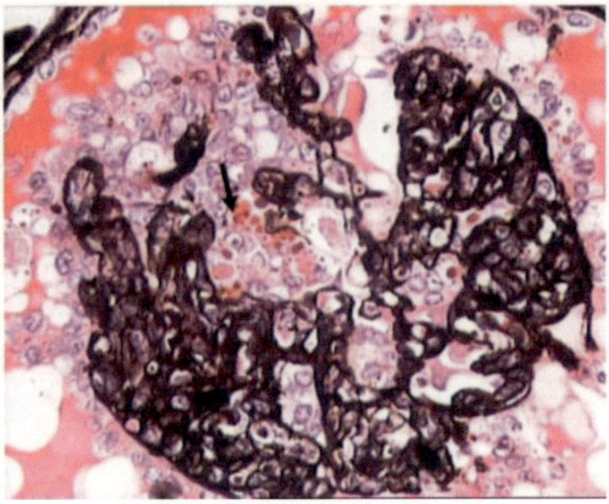

Fig. 5. High power photomicrograph showing global collapse of capillary tufts associated with marked hyperplasia and hypertrophy of podocytes. These show prominent cytoplasmic vacuolization and numerous hyaline, round to oval, protein resorption droplets (arrow). (Jones' methenamine silver, ×400)

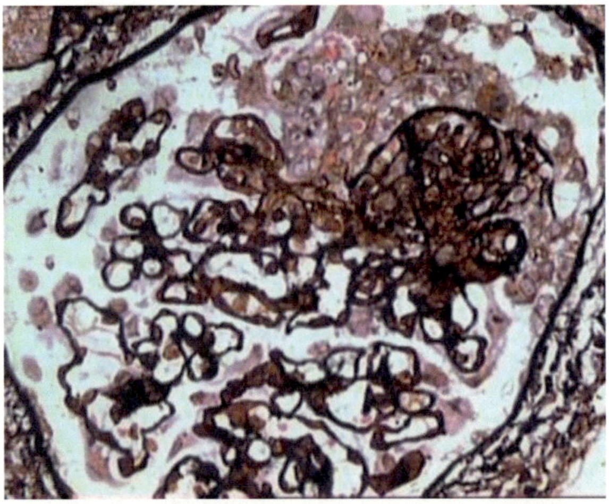

Fig. 6. High-power view showing segmental collapse of the capillary tufts associated with marked proliferation of the podocytes, forming a pseudo-crescent. The pseudo-crescent is separated from the Bowman's capsule by a cleft like space. There is no fibrinoid necrosis of the tuft, which distinguishes it from focal necrotizing lesion. (Jones' methenamine silver, ×400)

As is evident from the above discussion of pathology, the biopsy diagnosis of CG is based almost solely on LM study. Immunofluorescence microscopy (IF) for renal panel immunoglobulins and complement components is usually negative (Table 3) or shows only focal segmental positivity of IgM, C3, and occasionally C1q, in collapsed segments of the glomeruli in some cases (Fig. 10). The intensity of staining is usually mild, ranging from trace positivity to 1+ but may be up to 2+ on a scale of 0 to 3+.

**Light microscopic changes**

**Glomeruli**
Collapse: segmental or global wrinkling and folding of the GBM with occlusion or sub-occlusion of the capillary lumena
Pseudo-crescent formation: podocyte proliferation leading to multiple layers of cells located over collapsed tufts
Swollen podocytes with occasional large nuclei, the later usually in viral causes of CG
Protein reabsorption droplets and vacuolization in the cytoplasm of podocytes
In advanced stages: segmental and/or global sclerosis

**Tubulo-interstitial compartment**

**Acute changes:**
Interstitial edema
Interstitial inflammation
Acute tubular injury: flattening of the tubular epithelium, large epithelial cells, large, occasionally atypical, nuclei with prominent nucleoli

**Chronic changes:**
Tubular atrophy
Interstitial fibrosis
Microcysts: dilated, often angulated, tubules with flat epithelium containing eosinophilic proteinaceous casts with peripheral scalloping

**Vessels**
Nonspecific changes except for CG cases associated with vasculoapathy such as thrombotic microangiopathy

**Immunofluorescence**
Nonspecific segmental positivity of IgM and C3 in areas of collapse and/or sclerosis

**Electron microscopy**
Large cuboidal podocytes with pale cytoplasm
Retraction of primary processes
Diffuse and severe foot process effacement
Loss of detectable actin-based cytoskeleton
Electron dense protein resorption droplets in podocyte cytoplasm
Detachment of podocytes from underlying GBM and deposition of newly formed extracellular matrix in between GBM and podocytes
Absence of tubulo-reticular inclusions in idiopathic CG.

Table 3. The characteristic morphologic features of CG observed on renal biopsy examination by light microscopy, immunoflourescence, and electron microscopy.

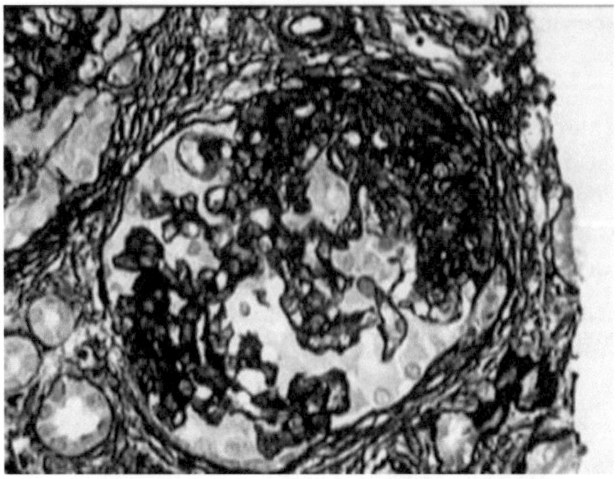

Fig. 7. High-power view showing a glomerulus exhibiting an admixture of segmental collapse on the left side and segmental scarring with adhesion formation with Bowman's capsule on the right, a not infrequent finding on renal biopsies at the time of primary diagnosis. Indeed, this concurrence of sclerotic and collapsing lesions has led the investigators to categorize the collapsing glomerulopathy as a variant of focal segmental glomerulosclerosis. (Jones' methenamine silver, ×400)

The main purpose of IF study is to rule out the secondary causes of CG. Similar to IF, electron microscopic (EM) features are also non-specific and consist of wrinkling and collapse of GBM in areas of collapse with little or no thickening of GBM. The overlying podocytes are greatly hypertrophied with diffuse foot process effacement with focal areas of separation from the underlying GBM. No electron dense deposits are observed. EM study also helps in excluding secondary causes of CG, such as HIVAN, which reveal characteristic tubuloreticular inclusions (D'Agati & Appel, 1998).

## 7. Differential diagnosis

The lesions of full-blown CG are so characteristic that they are rarely mistaken for any other renal glomerular diseases. Furthermore, there are very few histopathological lesions on renal biopsies which simulate CG and come in the differential diagnosis. These include other variants of FSGS as well as other forms of glomerular disease, most notably CresGN. Among the variants of FSGS, the closest differential diagnosis of CG is the cellular FSGS. Indeed, during 1980s, the term of "cellular lesion" was also used to denote some cases of typical CG (Schwartz & Lewis, 1985). Both the collapsing and cellular variants are characterized by marked hyperplasia and hypertrophy of podocytes. The discriminating features that separate the two variants are the implosive wrinkling and retraction of the GBM seen in CG associated with endocapillary hypocellularity as opposed to the expansile lesions of endocapillary hypercellularity seen in the cellular FSGS. All other variants of FSGS display segmental increase in mesangial matrix with consolidation and the obliteration of capillaries (segmental scars), hyalinosis, intracapillary foam cells, and adhesion formation with Bowman's capsule, lesions rarely seen in early stages of CG. Advanced cases of CG, however, may display segmental and/or global glomerulosclerosis. In many cases of CG, the podocyte proliferation may be so florid as to form a cellular

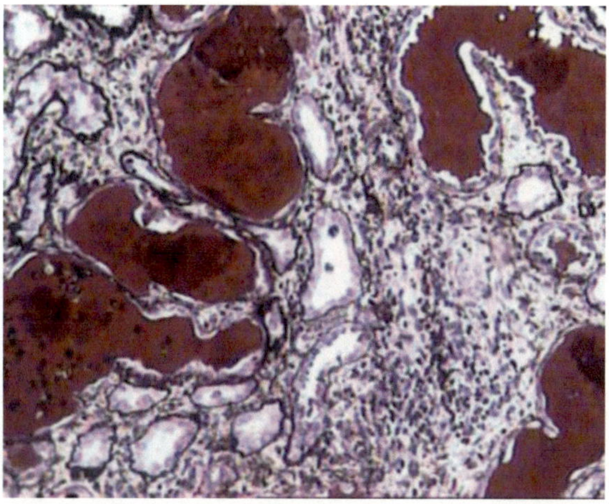

Fig. 8. Medium-power view showing moderate degree of tubular atrophy characterized by thickening and wrinkling of the tubular basement membranes, interstitial mononuclear inflammatory cell infiltration, and widespread microcystic transformation of tubules, the later filled with proteinaceous casts. The walls of many of the cystically dilated tubules are lined by flattened epithelium, which has resulted from degenerative changes. The changes in the tubulointerstitial compartment vary from case to case and some authors argue that these may be of differential diagnostic value regarding the underlying etiologic condition. It is suggested that these tubulointerstitial alterations are more important than the glomerular changes of collapsing glomerulopathy from poor prognostic point of view. (Jones' methenamine silver, ×200)

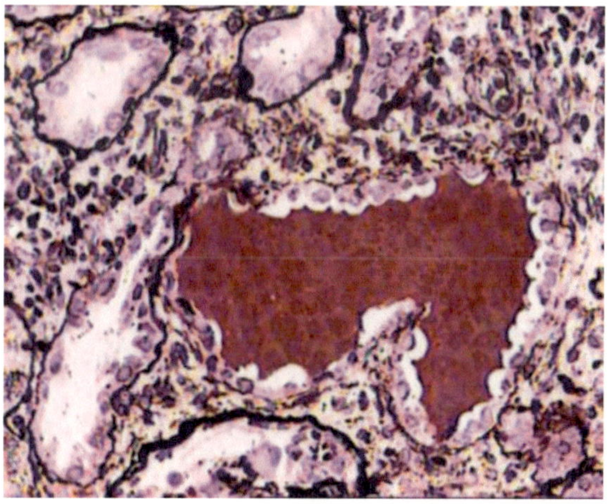

Fig. 9. High-power view showing marked tubular atrophy with irregular thickening and wrinkling of the tubular basement membranes and reduction in the diameter of the tubules. There is also patchy interstitial mononuclear inflammatory cell infiltration, and one tubule, which is cystically dilated and filled with proteinaceous cast with scalloped margins. This finding is highly characteristic of some forms of collapsing glomerulopathy. There are also marked degenerative changes in some of the tubular epithelial cells with shedding of cytoplasm and flattening of the cells (Jones' methenamine silver, ×400)

crescent like structure, known as pseudo-crescent, to differentiate it from true crescents. In such cases, the biopsy findings may be misdiagnosed as CresGN. A closer scrutiny of the lesions with special attention to the features described previously in pseudo-crescents, along with appropriate integration of the clinical history and LM, IF, and EM findings will aid in this differential diagnosis (Albaqumi et al., 2006; Schwimmer et al., 2003).

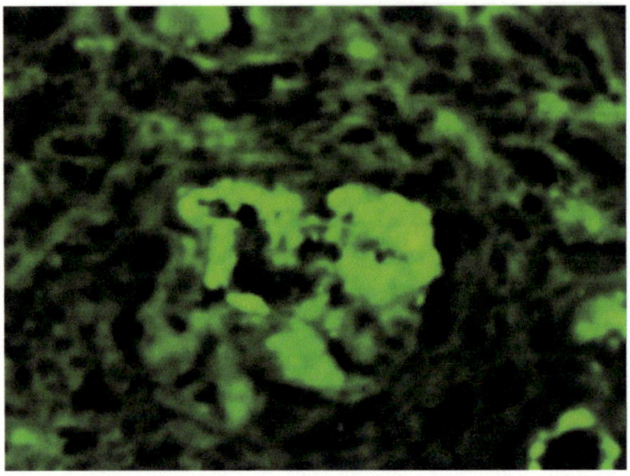

Fig. 10. Immunoflourescence on snap-frozen tissue showing segmental positivity of immunoglobulin M (IgM) in areas of segmental collapse. C3 also commonly accompanies IgM, whereas rest of the renal panel is usually negative. (Fluorescein isothiocyanate (FITC)-conjugated IgM, , ×200)

## 8. The clinical manifestations

The clinical spectrum of CG is also expanding with the expanding list of associated conditions and reflects to some extent the underlying causes. In general, the demographic, clinical and laboratory parameters resemble those observed in non-collapsing FSGS, but the disease is usually more severe. Idiopathic CG is typically a disease of young adults, with a median age of patients being 30 to 40 years, but a wide range of ages have been reported, with patients as young as 1.5 years and as old as 82 years. There are very few reports of CG in children (Singh et al., 2000; Gulati et al., 2008). Regarding gender distribution, most studies have reported a male predominance, although in one study, females predominated over males. CG is also notorious for its black racial predilection. Since Weiss et al's original report (1986), in which all six patients with CG were black, a predominance of black patients in the United States has been noted (Detwiler et al., 1994; Valeri et al., 1996). A study of eight patients in France by Bariety et al. also noted a predominance of black patients (1998). A review of all published series on CG has shown that, around 50% of the reported cases in the literature belong to black race (Albaqumi & Barisoni, 2006).

On presentation, a majority (>80%) of patients with CG have nephrotic range proteinuria, and studies have documented a significantly greater frequency of nephrotic syndrome (NS) and higher levels of proteinuria in patients with CG compared with patients with non-collapsing FSGS. There is also significantly greater renal functional impairment in patients with CG at presentation than patients with non-collapsing FSGS (Schwimmer et al., 2003). Other severe manifestations of NS are frequent, including hypoalbuminaemia, hypercholesterolemia, and edema, but these manifestations are not significantly different from patients with non-collapsing FSGS. Most patients are hypertensive on presentation. Once a diagnosis of CG is rendered, the possibility of HIVAN must be ruled out, usually by negative HIV serological tests, corroborated by the absence of endothelial tubuloreticular inclusions on ultrastructural examination (Mubarak & Kazi, 2010).

## 9. Current and future therapeutic approaches

Currently, there is no specific treatment available for CG, and there are no prospective treatment trials of CG (Schwimmer et al., 2003). The therapeutic approaches used at present are empirical, and analogous to those used for non-collapsing FSGS, i.e., use of steroids or immunosuppressive agents (Albaqumi et al., 2006; Schwimmer et al., 2003). The particular therapeutic agents, their dosages, duration, and the definition of response vary among different studies, contributing to variable results in different studies. Recent studies in patients with non-collapsing FSGS using steroids, cyclosporine, and other immunosuppressive agents have shown that remissions were obtained in over 67% of cases, resulting in prolonged renal survival (Stirling et al., 2005; Stirling, 2006). In contrast, data from retrospective studies of CG suggest that the disease is relatively resistant to most immunosuppressive agents (Detwiler et al., 1994; Valeri et al., 1996). Although, variable rates of success have been reported, the overall results are poor, with a complete remission of 9.6% and a partial remission of 15.2% been reported (Schwimmer et al., 2003). A more specific approach involves the use of highly active anti-retroviral therapy (HAART) in cases of CG in HIV-1 positive patients. This has been shown to decrease the rate of progression of the disease to ESRD by 38% (Albaqumi et al., 2006).

In view of the present lack of effective therapeutic agents and the uniformly poor prognosis of the disease, there is an urgent need for the development of highly effective and targeted agents, based on the knowledge of the pathogenetic pathways of CG. Indeed, some progress has been made in this regard in animal models. The administration of small molecule inhibitors of cyclin-dependent kinases (CDKs) in small animals in preclinical trials has been shown to prevent the development, and retard the progression, of experimental lesions of CG. In addition, the use of differentiating agents such as retinoic acid derivatives, to inhibit the proliferation of podocytes and induce their differentiation to a mature, resting phenotype, has also been shown to ameliorate the lesions of experimental CG. Promising results have also been obtained in improving renal function in experimental forms of CG by the use of small molecule inhibitors of inflammatory pathways controlled by NF-κB and cyclooxygenase-2. These findings underscore the multiplicity of pathogenetic pathways for the proliferative phenotype of podocytes in CG, and signify the emergence of rational approaches to therapy for CG based on the understanding of pathogenesis in the near future (Albaqumi et al., 2006).

## 10. Natural history and prognosis

Due primarily to the relatively scant data and the retrospective nature of most studies on CG, only generalizations can be made about the natural history of the disease and its prognosis. Patients with CG are at high risk of progressing to ESRD. Even with the currently available treatment, the incidence of ESRD is 50% to 100% in most series (Agarwal et al., 2008; Deegans et al., 2008; Detwiler et al., 1994; Grcevska & Polenakovik, 1999; Kazi &

Mubarak, 2007; Laurinavicious et al., 1999; Meyrier, 1999; Mubarak & Kazi, 2010; Nada et al., 2009; Valeri et al., 1996; Weis et al., 1986). In all comparative studies, the renal survival of patients with CG was significantly worse than patients with non-collapsing FSGS. Multiple studies have explored the possible prognostic features in CG. Valeri et al. (1996) found that progression to ESRD was predicted by serum creatinine concentration at the time of biopsy ($P < 0.05$) and lack of remission of proteinuria ($P < 0.025$), but did not find a correlation between severity of proteinuria or other features of NS with the outcome. The rate of progression of renal failure in the collapsing FSGS group correlated highly with the severity of tubular degenerative and regenerative changes ($P < 0$ .02) but not with any other parameter of tubulointerstitial or glomerular change. The rate of progression of renal failure correlated strongly with male sex. Laurinavicius et al. (1999) reviewed retrospectively the data from 42 patients with CG and 18 patients with HIVAN to determine the predictors of serum creatinine level, proteinuria, and progression of renal disease. In their multivariate model, the risk for ESRD was increased significantly by interstitial fibrosis of >20%, creatinine level > 2.0 mg/dL, proteinuria >8 g/d, glomeruli with collapsing lesions >20%, and HIV infection ($P < 0.0001$). Similar to its ominous prognosis in native kidneys, the disease also leads to rapidly progressive graft failure, usually with in two years of diagnosis.

## 11. Conclusion

In conclusion, with increasing awareness and research, significant advances have been made in understanding the etiopathogenetic mechanisms underlying this mysterious renal disease. This is likely to open up the avenues for the development of rational and targeted therapy for this uniformly resistant form of disease. The success of preclinical testing of the novel therapeutic strategies based on the knowledge of pathogenetic pathways obtained from studies in humans and animal models holds promise that the presently poor prognosis of CG is likely to improve in the near future.

## 12. References

Agrawal V, Vinod PB, Krishnani N, & Sharma RK. (2008). A case of collapsing glomerulopathy associated with febrile illness. *Indian J Pathol Microbiol*, Vol. 51, No. 4, pp. 509-11.

Albaqumi M, Soos TJ, Barisoni L, & Nelson PJ. (2006). Collapsing glomerulopathy. *J Am Soc Nephrol*, Vol. 17, No. 10, pp. 2854-63.

Albaqumi M, & Barisoni L. (2006). Current views on collapsing glomerulopathy. *J Am Soc Nephrol*, Vol. 19, No. 7, pp. 1276-81.

Amoura Z, Georgin-Lavialle S, Haroche J, Merrien D, Brocheriou I, Beaufils H, & Piette J-C. (2006). Collapsing glomerulopathy in systemic autoimmune disorders: a case occurring in the course of full blown systemic lupus erythematosus. *Ann Rheum Dis*, Vol. 65, No. 2, pp. 277-8.

Bariety J, Nochy D, Mandet C, Jacquot C, Glotz D, & Meyrier A. (1998). Podocytes undergo phenotypic changes and express macrophagic-associated markers in idiopathic collapsing glomerulopathy. *Kidney Int*, Vol. 53, No. 4, pp. 918-25.

Barisoni L, Kriz W, Mundel P, & D'Agati V. (1999). The dysregulated podocyte phenotype: a novel concept in the pathogenesis of collapsing idiopathic focal segmental glomerulosclerosis and HIV-associated nephropathy. *J Am Soc Nephrol*, Vol.10, No. 1, pp. 51-61.

Barisoni L, Schnaper HW, & Kopp JB. (2007). A proposed taxonomy for the podocytopathies: a reassessment of the primary nephrotic diseases. *Clin J Am Soc Nephrol*, Vol. 2, No. 3, pp. 529-42.

Canaud G, Bruneval P, Noel L-H, Correas J-M, Audard V, Zafrani L, Rabant M, Timsit MO, Martinez F, Anglicheau D, Thervet E, Patey N, Legendre C, & Zuber J. (2010). Glomerular collapse associated with subtotal renal infarction in kidney transplant recipients with multiple renal arteries. *Am J Kidney Dis*, Vol. 55, No. 3, pp. 558-65.

D'Agati V, & Appel GB. (1998). Renal pathology of human immunodeficiency virus infection. *Semin Nephrol*, Vol. 18, No. 4, pp. 406-21.

D'Agati VD, Fogo AB, Bruijn JA, & Jennette JC. (2004). Pathologic classification of focal segmental glomerulosclerosis. A working proposal. *Am J Kidney Dis*, Vol. 43, No. 2, pp. 368-82.

Deegans JKF, Steenbergen EJ, Borm GF, & Wetzels JFM. (2008). Pathological variants of focal segmental glomerulosclerosis in an adult Dutch population-epidemiology and outcome. *Nephrol Dial Transplant*, Vol. 23, No.1, pp.186-92.

Detwiler RK, Falk RJ, Hogan SL, & Jennette JC. (1994). Collapsing glomerulopathy: a clinically and pathologically distinct variant of focal segmental glomerulosclerosis. *Kidney Int*, Vol. 45, No. 5, pp. 1416-24.

Grcevska L, & Polenakovik M. (1999). Collapsing glomerulopathy: clinical characteristics and follow-up. *Am J Kidney Dis*, Vol. 33, No. 4, pp. 652-7.

Gupta R, Sharma A, Agarwal SK, & Dinda AK. (2011). Collapsing glomerulopathy in renal allograft biopsies: a study of nine cases. *Indian J Nephrol*, Vol. 21, No. 1, pp. 10-3.

Haas M, & Spargo BH, Coventry S. (1995). Increasing incidence of focal segmental glomerulosclerosis among adult nephropathies: A 20-years renal biopsy study. *Am J Kidney Dis*, Vol. 26, No. 5, pp. 740-50.

Haas M, Meehan SM, Karrison TG, & Spargo BH. (1997). Changing etiologies of unexplained adult nephrotic syndrome: A comparison of renal biopsy findings from 1976-1979 and 1995-1997. *Am J Kidney Dis*, Vol. 30, No. 5, pp. 621-31.

Kazi JI, & Mubarak M. (2009). Collapsing FSGS: a need of awareness. *J Pak Med Assoc*, Vol. 59, No. 8, pp. 583.

Kazi JI & Mubarak M. (2011). Collapsing glomerulopathy: A novel association with patchy acute cortical necrosis secondary to postpartum hemorrhage in native kidneys. *NDT Plus* (in press).

Laurinavicius A, Hurwitz S, & Rennke HG. (1999). Collapsing glomerulopathy in HIV and non-HIV patients: a clinicopathological and follow-up study. *Kidney Int*, Vol. 56, No. 6, pp. 2203-13.

Laurinavicius A, & Rennke HG. (2002). Collapsing glomerulopathy: a new pattern of renal injury. *Semin Diagn Pathol*, Vol. 19, No. 3, pp. 106-15.

Meehan SM, Pascual M, Williams WW, Tolkoff-Rubin N, Delmonico FL, Cosimi AB, & Colvin RB. (1998). De novo collapsing glomerulopathy in renal allografts. *Transplantation*, Vol. 65, No. 9, pp. 1192-7.

Meyrier AY. (1999). Collapsing glomerulopathy: expanding interest in a shrinking tuft. *Am J Kidney Dis*, Vol. 33, No. 4, pp. 801-3.

Mubarak M, & Kazi JI. (2011). Collapsing focal segmental glomerulosclerosis: a morphological lesion in search of identity. *Nephrol Urol Mon* (in press).

Mubarak M, & Kazi JI. (2010). Collapsing FSGS: a clinicopathologic study of 10 cases from Pakistan. *Clin Exp Nephrol*, Vol. 14, No. 3, pp. 222-7.

Mubarak M. (2011). Collapsing glomerulopathy in renal allograft biopsies: a study of nine cases. *Indian J Nephrol* (in press).

Nada R, Kharbanda JK, Bhatti A, Minz RW, Sakhuja V, & Joshi K. (2009). Primary focal segmental glomerulosclerosis in adults: is the Indian cohort different? *Nephrol Dial Transplant*, Vol. 24, No. 12, pp. 3701-7.

Nadasdy T, Allen C, & Zand MS. (2002). Zonal distribution of glomerular collapse in renal allografts: possible role of vascular changes. *Hum Pathol*, Vol. 33, No. 4, pp. 437-41.

Schwimmer JA, Markowitz GS, Valeri A, & Appel GB. (2003). Collapsing glomerulopathy. *Sem Nephrol*, Vol. 23, No. 2, pp. 209-18.

Stirling CM, Mathieson P, Boulton-Jones JM, Feehally J, Jayne D, Murray HM, & Adu D. (2005). Treatment and outcome of adult patients with primary focal segmental glomerulosclerosis in five UK renal units. *Q J Med*, Vol. 98, No. 6, pp. 443-9.

Stirling CM. (2006). Focal segmental glomerulosclerosis-does treatment work? *Nephron Clin Pract*, Vol. 104, No. 2, pp. c83-84.

Stokes MB, Davis CL, & Alpers CE. (1999). Collapsing glomerulopathy in renal allografts: a morphological pattern with diverse clinicopathologic associations. *Am J Kidney Dis*, Vol. 33, No. 4, pp. 658-66.

Swaminathan S, Lager DJ, Qian X, Stegall MD, Larson TS, & Griffin MD. (2006). Collapsing and non-collapsing focal segmental glomerulosclerosis in kidney transplants. *Nephrol Dial Transplant*, Vol. 21, No. 9, pp. 2607-14.

Thadhani R, Pascual M, Tolkoff-Rubin N, Nickeleit V, & Colvin R. (1996). Preliminary description of focal segmental glomerulosclerosis in patients with renovascular disease. *Lancet*, Vol. 347, No. 8996, pp. 231-3.

Valeri A, Barisoni L, Appel GB, Seigle R, & D'Agati V. (1996). Idiopathic collapsing focal segmental glomerulosclerosis: a clinicopathologic study. *Kidney Int*, Vol. 50, No. 5, pp. 1734-46.

Weiss MA, Daquioag E, Margolin EG, & Pollak VE. (1986). Nephrotic syndrome, progressive irreversible renal failure, and glomerular "collapse." A new clinicopathologic entity? *Am J Kidney Dis*, Vol. 7, No. 1, pp. 20-8.

# Part 4

# Renal Transplant Pathology

# 10

# Pathology of Renal Transplantation

Javed I. Kazi and Muhammed Mubarak
*Sindh Institute of Urology and Transplantation, Karachi*
*Pakistan*

## 1. Introduction

Renal transplantation has become the treatment of choice for patients with end-stage renal disease (ESRD) resulting from a variety of causes. The short-term patient and graft outcomes have improved markedly over the recent years (Hariharan et al., 2000). Renal transplant recipients are subject to all those diseases which affect the general population. In addition, like all other allograft recipients, renal transplant recipients are also susceptible to a variety of unique pathological lesions not seen in the non-transplant population. These lesions may involve the transplanted organ or other native organs/systems of the transplant recipients. The focus of this chapter will be on the major pathological processes affecting the kidney allograft itself and are diagnosed on renal allograft biopsy. In this chapter we will present a brief but comprehensive overview of the pathology of the renal allograft seen on allograft biopsies supplemented by representative pictures.

## 2. Role of renal allograft biopsy in the management of renal transplant patients

The renal allograft biopsy plays an important role in the diagnosis and management of causes of renal allograft dysfunction (Al-Awwa et al., 1998; Colvin,1996; Gaber, 1998; Mazzali et al., 1999; Matas et al., 1983; Matas et al., 1985; Parfrey et al., 1984). Regarding biopsy indications, it is befitting to state that it is always indicated to answer a clinical question. The question is formulated by the transplant physicians with the knowledge of the patient's clinical scenario, the results of relevant laboratory and imaging studies, and the response to any therapeutic measures already instituted to remedy the problem. The established indications for performing renal allograft biopsies are shown in Table 1.

| |
|---|
| 1. Delayed graft function (DGF) if worsening is seen in the renogram or DGF lasts longer than 2-3 weeks. |
| 2. Graft function lower than expected based on donor characteristics. |
| 3. A sudden rise in serum creatinine attributable to kidney disease. |
| 4. A progressive increase in creatinine levels (>20% from creatinine nadir). |
| 5. Proteinuria > 1 g. |
| 6. Urine sediment changes without apparent urological causes. |
| 7. Prior to changes in immunosuppressive treatment. |

Table 1. Established indications of renal allograft biopsies.

As is obvious from the table, renal allograft biopsy is indicated in both the acute and late dysfunction of the allograft as well as the investigation of recurrent/de novo glomerular disease. The causes of allograft dysfunction vary depending on the post-transplant duration, living vs. cadaveric source of organ, type of immunosuppression, underlying or primary disease, etc (Kazi & Mubarak, 2012). It is estimated that 30-50% of allografts develop dysfunction during the early period (John & Herzenberg, 2010). An accurate diagnosis of these is essential for the optimal management of the patients, as each of the major causes of renal allograft dysfunction requires different therapeutic approach (Colvin,1996; Gaber, 1998).

## 3. Types of renal allograft biopsies

Three important types of allograft biopsies are regularly and widely used in clinical transplant practice. These include; implantation biopsies, indication biopsies, and protocol biopsies. Each of these types of biopsy plays an important role in the optimal management of transplant patients if properly procured and interpreted (Racusen et al., 1999).

### 3.1 Implantation biopsy, donor biopsy

This is usually done after the allograft is anastomosed to the recipient's vessels, but before the clamp is removed. The Banff scheme recommends its routine use all over the world. It provides baseline information on the status of the donor organ and helps in the interpretation of subsequent dysfunctional renal allograft biopsies. Individual zero time biopsies have been shown to correlate with the graft outcome.

### 3.2 Indication biopsy

#### 3.2.1 Dysfunctional allograft biopsy

These are the most common form of biopsies that are performed on the allograft and most challenging in their interpretation. These biopsies are most commonly performed during early post transplant period and their frequency decreases as the post transplant duration increases. The Banff schema has detailed guidelines on the processing and interpretation of morphological changes on renal allograft biopsies, which are periodically updated and revised.

#### 3.2.2 Allograft biopsy for proteinuria

Although, majority of indication biopsies are done for a rise in serum creatinine, a significant proportion of biopsies are also performed for the investigation of proteinuria. The proportion of these biopsies increases as the post transplantation duration increases. Their optimal evaluation requires an approach similar to that used for native renal biopsies for the investigation of glomerular diseases, i.e., the use of immunoflourescence (IF), and electron microscopy (EM) in addition to light microscopy (LM).

#### 3.2.3 Protocol biopsies

These are the renal allograft biopsies which are performed at pre-determined intervals after transplantation in normal functioning allografts. These biopsies have provided marked insights into the subclinical processes affecting the graft with implications for the long term graft outcome (Choi et al. 2005; Furness et al., 2003; Jain et al., 2000; Rush et al., 1998; Serón et al., 1997). Indeed, the concept of Banff classification of renal allograft pathology originated from the experience with the use of, and the publication of studies related to, protocol biopsies. However, these biopsies have been done at only a few centers in the world and are not universal.

## 4. Causes of renal allograft dysfunction

The causes of renal allograft dysfunction can be conveniently divided into two categories depending on the time after transplantation; early and delayed, and generally follow the same pattern of etiologic factors as observed in native kidneys; pre-renal, renal, and post-renal types. The causes of renal allograft dysfunction according to time after transplantation are shown in table 2.

Acute or subacute renal allograft dysfunction generally manifests in the form of a sudden rise of serum creatinine. It is quite common and occurs in roughly half of all patients with kidney transplants. In the immediate post-transplant period, ischemic injury is the major cause, but acute rejection may occur during this period, especially acute antibody-mediated rejection (ABMR) in pre-sensitized recipients. However, majority of acute rejections manifest after one week. Over the first month, the risk of rejection is high and it gradually decreases over the ensuing few months. Acute rejection is rare after six months of transplantation. In contrast, acute ischemic injury can continue to occur at any time. Drug toxicity caused by calcineurin inhibitors (CNI) can occur at any time after transplantation and should always be in the differential diagnosis. Rarely, thrombotic microangiopathy (TMA) may occur, mainly caused by CNI toxicity, but has many other causes (Bergstrand et al., 1985: Pascual et al., 1999).

| |
|---|
| Acute (0-6 months after transplant) |
| Acute cellular rejection |
| Acute humoral rejection |
| Acute calcineurin inhibitor toxicity |
| Acute pyelonephritis |
| Acute ischaemic injury |
| |
| Chronic (>6 months after transplant) |
| Chronic cellular rejection |
| Chronic humoral rejection |
| Chronic calcineurin inhibitor toxicity |
| Hypertension |
| Chronic obstruction/reflux |
| Chronic pyelonephritis |
| Polyomavirus nephropathy |
| Glomerular disease |
| Recurrent |
| De novo |
| Graft ageing, including: |
| Donor-related changes |
| Progression of perioperative injury |
| Post-transplant lymphoproliferative disorder |
| Interstitial fibrosis / tubular atrophy, not otherwise specified |

Table 2. Causes of renal allograft dysfunction categorized according to time after transplantation.

Late or chronic allograft dysfunction is usually labeled when graft dysfunction develops after six months of transplantation, and generally presents with a slowly rising serum creatinine. It is often also accompanied by low grade proteinuria and hypertension as the post transplant duration increases. This chronic allograft loss occurs at a relatively constant rate of 2-4% per year and is the major cause of graft failure throughout the world. It is caused by a multitude of causes; both the allo-immune and the non-immune causes contribute to this process. Chronic CNI toxicity and hypertension are among the major etiologic factors leading to chronic graft loss. In addition, chronic obstruction, reflux, and hyperlipidemia are also contributing factors. As post transplant duration increases, the risk of recurrence of original renal disease or de novo occurrence of the same also increases. More recently, chronic allo-immune injury has been identified as a major cause of chronic graft loss. An acute rise in serum creatinine may occur during late post transplant period, and in most instances is caused by stopping the drugs by the patients. Similarly, a chronically failing allograft may show an apparent acute rise in serum creatinine, resulting from diminished functional reserve, and precipitated by some acute insult (John & Herzenberg, 2010).

It is worth reiterating that the causes of renal allograft dysfunction vary depending on the induction protocol, maintenance immunosuppression, living vs. cadaveric organ source, and many other factors (D'Alessandro et al., 1995; Farnsworth et al., 1984; Matas et al., 2001; Mihatsch et al., 1985; Mishra et al., 2004; Ratnakar et al., 2002; Rizvi et al., 2011; Verma et al., 2007).

## 5. Procurement of renal allograft biopsy

Renal allograft biopsy procurement should follow the same methodology, as the native renal biopsy, discussed previously in chapter 1, especially, if ABMR is suspected or proteinuria is the clinical indication. The timing of obtaining biopsy is also important, especially for dysfunctional graft biopsies. Ideally, the biopsy should be obtained before any attempt at treatment of the suspected rejection process. It should be planned as an elective procedure, and a technician from the histopathology department should be present in the biopsy suite to examine the removed tissue under the dissection microscope for the adequacy of the tissue removed and for apportioning the removed tissue for immunoflourescence (IF) and EM study, if the later are required. This allows fulfillment of adequacy criteria for the proper histopathological evaluation of the biopsy material and complete pathologic evaluation including IF study for complement fragment C4d and renal panel IF. Two cores of renal graft tissue including both cortex and medulla should be obtained. The sensitivity of rejection diagnosis increases with increasing number of cores. The rejection process can be patchy and can be missed if only a single core is obtained. The sensitivity for rejection diagnosis is estimated to be around 90% with one core, and reaches 99% if two cores of renal cortex are obtained. The sensitivity for rejection diagnosis varies from 75 to 80% if medulla alone is received. The specificity of diagnosis of rejection in the medullary tissue is even lower, as other causes of graft dysfunction such as infection, obstruction, or drug hypersensitivity may present with infiltrates and even tubulitis in the medulla (John & Herzenberg, 2010).

## 6. Preparation of the biopsy for evaluation

After the adequacy criteria are fulfilled, the graft biopsy material should be prepared with great care and dexterity. The biopsy should be processed and prepared according to the guidelines for allograft biopsy handling by the most experienced technologists. The quality of biopsy material available for pathologic study is of utmost importance in the correct interpretation of the abnormalities in the tissue (Serón et al., 2008). Many centers process the biopsy by urgent methods, including microwave oven method (John & Herzenberg, 2010). We also process the allograft biopsies by the rapid method using auto-processor and report the biopsies on the same day. The quality of reagents is also very important. According to Banff schema, it is recommended to prepare at least seven slides, with multiple sections mounted on each slide. Three of these should be stained with hematoxylin and eosin (H&E), three with periodic acid-Schiff reagent (PAS), and one with a Masson's trichrome stain. The PAS and/or silver stains are very useful in delineating tubular basement membranes (TBMs) and in defining the severity of tubulitis, and for evaluating glomerulitis. The PAS stain is also useful in the identification of arteriolar hyalinosis (ah) and tubular atrophy and their semi-quantitative scoring. Trichrome stains help in assessing the chronic sclerosing changes in the interstitium and in the arterial intima. Banff schema recommends cutting tissue sections at a thickness of 3 to 4 microns for an accurate semiquantitative assessment of the morphological lesions in the biopsy sections (Racusen et al., 1999).

## 7. Pathologic evaluation of allograft biopsy

The accurate pathologic evaluation of renal allograft biopsy requires a well trained renal pathologist with a thorough knowledge of renal transplant pathology, and also of renal and transplant medicine in order to correlate the morphologic abnormalities with the detailed clinical information. The importance of correlation of morphological findings on the renal allograft biopsy with clinical data and a close liaison between the nephrologists and pathologists cannot be overemphasized and is self-explanatory. However, the biopsy should be examined by the pathologist initially, without reference to the available clinical information and a morphological diagnosis formulated. This morphological diagnosis should be an objective and unbiased record of all abnormalities seen under the microscope. An attempt should then be made to correlate the clinical details provided with the morphological changes and preferably following discussion with the clinicians. A final diagnosis is then made and any treatment available, given. Further, in an ideal situation a follow up on the patient's progress is also communicated to the pathologist so that the predictions made from the biopsy can be confirmed or corrected if possible. Renal allograft biopsy interpretation is therefore developed out of a discussion between a clinician and the renal pathologist and is a learning process for both based on the patient's clinical course. In this context, it is worth emphasizing that transplant pathology is the youngest discipline of surgical pathology and is continuously evolving rapidly (John & Herzenberg, 2010).

## 8. Diagnosis of acute graft dysfunction

Acute graft dysfunction may be caused by acute ischemic injury, acute rejection, or drug toxicity. Rare causes include; infections, surgical complications, vascular complications, or obstruction. Acute ischemic injury with delayed graft function (DGF) is more common in the cadaveric setting and is recognized by degenerative and regenerative changes in the tubular epithelium.

Renal graft biopsy is the gold standard test to identify many of these lesions. However, it is invasive, and not without risks (Vidhun et al., 2003; Wilckzek, 1990). Renal allograft biopsies are of three major types according to their indications: time zero biopsies or implantation biopsies; dysfunctional graft biopsies; and protocol biopsies. Among these, the second category is obviously the most common type in most of the centers around the world. Many centers do not perform routine implantation or protocol biopsies.

### 8.1 Diagnosis of acute rejection

Renal allograft biopsy is the gold standard procedure for the diagnosis of acute rejection. Acute rejection was traditionally classified on the basis of rapidity and severity of the process, as hyperacute, acclerated acute, and acute rejection. Banff classification tried to classify the rejection on the basis of pathological and pathogenetic mechanisms with considerable refinements in the classification over the past 20 years (Solez et al., 1993; Racusen et al., 1999; Racusen et al., 2003; Solez et al., 2007; Solez et al., 2008). More recently, the Banff classification has categorized acute rejection on pathogenetic mechanisms, as acute ABMR and acute T cell mediated rejection (TCMR). Each of these types of rejection has unique morphological, immunohistochemical, and clinical features and different responses to therapy. Acute TCMR is diagnosed on the concurrent fulfillment of two key thresholds: significant interstitial lymphocytic infiltration (i2) associated with significant tubulitis (t2). If only one of these features is present, the diagnosis is made of borderline rejection. The borderline category exists only in type I or TCMR. Once a diagnosis of acute TCMR is made, its severity is assessed mainly on the basis of severity of tubulitis as Type IA and IB. Acute TCMR may also manifest as varying degrees of arterial inflammation and necrosis. It most often causes intimal arteritis, but occasional cases may manifest as V3 lesion. Often the vascular involvement is accompanied by tubulo-interstitial inflammation.

### 8.2 Mechanisms of rejection

Rejection is a complex and somewhat redundant response of the specific and innate immune systems to the allograft tissue. The major targets of this response are the major histocompatibility complex (MHC) antigens, which are known as human leukocyte antigens (HLAs) in humans. The HLA genes on the short arm of chromosome 6 encode two structurally distinct classes of cell-surface antigens, known as class I (HLA-A, -B, and -C) and class II (-DR, -DQ, -DP). The T lymphocytes recognize allograft antigens by one of two mechanisms; direct and indirect allorecognition. In the direct pathway, T cells recognize intact allogenic MHC molecules on the surface of allogenic donor cells. The T-cell response that results in early acute TCMR is caused mainly by direct allorecognition. In the indirect pathway, T cells recognize processed alloantigens in the context of self antigen presenting cells (APCs). Indirect presentation may be important in maintaining and amplifying the rejection response, especially in chronic rejection.

In both pathways, T lymphocytes recognize foreign antigen only when the antigen is associated with HLA molecules on the surface of APCs. Helper T lymphocytes (CD4) are activated and they proliferate, differentiate, and secrete a variety of cytokines. These cytokines increase expression of HLA class II antigens on the allograft tissues, stimulate B lymphocytes to produce antibodies against the graft antigens, and help cytotoxic T cells (CD8), macrophages, and natural killer cells to develop effective specific and innate immunity against the graft (Nankivell & Alexander, 2010).

### 8.3 Semiquantitative assessment of histological changes – The mainstay of Banff schema

The semiquantitative scoring of the acute and chronic structural changes in different compartments of the graft parenchyma forms the mainstay for the Banff classification of renal allograft pathology (Solez et al., 1993; Racusen et al., 1999; Racusen et al., 2003; Solez et al., 2007; Solez et al., 2008). Altogether, five categories of acute and four of chronic changes are assessed. These are given in table 3.

| | | |
|---|---|---|
| **Acute changes:** | | |
| g | 0, 1, 2, 3 | No, mild, moderate, severe glomerulitis (g3 = mononuclear cells in capillaries of all or nearly all glomeruli with endothelial enlargement and luminal occlusion) |
| i | 0, 1, 2, 3 | No, mild, moderate, severe interstitial mononuclear cell infiltration (in rejection edema & lymphocyte activation usually accompany mononuclear cell infiltration: i3 = >50% pf parenchyma inflamed) |
| t | 0, 1, 2, 3 | No, mild, moderate, severe tubulitis (t3 = >10 mononuclear cell per tubule or per 10 tubular cells in several tubules) |
| v | 0, 1, 2, 3 | No, mild, moderate, severe intimal arteritis (assessed in most involved vessel) (v3 = severe intimal arteritis and / or transmural arteritis and / or hemorrhage and recent infarction) |
| ah | 0, 1, 2, 3 | No, mild, moderate, severe nodular hyaline afferent arteriolar thickening suggestive of cyclosporine toxicity (ah3 = severe PAS-positive thickening in many arterioles) |
| **Chronic changes:** | | |
| cg | 0, 1, 2, 3 | No, mild, moderate, severe chronic transplant glomerulopathy (% glomeruli). |
| ci | 0, 1, 2, 3 | No, mild, moderate, severe interstitial fibrosis, often with mononuclear cell inflammation (% total interstitial area). |
| ct | 0, 1, 2, 3 | No, mild, moderate, severe tubular atrophy and loss (% tubular area). |
| cv | 0, 1, 2, 3 | No, mild, moderate, severe fibrous intimal thickening often with elastica fragmentation (cv3 indicates occlusion( (cg and cv lesions suggest the presence of chronic rejection) (assessed in most damaged vessels). |

Table 3. Semiquantitative scoring of acute and chronic changes in different compartments of renal graft parenchyma.

The focus of acute rejection diagnosis in Banff schema is on the tubulitis and intimal arteritis. However, it is worth emphasizing that with the exception of arteritis, there is no single specific feature of rejection. The diagnosis of rejection depends on the concurrence of interstitial inflammation of at least i2 (>25% to <50% of the unscarred parenchyma) and a tubulitis of grade t2 (4 -10 lymphocytes invading the tubule), as shown in Figures 1 and 2.

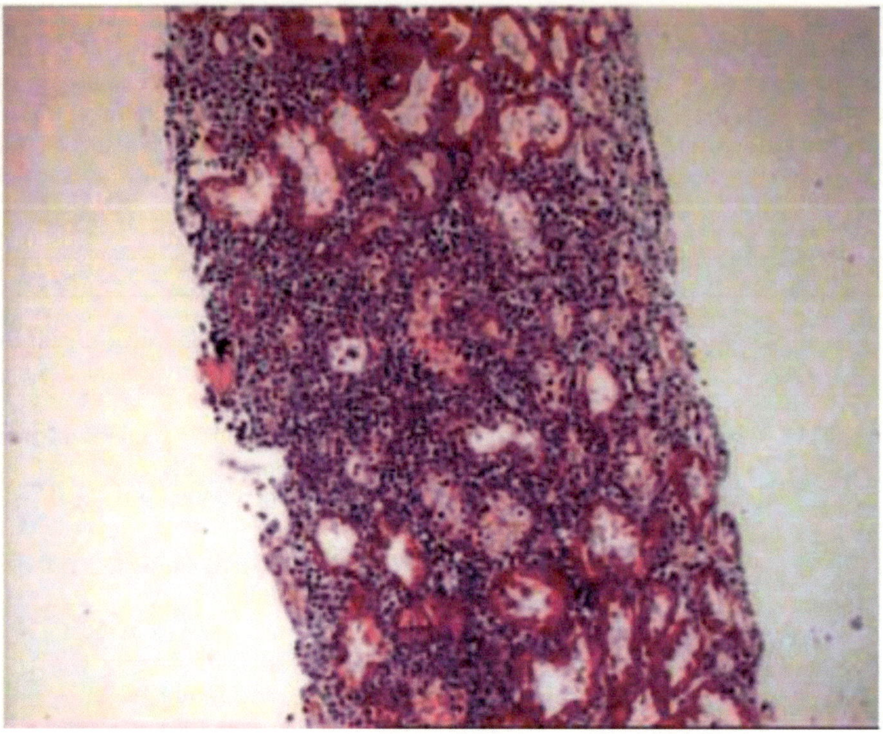

Fig. 1. Low-power view showing almost diffuse, dense, lymphocytic infiltrate in the interstitium. This is highly suggestive of acute T cell mediated rejection. (H&E, ×100).

The tubulitis grading is carried out on the most severely involved tubule. Most difficulty is encountered in the diagnosis of Type I acute cellular rejection, ie., the tubulo-interstitial type, especially during very early stages of the process. The process starts and builds gradually with interstitial accumulation of progressively increasing numbers of inflammatory cells which later invade and attack the tubules. Thus if the biopsy is done at very early stage, tubulitis may not be found (Kazi et al., 1998). The rejection also begins as a patchy process, which in later stages becomes diffuse. The clearly defined threshold of rejection diagnosis, especially interstitial inflammation and tubulitis, has helped in improving the interobserver reproducibility of diagnosis (Furness et al., 1997; Furness et al., 1999). The rationale behind this threshold setting is that some inflammatory changes are to be expected in any allograft, but do not signal rejection. At the same time, this has resulted in lower sensitivity of diagnosis of very early acute TCMR. For this reason, various investigators have tried alternative approaches for increasing the sensitivity of diagnosis of early acute TCMR. One such approach involves the use of a computer program, known as Baysian Belief Network (BBN) to record and analyze multiple biopsy features to diagnose more accurately the cases of early acute rejection. In one study involving 21 difficult cases of early acute rejection, the use of computer program resulted in higher correct diagnoses than any of the pathologists using the Banff criteria (Furness et al., 1999; Kazi et al., 1998). Moreover, there are interinstitutional differences in the quality and quantity of inflammatory infiltrates of rejection (Furness & Taub, 2001; Furness et al., 2003; Kazi et al., 1999). In spite of these limitations, Banff schema has become the international benchmark for the pathologic interpretation of renal allograft biopsies.

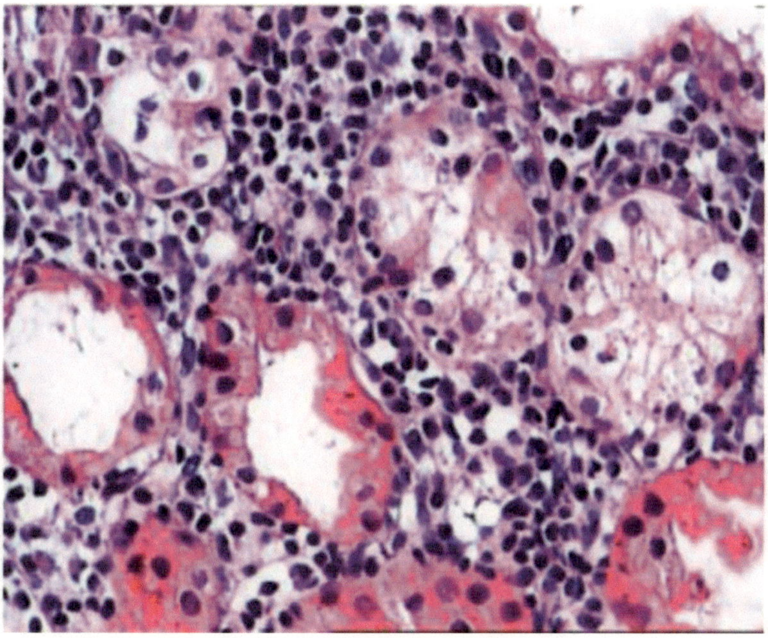

Fig. 2. Medium-power view showing almost diffuse, dense, lymphocytic infiltrate in the interstitium associated with foci of significant tubulitis (t2). This is highly suggestive of acute T cell mediated rejection. (H&E, ×200).

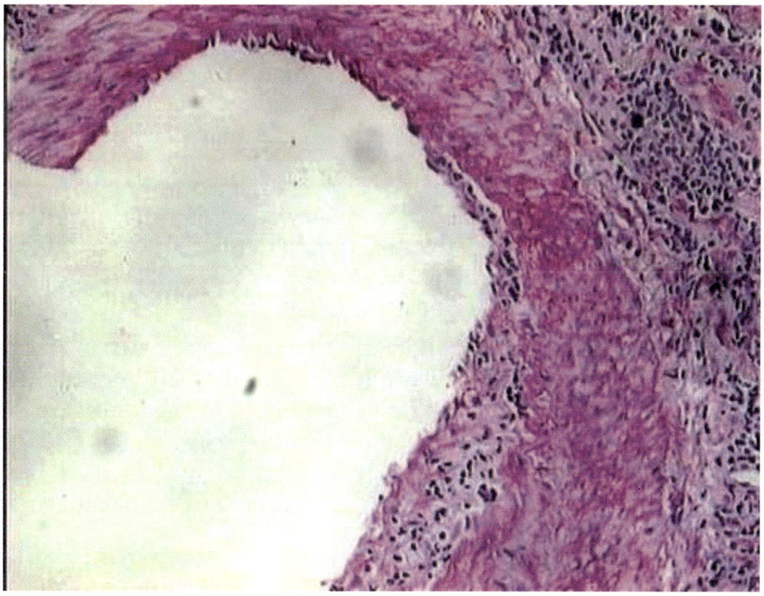

Fig. 3. Medium-power view showing part of wall of artery with focal intimal arteritis consistent with acute vascular rejection: Banff category, IIA. There is also dense lymphocytic infiltrate in the surrounding interstitium. (PAS stain, ×200).

The diagnosis of acute vascular rejection (AVR) is most often straight forward. Detection of even a single lymphocyte in the arterial intima (intimal arteritis) is sufficient to diagnose a case as AVR. The severity of rejection is also graded on the basis of V scores. AVR may be a manifestation of TCMR or antibody-mediated rejection (ABMR). The later mechanism of rejection most often results in V3 lesions, while the former pathway causes V1 and V2 lesions (Figures 3 to 7).

Significant tubulointerstitial inflammation and vasculitis may also be a manifestation of recurrent or de novo development of renal disease in the allograft. A good pretransplant clinical history is highly valuable in resolving this differential, the occurrence of which increases with increased post-transplant duration.

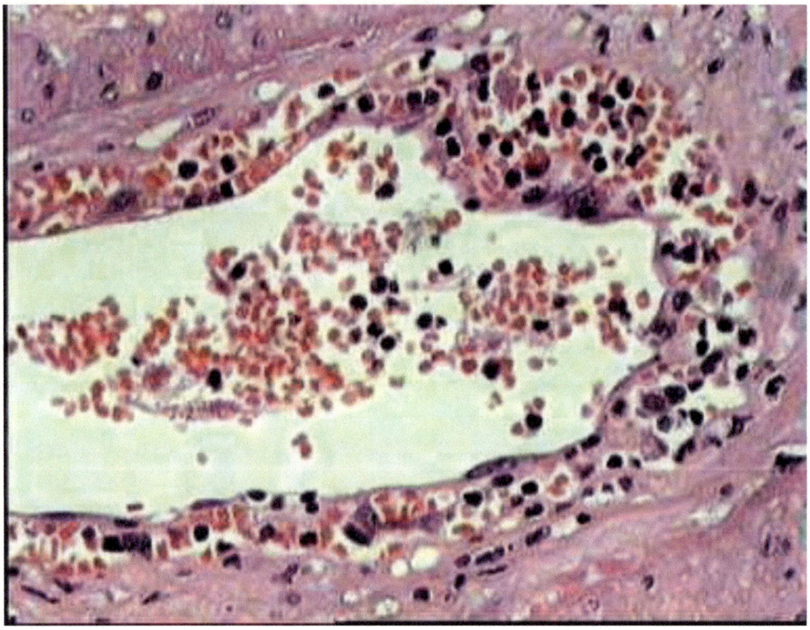

Fig. 4. High-power view showing numerous lymphocytes invading the arterial intima. Many red blood cells are also seen in the intima. (H&E stain, ×400).

### 8.4 Antibody-mediated rejection (ABMR)

Recently, more attention is focused on antibody mediated rejection (ABMR) as a common cause of graft loss, and it is increasingly being recognized as an important cause of both acute and chronic renal allograft injury (Mauiyyedi et al., 2001;Mauiyyedi et al., 2002). This has been made possible with the discovery and the widespread use of C4d as a marker of ABMR. The detailed diagnostic criteria and classification of ABMR have been developed during recent updates of the Banff classification. A category of C4d negative ABMR has also been included in Banff 07 classification.

The definite diagnosis of ABMR requires fulfillment of three criteria; the histological evidence of graft injury, the immunohistochemical evidence of C4d positivity, and the presence of donor specific antibodies (DSA). If only two of these criteria are present, the case is labeled as presumptive ABMR. The pathological changes of ABMR may coexist with other categories of alloimmune or non-immune injuries of the graft (Racusen et al., 1999; Racusen et al., 2003; Solez et al., 2007; Solez et al., 2008).

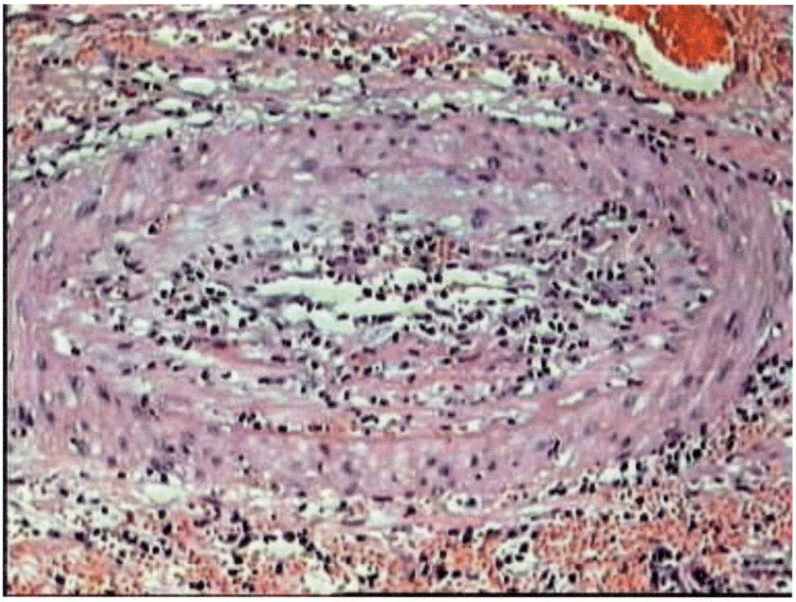

Fig. 5. Medium-power view showing severe/circumferential intimal arteritis, consistent with acute vascular rejection; Banff category, IIA. (H&E, ×200).

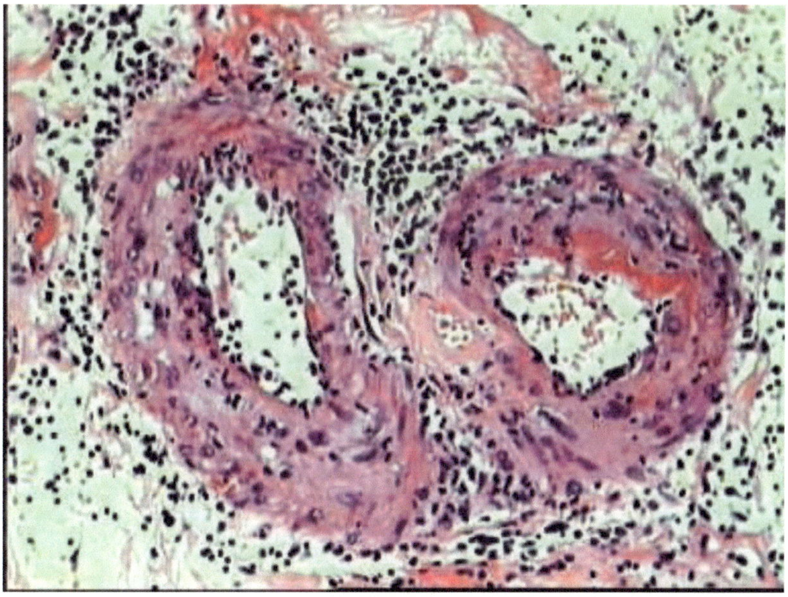

Fig. 6. Medium-power view showing two small arteries showing transmural arteritis along with a small area of fibrinoid necrosis in one of the arteries. This is consistent with V3 lesion and is categorized as acute vascular rejection; Banff category, III. Although, this morphological change may be seen in acute cellular rejection, this lesion is typically seen in cases of antibody mediated rejection (H&E, ×200).

A variety of morphological changes have been described, which, although, not entirely specific, are found more commonly in cases of ABMR. These changes include; polymorphonuclear glomerulitis, peritubular capillaritis, fibrin thrombi in glomerular capillaries, and fibrinoid necrosis of arteries. More recent Banff updates have formulated criteria for scoring the peritubular capillaritis and C4d positivity. These are undergoing clinical validation studies in many transplant centers in the world (Racusen et al., 1999; Racusen et al., 2003; Solez et al., 2007; Solez et al., 2008).

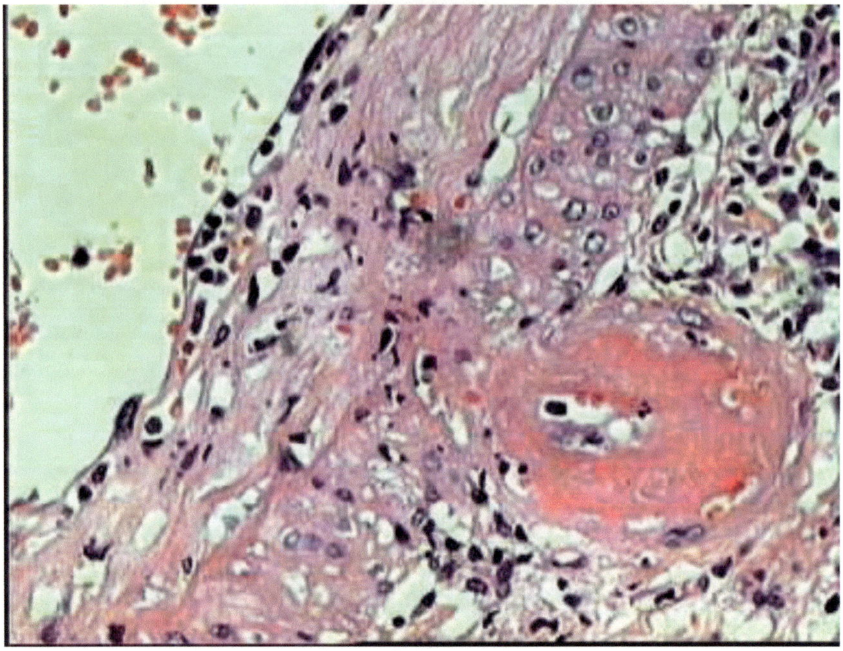

Fig. 7. Medium-power view showing fibrinoid necrosis of the wall of one small artery, characteristic of antibody mediated rejection. The wall of adjacent large artery shows intimal arteritis. (H&E, ×200).

## 9. Pathological changes not related to allo-immune mechanisms

### 9.1 Calcineurin inhibitor (CNI) drug toxicity

Calcineurin inhibitors (CNIs) including cyclosporine (CsA) and tacrolimus form the mainstay of maintenance immunosuppression. The discovery of CsA in 1979 has revolutionized the iatrogenic immunosuppressive protocols and the overall success rate of solid organ transplantation. However, the drugs are also potentially nephrotoxic, causing both acute and chronic nephrotoxicity. Acute CNI toxicity is one of the important causes of acute graft dysfunction. It also frequently poses differential diagnostic problems with acute TCMR. Toxic effects of CsA have been studied in detail, however, the toxicity profile of tacrolimus is still being defined. Both the mechanism of action and the toxicity profile of the two drugs also shows overlapping features (Figures 8 to 10). Acute tubular injury (ATI) is the most common lesion, accompanied by isometric vacuolization of tubular epithelial cell cytoplasm. This change is observed in both the proximal and distal convoluted tubules, and focal coalescence of vacuoles may yield larger vacuoles. Both the drugs are also associated with microvascular toxicity characterized by damage to glomerular capillaries and renal arterioles. Acute arteriolar damage manifests in a variety of ways: there may be endothelial cell swelling, mucinous intimal thickening, nodular hyalinosis, and focal medial necrosis. Marked vacuolization of media of arterioles is also frequently observed (Figure 9). Sometimes, CNI toxicity manifests itself in the form of thrombotic microangiopathy (TMA). Chronic CNI toxicity results in nodular arteriolar hyalinosis, characterized by hyaline, eosinophilic deposits encroaching onto the media. These deposits consist of fibrin, IgM, C3, and C1q. This nodular hyalinosis differs from the circumferential arteriolar hyalinosis limited to the intima, and found in aging, hypertension, and diabetes mellitus. We have observed nodular arteriolar hyalinosis in CNI toxicity as early as one week after transplantation (unpublished data). Drug induced vasculopathy leads to ischemic injury accentuated in the medullary rays, leading to striped or diffuse interstitial fibrosis (Myers et al., 1984).

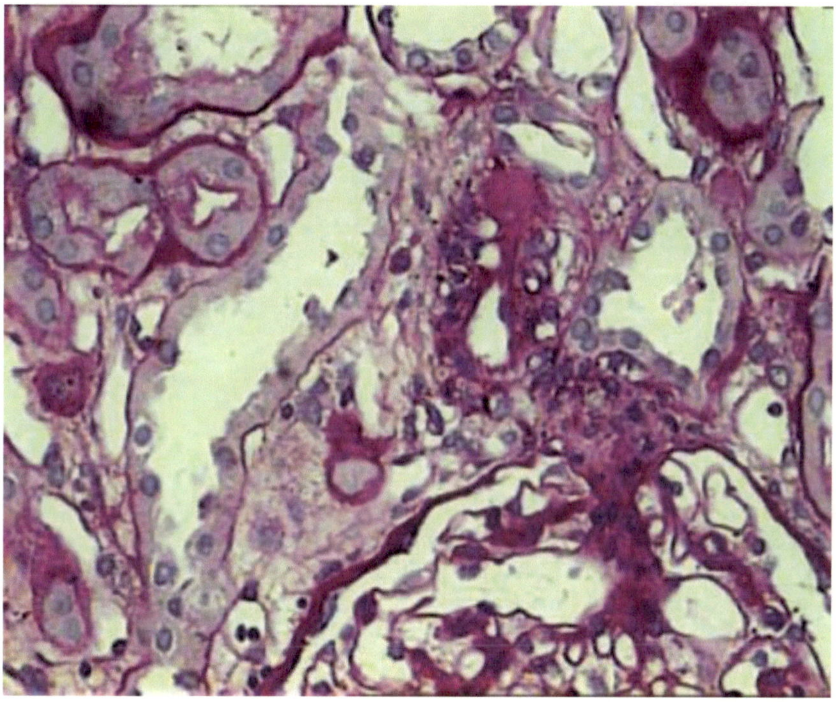

Fig. 8. Medium-power view showing part of a glomerulus with an arteriole, showing nodular hyalinosis. The hyaline is replacing the media and adventitia. This is highly suggestive of cyclosporine toxicity. (PAS, ×200).

### 9.2 Infections

The iatrogenic immunosuppression induced in renal transplant patients predisposes these patients to a variety of infections. The etiologic agents and the site of infections varies depending on a number of factors. Among the different infective agents affecting renal transplant recipients, bacterial, fungal, protozoal, and viral infections are common. Urinary tract infections are common in renal transplant patients in the early post-transplant period. The infective agents may affect the allograft or the native organs of the recipient. Bacterial infections may involve the graft and may be diagnosed on renal allograft biopsy. Bacterial

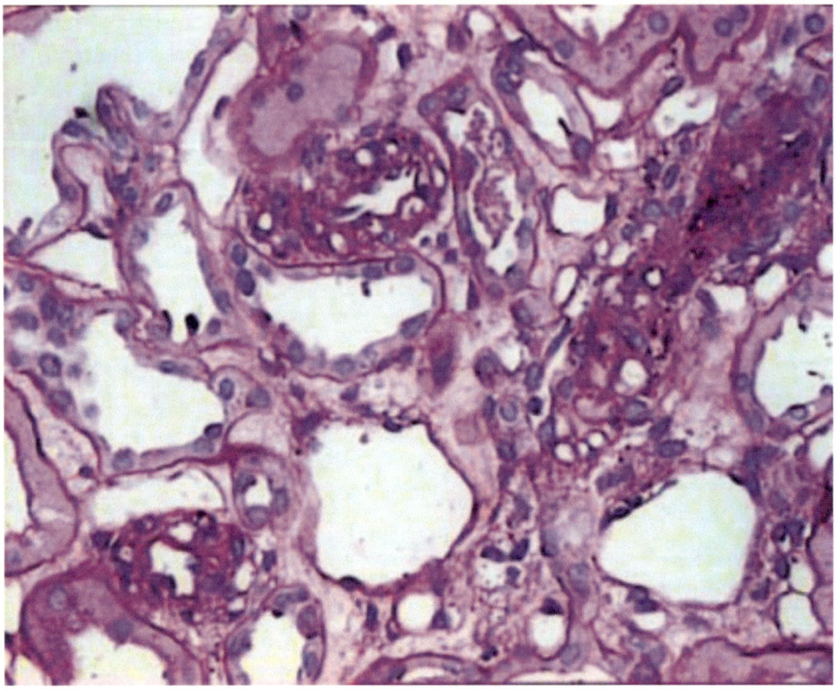

Fig. 9. Medium-power view showing three arterioles with marked vacuolization of medial muscle fibers. This change is also suggestive of cyclosporine toxicity. (PAS, ×200).

infections result in a mixed inflammatory cell infiltrate in the interstitium with a predominance of neutrophils, associated with tubular microabscesses (Figures 11 and 12). The infiltrate is usually localized in the medulla but may be found in the cortex. Sometimes, the infection may not be picked up on urine culture (Imtiaz et al., 2000; Oguz et al., 2002). Among the viral infections affecting the graft, CMV and polyoma viruses are of paramount importance (Nickeleit et al., 1999).

### 9.3 Posttransplant Lymphoproliferative Disorder (PTLD)

Although rare, this disorder is an important differential diagnosis with acute cellular rejection, especially as the posttransplant duration increases. An early diagnosis of this complication is necessary for its successful management. Although, typically the disorder occurs many months to years after transplantation, there are many examples of its occurrence during early posttransplant period.

On light microscopy, PTLD is characterized by a monomorphic or polymorphic lymphocytic infiltrate containing plasma cells, many of which are atypical. There is typically a diffuse interstitial infiltrate without associated tubulitis or arteritis, the later features help in its differential diagnosis from rejection. Occasionally, the two processes may be concurrent. Immunophenotyping of lymphocytes helps in the definite diagnosis of this concurrence.

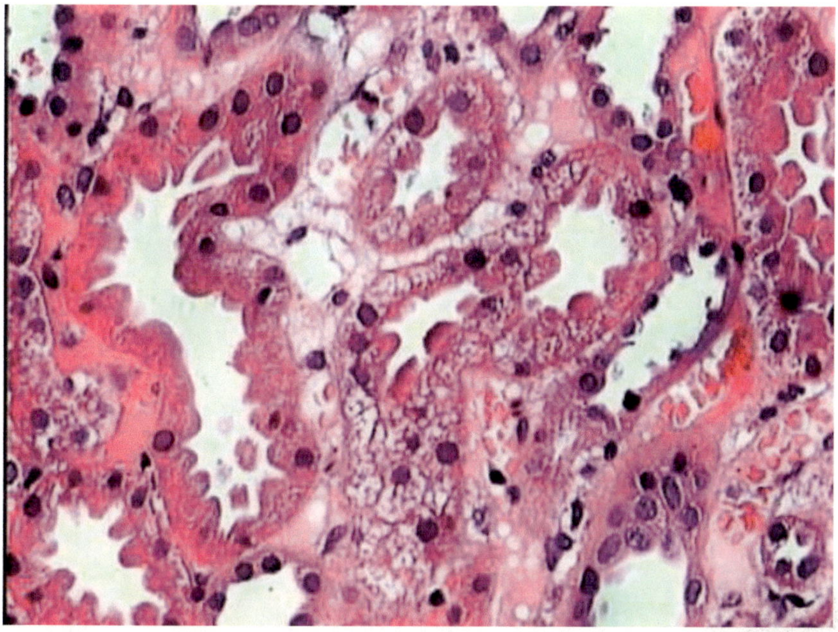

Fig. 10. High-power vies showing prominent isometric vacuolization of tubular epithelial cells in two tubules in the center of the field. Although, no specific, this is highly suggestive of cyclosporine toxicity. (H&E, ×400).

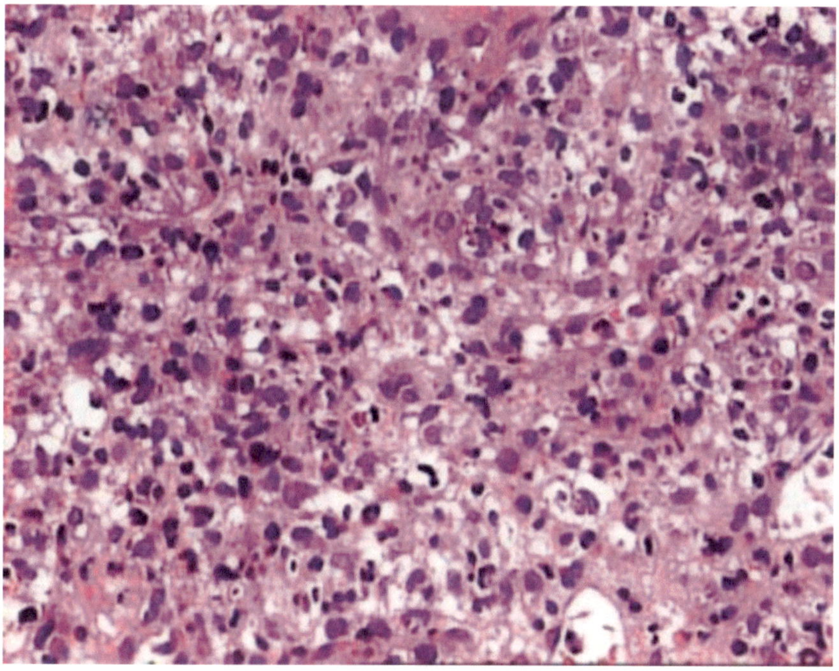

Fig. 11. Medium-power view showing dense, mixed inflammatory cell infiltrate with predominnat neutrophils. This is strongly suggestive of infection. (H&E, ×200).

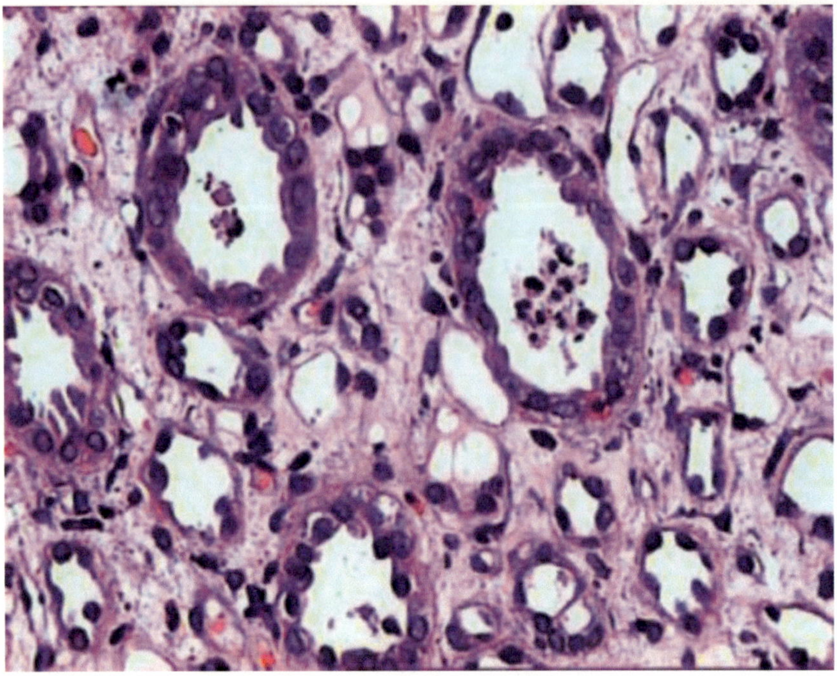

Fig. 12. High-power view showing accumulation of polymorphonuclear neutrophils in the tubular lumina, so called tubular microabscesses. These are highly suggestive of infection. (H&E, ×400).

### 9.4 Acute Tubular Necrosis (ATN)

Acute tubular injury (ATI) or ATN is a common finding in renal biopsies from transplanted kidneys, especially in the cadaveric setting. It is the main cause of primary nonfunction of the allograft in this setting. ATI results from a multitude of causes and situations, including in situ injury in the donor; ischemia during organ harvesting, storage, or transportation of the organ; and ischemic injury incurred perioperatively in the recipient. The morphological picture is similar to that seen in the native kidneys and spans the whole spectrum from mild injury, which is difficult to identify, to severe flattening and loss of tubular epithelium from the tubular basement membrane. These degenerative changes in the tubular epithelial cells are accompanied by signs of regeneration, including mitoses. There may be accompanying interstitial edema, and mild mixed inflammatory cell infiltration. Tubulitis is typically absent or only trivial. Other changes include tubular cell vacuolization and blebbing, and tubular dilatation reflecting downstream tubular obstruction. There are also deposits of calcium salts in tubular lumina in the form of dystrophic calcification.

There is a poor correlation between the morphological changes of ATN and the allograft function. Although, the morphological lesions of ATI or ATN in the transplanted kidneys are similar to those of native kidneys, some authors have noted a few differences in the morphological profile.

### 9.5 Acute Tubulointerstitial Nephritis (ATIN)

Non-immune related ATIN may occur in the transplanted kidneys and may be very difficult to distinguish from the tubulointerstitial rejection. The disorder may result from a variety of insults to the transplanted kidneys, such as infection, drug hypersensitivity, viral infection, etc. A predominance of neutrophils in the mixed inflammatory cell infiltrate in the interstitium, especially if associated with tubular microabscesses or leucocyte casts favor the possibility of infection. A predominance of eosinophils raises the possibility of drug hypersensitivity. Viral infections are accompanied by appropriate viral cytopathic effects in addition to the infiltrate. It may be reiterated here that neutrophils and eosinophils may also be seen in rejection, and sometimes the above lesions are superimposed on underlying rejection reaction.

## 10. Diagnosis of chronic allograft dysfunction

As is evident in table 2, the causes of late allograft dysfunction are more varied that those of acute allograft dysfunction. The late graft dysfunction may manifest as an acute rise in serum creatinine or a slowly increasing serum creatinine, and the causes vary accordingly. An advanced failing allograft may show an apparent acute decline of graft function due to diminished renal reserve, as in native kidneys. Renal allograft biopsy is essential to diagnose the causes of late allograft dysfunction.

In the past, all cases of chronic allograft dysfunction were labeled as "chronic allograft nephropathy" by the pathologists, a "paper wastebasket" for all forms of chronic allograft damage (Cornell & Colvin, 2005; Ivanyi et al., 2001; Nankivell et al., 2003). This was mainly because the morphological features of various diseases were not clearly defined, as well as, the loss of features of primary pathology in advanced stages of sclerosing process. The main morphological changes of specific causes of chronic allograft dysfunction are shown in table 4.

The diagnosis of interstitial fibrosis/tubular atrophy, not otherwise specified, is reserved only for those cases, which show no evidence of specific causes after a detailed and meticulous investigation of the allograft biopsy by morphology, immunohistochemistry, electron microscopy, and molecular genetic methods.

## 11. Recurrent and de novo renal diseases

There are many renal diseases, especially glomerular diseases, which can recur in the transplanted kidneys after a variable period of time (Hariharan, 2000). Currently, glomerular diseases account for approximately 10-20% of cases of ESRD undergoing transplantation, and overall approximately 20% of these patients experience recurrence. The same disease can also occur as de novo disease in the transplanted kidneys. Disease characteristics of the recurrent disease are similar to those of the original disease, but are usually mild in nature. This may be due in part to the use of immunosuppressive agents in the transplant patients. De novo diseases generally occur later than the recurrent diseases. Almost all diseases that occur in the native kidneys can occur de novo in transplant kidneys. However, the two most common diseases are membranous glomerulonephritis and focal segmental glomerulosclerosis. The work up of renal allograft biopsies in cases suspicious for recurrent or de novo glomerulopathies should follow the approach used in native renal biopsy investigation.

One important non-glomerular disease that frequently recurs in transplanted kidneys is the primary hyperoxaluria, if kidney transplantation is carried out without concomitant liver transplantation.

| |
|---|
| **Chronic hypertension:** fibrous thickening of the arterial intima with reduplication of elastic lamina, and arteriolar hyalinosis. |
| **Chronic calcineurin inhibitor toxicity:** nodular peripheral arteriolar hyalinosis, and striped interstitial fibrosis |
| **Chronic obstruction:** prominent tubular dilation, and ruptured tubules with extravasated casts |
| **Chronic pyelonephritis:** chronic interstitial inflammation and fibrosis, out of proportion to vascular or glomerular changes, in the context of clinical history of recurrent urinary tract infections |
| **Polyomavirus nephropathy:** tubular epithelial viral infection evidenced by typical viral inclusions on H&E stain, or positive staining for SV40-large T antigen |
| **De novo/recurrent renal diseases:** morphological features of respective diseases |

Table 4. The morphological features of specific causes of chronic allograft dysfunction, other than chronic allo-immune causes.

## 12. Conclusion

In conclusion, renal transplant pathology is a complex and rapidly evolving field, in which significant improvements have taken place in recent years in both the characterization and categorization of allo-immune mechanisms of injury. More refinement is expected to take place in near future with the inclusion of molecular genetic and image analysis techniques into the Banff classification.

## 13. References

Al-Awwa I, Hariharan S, & First M. (1998). The importance of allograft biopsy in renal transplant recipients. *Am J Kidney Dis,* Vol. 31, No.6, pp. S15–S18.

Bergstrand A, Bohman SO, Farnsworth A, Gokel JM, Krause PH, Lang W, Mihatsch MJ, Oppedal B, Sell S, & Sibley RK. (1985). Renal histopathology in kidney transplant recipients immunosuppressed with cyclosporine A: results of an international workshop. *Clin Nephrol,* Vol. 24, No. 3, pp.107-19.

Choi BS, Shin MJ, Shin SJ, Kim YS, Choi YJ, Kim YS, Moon IS, Kim SY, Koh YB, Bang BK, & Yang CW. (2005). Clinical significance of an early protocol biopsy in living-donor renal transplantation: ten-year experience at a single center. *Am J Transplant,* Vol. 5, No. 6, pp. 1354-60.

Colvin RB. The renal allograft biopsy. (1996). *Kidney Int,* Vol. 50, No. 3, pp. 1069-82.

Colvin RB, Cohen AH, Saiontz C, Bonsib S, Buick M, Burke B, Carter S, Cavallo T, Haas M, Lindblad A, Manivel JC, Nast CC, Salomon D, Weaver C, & Weiss M. (1997). Evaluation of pathologic criteria for acute renal allograft rejection: Reproducibility, sensitivity, and clinical correlation. *J Am Soc Nephrol,* Vol. 8, No. 12, pp.1930-41.

Cornell LD, & Colvin RB. Chronic allograft nephropathy. (2005). *Curr Opin Nephrol Hypertens,* Vol. 14, No. 3, pp. 229-34.

D'Alessandro AM, Sollinger HW, Knechtle SJ, Kalayoglu M, Kisken WA, Uehling DT, Moon TD, Messing EM, Bruskewitz RC, Pirsch JD, & Belzer FO. (1995). Living related and unrelated donors for kidney transplantation- a 28-year experience. *Ann Surg,* Vol. 222, No. 3, pp. 353-64.

Farnsworth A, Hall BM, Ng AB, Duggin GG, Horvath JS, Sheil AG, & Tiller DJ. (1984). Renal biopsy morphology in renal transplantation. A comparative study of the light-microscopic appearances of biopsies from patients treated with cyclosporin A or azathioprine prednisone and antilymphocyte globulin. *Am J Surg Pathol,* Vol. 8, No. 4, pp. 243-52.

Furness PN, Kirkpatrick U, Taub N, Davies DR, & Solez K. (1997). A UK-wide trial of the Banff classification of renal transplant pathology in routine diagnostic service. *Nephrol Dial Transplant,* Vol. 12, No. 5, pp. 995-1000.

Furness PN, Kazi JI, Levesley J, Taub N, & Nicholson M. (1999). A neural network approach to the diagnosis of early acute allograft rejection. *Transplant Proc,* Vol. 31, No. 8, pp. 3151.

Furness PN, Levesley J, Luo Z, Taub N, Kazi JI, Bates WD, & Nicholson ML. (1999). A neural network approach to the diagnosis of early acute renal transplant rejection. *Histopathology,* Vol. 35, No. 5, pp. 461-7.

Furness PN, & Taub N: Convergence of European Renal Transplant Pathology Assessment Procedures (CERTPAP) Project. (2001). International variation in the interpretation of renal transplant biopsies: report of the CERTPAP Project. *Kidney Int,* Vol. 60, No.5, pp. 1998-2012.

Furness PN, Philpott CM, Chorbadjian MT, Nicholson ML, Bosmans JL, Corthouts BL, Bogers JJ, Schwarz A, Gwinner W, Haller H, Mengel M, Seron D, Moreso F, & Cañas C. (2003). Protocol biopsy of the stable renal transplant: a multicenter study of methods and complication rates. *Transplantation,* Vol. 76, No. 6, pp. 969-73.

Furness PN, Taub N, Assmann KJ, Banfi G, Cosyns JP, Dorman AM, Hill CM, Kapper SK, Waldherr R, Laurinavicius A, Marcussen N, Martins AP, Nogueira M, Regele H, Seron D, Carrera M, Sund S, Taskinen EI, Paavonen T, Tihomirova T, & Rosenthal R. (2003). International variation in histologic grading is large, and persistent feedback does not improve reproducibility. *Am J Surg Pathol,* Vol. 27, No. 6, pp. 805-10.

Gaber LW. (1998). Role of renal allograft biopsy in multicentre clinical trials in transplantation. *Am J Kidney Dis,* Vol. 31, No. 6, pp.S19–S25.

Hariharan S, Johnson CP, Bresnahan BA, Taranto SE, Mcintosh MJ,& Stablein D. (2000). Improved graft survival after renal transplantation in United States; 1988-1996. *N Eng J Med,* Vol. 342 No. 9, pp. 605-12.

Hariharan S. (2000). Recurrent and de novo diseases after renal transplantation. *Semin Dial,* Vol. 13, No. 3, pp. 195-9.

Imtiaz S, Akhtar F, Ahmed E, Khan M, Kazi JI, Naqvi A, & Rizvi A. (2000). Acute graft dysfunction due to pyelonephritis, value and safety of graft biopsy. *J Nephrol Urol Transpl,* Vol. 1, No. 1: 127-9.

Ivanyi B, Kemeny E, Szederkenyi E, Marofka F, & Szenohradszky P. (2001). The value of electron microscopy in the diagnosis of chronic renal allograft rejection. *Mod Pathol,* Vol. 14, No.12, pp. 1200-8.

Jain S, Curwood V, Kazi JI, White SA, Furness PN, & Nicholson M. (2000). Acute rejection in protocol renal transplant biopsies-institutional variations. *Transplant Proc,* Vol. 32, No. 3, pp. 616.

John R, & Herzenberg AM. (2010). Our approach to a renal transplant biopsy. *J Clin Pathol,* Vol. 63, No. 1, pp. 26-37.

Kazi JI, Furness PN, & Nicholson M. (1998). Diagnosis of early acute renal allograft rejection by evaluation of multiple histological features using a Bayesian Belief Network. *J Clin Path,* Vol. 51, No. 2, pp. 108-13

Kazi JI, Furness PN, Nicholson M, Ahmed E, Akhtar E, Naqvi A, & Rizvi A. (1999). Interinstitutional variation in the performances of Bayseian Belief Network for the diagnosis of acute renal graft rejection. *Transplant Proc,* Vol. 31, No. 8, pp. 3152.

Kazi JI, & Mubarak M. (2012). Biopsy findings in renal allograft dysfunction in a live related renal transplant program. *J Transplant Technol Res,* Vol. 2, No. 1, pp. 108. doi:10.4172/2161-0991.1000108

Matas AJ, Sibley R, Mauer M, Sutherland DE, Simmons RL, & Najarian JS. (1983). The value of needle renal allograft biopsy. I. A retrospective study of biopsies performed during putative rejection episodes. *Ann Surg,* Vol. 197, No. 2, pp. 226–37.

Matas AJ, Tellis VA, Sablay L, Quinn T, Soberman R, & Veith FJ. (1985). The value of needle renal allograft biopsy. III. A prospective study. *Surgery,* Vol. 98, No. 5, pp. 922–6.

Matas AJ, Payne WD, Sutherland DE, Humar A, Greessner RW, Kandaswamy R, Dunn DL, Gillingham KJ, & Najarian JS. (2001). 2,500 living donor kidney transplants: a single-center experience. *Ann Surg,* Vol. 234, No. 2, pp. 149-64.

Mauiyyedi S, Crespo M, Collins AB, Schneeberger EE, Pascual MA, Saidman SL, Tolkoff-Rubin NE, Williams WW, Delmonico FL, Cosimi AB, & Colvin RB. (2002). Acute humoral rejection in kidney transplantation: II. Morphology, immunopathology, and pathologic classification. *J Am Soc Nephrol,* Vol. 13, No. 3, pp. 779-87.

Mauiyyedi S, Pelle PD, Saidman S, Collins AB, Pascual M, Tolkoff-Rubin NE, Williams WW, Cosimi AA, Schneeberger EE, & Colvin RB. (2001). Chronic humoral rejection: identification of antibody-mediated chronic renal allograft rejection by C4d depositsin peritubular capillaries. *J Am Soc Nephrol,* Vol. 12, No. 3, pp. 574-82.

Mazzali M, Ribeiro-alves MA, & Alves FG. (1999). Percutaneous renal graft biopsy: a clinical, laboratory and pathological analysis. *Sao Paulo Med J,* Vol. 117, No. 2, pp. 57-62.

Mihatsch MJ, Thiel G, Basler V, Ryffel B, Landmann J, von Overbeck J, & Zollinger HU. (1985). Morphological patterns in cyclosporine-treated renal transplant recipients. *Transplant Proc,* Vol. 17, No. 4 (suppl 1), pp. 101-16.

Mishra MN, Saxena VK, Narula AS. (2004). Differences in renal transplantation in India and first world countries. *Int J Hum Genet,* Vol. 4, No. 2, pp. 161-5.

Myers BD, Ross J, Newton L, Luetscher J, & Perlroth M. (1984). Cyclosporine-associated chronic nephropathy. *N Engl J Med,* Vol. 311, No. 11, pp.699-705.

Nankivell BJ, & Alexander SI. (2010). Rejection of the kidney allograft. *New Engl J Med,* Vol. 363, No. 15, pp. 1451-62.

Nankivell BJ, Borrows RJ, Fung CL, O'Connell PJ, Allen RD, & Chapman JR. (2003). The natural history of chronic allograft nephropathy. *N Engl J Med,* Vol. 349, No. 24, pp. 2326-33.

Nickeleit V, Hirsch HH, Binet IF, Gudat F, Prince O, Dalquen P, Thiel G, & Mihatsch MJ. (1999). Polyomavirus infection of renal allograft recipients: From latent infection to manifest disease. *J Am Soc Nephrol,* Vol.10, No. 5, pp.1080-9.

Oguz Y, Doganci L, Bulucu F, Can C, Oktenli C, Yenicesu M, & Vural A. (2002). Acute pyelonephritis causing acute renal allograft dysfunction. *Int Urol Nephrol,* Vol. 34, No.3, pp. 299-301.

Parfrey P, Kuo Y, Hanley J, Knaack J, Xue Z, Lisbona R, & Guttmann RD. (1984). The diagnostic and prognostic value of renal allograft biopsy. *Transplantation,* Vol. 38, No. 6, pp. 586–90.

Pascual M, Vallhonrat H, Cosimi AB, Tolkoff-Rubin N, Colvin RB, Delmonico FL, Ko DS, Schoenfeld DA, & Williams WW Jr. (1999). The clinical usefulness of the renal allograft biopsy in the cyclosporine era: a prospective study. *Transplantation,* Vol. 67, No. 5, pp.737–41.

Ratnakar KS, George S, Datta BN, Fayek AH, Rajagopalan S, Fareed E, Al Tantawi M, Al Arrayed S, & Al Arrayed A. (2002). Renal transplant pathology: Bahrain experience. *Saudi J Kidney Dis Transplant,* Vol. 13, No. 1, pp.71-6.

Rizvi SAH, Naqvi SAA, Zafar MN, Hussain Z, Hashmi A, Hussain M, Akhter SF, Ahmed E, Aziz T, Sultan G, Sultan S, Mehdi SH, Lal M, Ali B, Mubarak M, & Faiq SM. (2011). A renal transplantation model for developing countries. *Am J Transplant,* doi: 10.1111/j.1600-6143.2011.03712.x

Serón D, Anaya F, Marcén R, del Moral RG, Martul EV, Alarcón A, Andrés A, Burgos D, Capdevila L, Molina MG, Jiménez C, Morales JM, Oppenheimer F, Pallardó L, Fructuoso AS. (2008). Guidelines fro indicating, obtaining, processing, and evaluating kidney transplant biopsies. *Nefrologia,* Vol. 28, No. 4, No. pp. 385-96.

Racusen LC, Solez K, Colvin RB, Bonsib SM, Castro MC, Cavallo T, Croker BP, Demetris AJ, Drachenberg CB, Fogo AB, Furness P, Gaber LW, Gibson IW, Glotz D, Goldberg JC, Grande J, Halloran PF, Hansen HE, Hartley B, Hayry PJ, Hill CM, Hoffman EO, Hunsicker LG, Lindblad AS, Marcussen N, Mihatsch MJ, Nadasdy T, Nickerson P, Olsen TS, Papadimitriou JC, Randhawa PS, Rayner DC, Roberts I, Rose S, Rush D, Salinas-Madrigal L, Salomon DR, Sund S, Taskinen E, Trpkov K, & Yamaguchi Y. (1999). The Banff 97 working classification of renal allograft pathology. *Kidney Int,* Vol. 55, No. 2, pp. 713-23.

Racusen LC, Colvin RB, Solez K, Mihatsch MJ, Halloran PF, Campbell PM, Cecka MJ, Cosyns JP, Demetris AJ, Fishbein MC, Fogo A, Furness P, Gibson IW, Glotz D, Hayry P, Hunsickern L, Kashgarian M, Kerman R, Magil AJ, Montgomery R, Morozumi K, Nickeleit V, Randhawa P, Regele H, Seron D, Seshan S, Sund S, & Trpkov K. (2003). Antibody-mediated rejection criteria —an addition to the Banff 97 classification of renal allograft rejection. *Am J Transplant,* Vol. 3, No. 6, pp. 708-14.

Rush D, Nickerson P, Gough J, McKenna R, Grimm P, Cheang M, Trpkov K, Solez K, & Jeffery J. (1998). Beneficial effects of treatment of early subclinical rejection: a randomized study. *J Am Soc Nephrol,* Vol. 9, No. 11, pp. 2129-34.

Serón D, Moreso F, Bover J, Condom E, Gil-Vernet S, Cañas C, Fulladosa X, Torras J, Carrera M, Grinyó JM, & Alsina J. (1997). Early protocol renal allograft biopsies and graft outcome. *Kidney Int,* Vol. 51, No. 1, pp. 310-6.

Solez K, Axelsen RA, Benediktsson H, Burdick JF, Cohen AH, Colvin RB, Croker BP, Droz D, Dunnill MS, Halloran PF, Hayry P, Jennette CJ, Keown PA, Marcussen N, Mihatsch MJ, Morozumi K, Myers BD, Nast CC, Olsen S, Racusen LC, Ramos EL, Rosen S, Sachs DH, Salamon DR, Sanfilippo F, Verani R, Willebrand EV, & Yamaguchi Y. (1993). International standardization of criteria for the histologic diagnosis of renal allograft rejection: the Banff working classification of kidney transplant pathology. *Kidney Int,* Vol. 44, No. 2, pp. 411-22.

Solez K, Colvin RB, Racusen LC, Sis B, Halloran PF, Birk PE, Campbell PM, Cascalho M, Collins AB, Demetris AJ, Drachenberg CB, Gibson IW, Grimm PC, Haas M, Lerut E, Liapis H, Mannon RB, Marcus PB, Mengel M, Mihatsch MJ, Nankivell BJ, Nickeleit V, Papadimitriou JC, Platt JL, Randhawa P, Roberts I, Salinas-Madriga L, Salomon DR, Seron D, Sheaff M, & Weening JJ. (2007). Banff '05 Meeting Report: differential diagnosis of chronic allograft injury and elimination of chronic allograft nephropathy (CAN). *Am J Transplant,* Vol. 7, No. 3, pp. 518-26.

Solez K, Colvin RB, Racusen LC, Haas M, Sis B, Mengel M, Halloran PF, Baldwin W, Banfi G, Collins AB, Cosio F, David DS, Drachenberg C, Einecke G, Fogo AB, Gibson IW, Glotz D, Iskandar SS, Kraus E, Lerut E, Mannon RB, Mihatsch M, Nankivell BJ, Nickeleit V, Papadimitriou JC, Randhawa P, Regele H, Renaudin K, Roberts I, Seron D, Smith RN, & Valente M. (2008). Banff' 07 classification of renal allograft pathology: updates and future directions. *Am J Transplant,* Vol. 8, No. 4, pp. 753-60.

Verma PP, Hooda AK, Sinha T, Chopra GS, Karan SC, Sethi GS, Badwal S, & Kotwal A. (2007). Renal transplantation- an experience of 500 patients. MJAFI, Vol. 63, No. pp. 107-11.

Vidhun J, Masciandro J, Varich L, Salvatierra O, Jr., Sarwal M. (2003). Safety and risk stratification of percutaneous biopsies of adult-sized renal allografts in infant and older pediatric recipients. *Transplantation,* Vol. 76, No. 3, pp. 552-7.

Wilckzek HE. (1990). Percutaneous needle biopsy of the renal allograft. A safety evaluation of 1129 biopsies. *Transplantation,* Vol. 50, No. 5, pp. 790-7.

# Part 5

# Pathophysiology and Renal Diseases

# 11

# Acute Kidney Injury (AKI) and Management of Renal Tumors

Yoshio Shimizu and Yasuhiko Tomino
*Division of Nephrology, Department of Internal Medicine,*
*Juntendo University Faculty of Medicine*
*Japan*

## 1. Introduction

Acute kidney injury (AKI) is characterized by a rapid decline in kidney function within a few hours or a few days. AKI is an independent risk factor for mortality in critically ill patients. Determination of the prevalence of AKI depends on the definition employed and on methods used for definite diagnosis. The incidence and prevalence of AKI vary with the clinical setting, based on separately addressed community-based, hospital-based or intensive care unit (ICU)-based AKI [Himmelfaub, Ikizler 2007]. The epidemiology of AKI has been made unclear in the past because of the use of different definitions across various studies. The lack of a uniform definition may results in many differences in the reported incidences and outcomes of AKI in the literature.

## 2. Definition of AKI

### 2.1 RIFLE criteria

In 2004, a group of experts on acute renal failure (Acute Dialysis Initiative, ADQI) stated that the name should be changed from "acute renal failure" to "acute kidney injury (AKI)" [Bellomo, Ronco, Kellum et al. 2004]. This group developed criteria for standardizing and staging AKI, which consist of Risk, Injury, Loss and End-stage Renal Failure (RIFLE). The aim of this classification was to standardize the definition of AKI in the same way as the two other common ICU syndromes (sepsis and ARDS). In the RIFLE criteria, serum creatinine and urine output were adopted as clinical parameters to formulate three severity categories (Risk, Injury and Renal Failure) of AKI and two clinical outcome categories (Loss and Renal Failure) (Table 1). At present, RIFLE criteria have been validated in more than 550,000 patients around the world [Srisawat, Hoste, Kellum et al. 2010]. The problems in adopting the criteria were using 1) very small alterations in serum creatinine and urine output, 2) an acronym instead of numerical stages such as with chronic kidney disease (CKD) and 3) a 50% increase of serum creatinine for categorizing as Risk. Recent investigations revealed that an alteration of less than 50% of serum creatinine was important [Chertow, Burdick, Honour 2005].

### 2.2 AKIN criteria

In 2007, the RIFLE criteria were revised by members of the Acute Kidney Injury Network (AKIN), a multi-disciplinary international group to increase their sensitivity [Mehta,

Kellum, Shah et al. 2007]. These modifications are summarized as follows: 1) broadening of the 'risk' category of RIFLE to include an increase in serum creatinine of at least 0.3mg/dL even it this does not reach the 50% of the basal creatinine level; 2) setting a 48-hour window on the first documentation of any criteria; 3) categorizing all patients as 'failure' if they are undergoing renal replacement therapy (RRT) regardless of what their serum creatinine or urine output is at the point of initiation and 4) using stages 1, 2 and 3 were used instead of R, I and F (Table 1).

## 3. Etiology of AKI in patients with neoplasms

The etiology of AKIs is classified into three types: pre-renal, intrinsic renal injury and post-renal causes [Denker, Robles-Osorio, Sabath 2011]. AKI in patients with neoplasms is most often multifactorial. Clinicians may experience each type or combinations of AKI during treatment of these patients.

### 3.1 Pre-renal causes

Pre-renal causes are common in patients with malignancies because these patients suffer from anorexia, nausea and vomiting or diarrhea as malignancy-related symptoms together with side effects of treatments. It is often difficult to diagnose in the pre-renal phase during which recovery of kidney function is possible with adequate fluid supplementation and also difficult to differentiate from the intrinsic renal renal phase during which AKI has been established [Lameire, Van Biesen, Vanholder 2010]. Moreover, electrolyte disturbances are frequently observed in patients with malignancies and they can aggravate AKI. Electrolyte and acid base disturbances are consequences of neoplastic spread, anticancer treatment or paraneoplastic phenomena of tumors.

### 3.2 Intrinsic renal causes

Most intrinsic renal injury is classified as acute tubular necrosis (ATN), acute interstitial nephritis, vasculopathy and glomerulopathy.

#### 3.2.1 Acute tubular necrosis (ATN)

ATN is defined by AKI and tubular damage in the absence of significant glomerular or vascular pathology [John, Herzenberg 2009]. The presentation of ATN is a sudden rise of serum creatinine, sometimes with microscopic hematuria and small amounts of proteinuria. The presence of tubular epithelial enzymes in the urine is a valuable indicator of detect damage. Microscopically, ATN is recognized by a combination of degenerative tubular changes. The mildest change is apical blebbing and the most severe is cellular necrosis, which is rare. The presence of sloughed epithelium and casts is a common finding. Mild interstitial inflammatory cell infiltration is commonly observed around the damaged tubular segments. Tamm-Horsfall mucoprotein can elicit an exuberant inflammatory reaction. Isometric vacuolization is a form of tubular injury characterized by numerous small vacuoles filling the cytoplasm. The pathogenetic mechanism of ATN is still unclear. The two major causes of ATN are ischemic and toxic factors. Both lead to ATN via tubular epithelial cell damage. Prolonged renal ischemia is the most common cause of ATN. While sepsis, commonly observed in critically ill patients with malignancy, is a cause of hypotension and renal ischemia, a recent investigation using sepsis models suggested that reactions between Gram-negative toxins and toll-like receptors including their effector

| | RIFLE | | AKIN | | |
|---|---|---|---|---|---|
| Category | Creatinine/GFR | Urine output (UO) | Stage | Creatinine | Urine output (UO) |
| Risk | Cr increase by 1.5 times or GFR decrease by ≧25% | UO≦0.5mL/kg/hr for 6hrs | Stage 1 | Cr increase by ×1.5 times or ≧26μmol/L | UO≦0.5mL/kg/hr for 6hrs |
| Injury | Cr increase by ×2 times or GFR decrease by ≧50% | UO≦0.5mL/kg/hr for 12hrs | Stage 2 | Cr increase by ×2 | UO≦0.5mL/kg/hr for 12hrs |
| Failure | Cr increase by ×3 times or GFR decrease by 75% or Cr≧354μmol/L (with acute rise≧ 44μmol/L | UO≦0.3mL/kg/hr for 24hrs or anuria for 12hrs | Stage 3 | Cr increases by ×3 or Cr ≧354μmol/L (with acute rise 44μmol/L) or RRT | UO≦0.3mL/kg/hr for 24hrs or anuria for 12hrs |
| Loss (outcome) | Persistent ARF = compete loss of renal function > 4 weeks ( but > 3 months | N/A | Nil | | |
| ESRD (outcome) | | N/A | Nil | | |

Table 1. RIFLE and AKIN criteria

Patients requiring RRT are automatically classified as Stage 3 AKIN regardless of stage at time of RRT initiation.

proteins such as MyD88 were also involved in ATN [Goncalves, Zamboni , Camara 2010, Li, Khan, Maderdrut et al. 2010].

### 3.2.2 Tubulointerstitial nephritis

Tubulointerstitial nephritis is defined as inflammation of the renal interstitium and tubules either with interstitial edema and acute tubular damage or with interstitial fibrosis and tubular atrophy. Acute interstitial nephritis (AIN) is clinically similar to ATN. Signs suggesting systemic hypersensitivity such as rash or eosinophilia are sometimes present. The major causes of AIN include drugs, infection, autoimmune diseases and cancer infiltration. The most frequent cause is drugs, which account for two thirds of all AIN [Baker, Pusey2004]. The onset of symptom after administration of a drug that can induce AIN is on average 2-3 weeks, but this interval varies widely [Rossert 2000]. While eosinophilia has been suggested to predict drug-induced AIN, good evidence is lacking for diagnosis of AIN based on the presence or absence of eosinophilia [Nolan, Anger, Kelleher 1986]. AIN shows interstitial edema, tubular damage and mixed infiltration of mononuclear cells. Eosinophilic infiltration is common drug-induced AIN, but it shows low sensitivity. An immunological basis for drug-induced AIN is apparent in most cases. Drugs act as haptens and create antigenicity after binding to tubular basement membrane or interstitial matrices [Rossert 2000].

### 3.2.3 Thrombotic microangiopathy

The association between thrombotic microangiopathy (TMA) and cancer was first described in 1973. TMA may be associated with cancer itself, with cancer chemotherapy or with allogenic bone marrow transplantation (BMT) [Kwaan, Gordon 2001]. Thrombocytopenia with microangiopathic hemolytic anemia (peripheral non-autoimmune anemia with schizocytes) and no alternative diagnosis is sufficient to establish a presumptive diagnosis of TMA [Darmon, Ciroldi, Thiery et al. 2006]. Intravascular coagulation (DIC) must be ruled out in this setting. Most TMA occurs in patients with solid tumors, the most common type being adenocarcinoma (stomach, breast and lungs) although TMA has been reported in patients with other solid tumors or hematological malignancies [Gordon, Kwaan 1997]. While the pathophysiology of malignancy-related TMA remains controversial, recent studies have shown that disseminated cancer is associated with decreased ADAMTS 13 activity, without anti-ADAMTS 13 antibodies [Oleksowicz, Bhagwati, DeLeon-Fernandez 1999].
The link between TMA and cancer chemotherapy was first described for mitomycin C. Subsequently, TMA has been reported in connection with many anti-cancer agents, including gemcitabine, bleomycin, cisplatin, cytosine arabinoside, daunorbicin, deoxycoformycin, 5-FU, azathioprine and interferon α[Kwaan, Gordon 2001]. The association between TMA and bone marrow transplantation (BMT) has been reported since the 1980s. Typically, TMA starts from 2 to 12 months after BMT and is unresponsive to plasma exchange. BMT associated TMA has been reported to be related to total body irradiation, graft-vs-host disease and cytomegalovirus infection. Treatment of TMA has not been established. Although plasma exchange has been shown to improve patients without malignancies [Rock, Shumak, Buskard et al. 1991], it is possible that plasmatherapy harms TMA patients with malignancies [Penne, Vignau, Auburtin et al. 2005].

## 3.3 Toxicity related to cancer treatment

### 3.3.1 Contrast-induced AKI (CI-AKI)

CI-AKI accounts for approximately 10% of all cases of hospital-acquired AKI. CI-AKI may lead to increased morbidity and mortality rates in the selected at-risk population including critically ill patients with cancer [Briguori, Tavano, Colombo2003]. Hemodynamic changes in renal blood flow, which lead to hypoxia of the renal medulla and direct toxic effects of contrast media on renal cells are thought to contribute to the pathogenesis of CI-AKI [Briguori, Quintavalle, De Micco et al. 2011].

### 3.3.2 Cisplatin-induced renal toxicity

Metastatic renal pelvic cancers, like those of the bladder, are generally highly chemosensitive diseases. At present, a combination of cisplatin, methotrexate, doxorubicin and vincristine (M-VAC) is most widely used for the treatment of metastatic urothelial carcinoma [Sternberg, Yagoda, Scher et al. 1989, Tannock, Gospodarowicz, Connolly. 1989]. The dismal results obtained with M-VAC have prompted efforts to determine new regimens against urothelial carcinoma. Combined chemotherapy with gemcitabine and cisplatin is now widely considered to be first-line chemotherapy against metastatic renal pelvic cancer [von der Maase, Hansen, Roberts et al. 2000, Tanji, Ozawa, Miura et al. 2010].

Cisplatin has direct toxicity and causes AKI. Cisplatin is also associated with chronic dose-dependent reduction of the glomerular filtration rate (GFR) [Arany, Safirstein 2003]. The most widely used protective measurement is saline infusion to induce solute diuresis. Since amifostine (an inorganic thiophosphate) has been found to be effective for prevention of AKI, the American Society of Clinical Oncology recommended use of amifostine for the prevention of AKI in patients receiving cisplatin-based chemotherapy (grade A recommendation) [Schuchter, Hensley, Meropol et al. 2002].

Metastatic renal cell carcinoma (RCC) is highly resistant to both conventional chemotherapy and radiotherapy. During the last decade, several new targeted drugs (sorafenib, sunitinib, everolimus and temsirolimus) have been used for the treatment of advanced RCC [Tanji, Yokoyama 2011]. Molecular targeted drugs are associated with adverse events different from those of classical anticancer agents. AKI has been reported in patients with advanced RCC administered anti-vascular endothelial growth factor (VEGF) agents, including sorafenib and sunitinib. Proteinuria and hypertension are often observed in the patients treated with these agents and pathologically, various kidney lesions, including thrombotic microangiopathy, focal segmental glomerulosclerosis, mesangial proliferative glomerulonephritis, cyroglobulinemic glomerulonephritis, immune complex glomerulonephritis, glomerular endotheliosis and AIN, are detected [Gurevich, Parazella 2009]. A patient contracting AKI after using temsirolimus has been reported [Kwitkowski, Prowell, Ibrahim 2010].

## 3.4 Intra- or extra-renal obstruction

### 3.4.1 Acute tumor lysis syndrome

Tumor lysis syndrome (TLS) is a potentially life-threatening complication of cancer treatments in patients with extensive growing and chemosensitive malignancies. TLS results from degenerated cells, which rapidly release intracellular electrolytes, proteins and metabolites into the extracellular space. TLS often causes AKI by renal tubular occlusion resulting from uric acid crystal formation secondary to hyperuricemia [Jasek, Day 1994]. Another cause is calcium phosphate deposition by hyperphosphatemia [Darmon, Ciroldi, Thiery et al. 2006]. Although TLS typically occurs in patients with hematological malignancies, it has been reported in patients with RCC and pelvic cancer [Lin, Lim , Chen 2007, Persons, Garst, Vollmer et al. 1998]. Volume expansion and recombinant urate oxidase (rasburicase), which reduce uric acid levels, diminish the risk of uric acid deposition nephropathy. Urine alkalization, which was previously recommended to prevent uric acid precipitation within renal tubules, is controversial since urine alkalization induces calcium phosphate deposition [Baeksgaard, Sorensen 2003].

### 3.5 Post-renal causes

Post-renal causes of AKI are based on obstruction of the outflow tracts of the kidneys. Causes include prostatic hypertrophy, catheters, tumors, strictures and crystals. Neurogenic bladder also causes an obstruction. Clinical manifestations of post-renal obstructive uropathy vary with the site, degree and rapidity of obstruction [Kapoor, Chan 2001].
B-mode ultrasonography is a very useful imaging tool to rule out the possibly of urinary tract obstruction as a cause of AKI [Kalantarinia 2009]. Early detection of urinary tract obstruction may prevent patients from progressing to established AKI by early release of urinary obstruction [Choudhury 2010].
Release of obstruction, either by percutaneous nephrostomy or through a ureteral stent, is the fundamental treatment. Recovery of renal function depends on the severity and duration of the obstruction [Kapoor and Chan 2001]. Thus, early discovery and treatment are crucial.

## 4. Biomarkers of AKI

Although serum creatinine and blood urea nitrogen have been used as standard biomarkers, they are not sufficiently specific and sensitive to detect AKI in the early phase [Choudhury 2010]. Moreover, the resultant inability to meaningfully segregate critical aspects of injury such as type, onset, propagation and recovery from ongoing renal function has hindered successful translation of promising therapeutics. Recently, efforts to identify novel plasma or urine biomarkers for AKI have resulted in discovery about 20 potential candidates. Promising markers include urine or plasma neutrophil gelatinase-associated lipocalin (NGAL), kidney injury molecule-1 (KIM-1), IL-18, cystatin C and liver fatty-acid binding protein (L-FABP) [Malyszko 2010].

### 4.1 NGAL

Human NGAL is a 25-kDa protein expressed by neutrophils and various epithelial cells including cells of the proximal convoluted tubules [Goetz, Holmes, Borregaad et al. 2002]. Urinary NGAL is up-regulated within 2 hours after acute renal cellular injury. Microarray analysis identified NGAL as one of the earliest and most prominently induced genes in the kidneys after ischemic or nephrotoxic renal injury in mouse models and humans [Schmidt-Ott, Mori, Kalandadze 2006, Cowland, Borregaad 1997]. In one study, patients in an intensive care unit with AKI had more than 10-fold increases in plasma NGAL and more than 100-fold increases in urine NGAL levels, when compared with controls [Mori, Lee, Rapoport et al. 2005]. Other studies demonstrated the ability of serum and/or urine NGAL to predict the development of postsurgical AKI before elevation of serum creatinine [Mishra, Dent, Tarabishi et al. 2005, Dent, Ma, Dastrala et al. 2007].

### 4.2 KIM-1

Kidney injury molecule-1 (KIM-1) is a transmembrane protein overexpressed in proximal tubule cells of the kidneys in response to ischemic or nephrotoxic injury and has a potential role as a predictive marker of AKI [Ichimura, Bonventre, Bailly et al. 1998]. In a cross-sectional study, the area under the curve (AUC) of KIM-1 for differentiating patients with AKI from controls was 0.9 [Han, Waikar, Johnson et al. 2008]. A prospective study of 90 adult patients undergoing cardiac surgery indicated that the AUC of urinary KIM-1 was higher than those of NGAL and NAG. Several studies demonstrated that urinary KIM-1 can differentiate ischemic AKI from pre-renal azotemia and CKD and may be useful for differentiating among various subtypes of AKI [Han, Waikar, Johnson 2008].

### 4.3 Cystatin C

Cystatin C is a low molecular weight cysteine protease inhibitor. The serum level of cystatin C is determined by the glomerular filtration rate (GFR), indicating that serum and urine levels of cystatin C reflect changes in the GFR [Villa, Jimenez, Soriano et al. 2005]. Although serum creatinine levels do not rise until GFR drops to under 50 ml/min (creatinine blind area), serum cystatin C increases at a GFR of around 70ml/min [Shimizu-Tokiwa, Kobata, Io et al. 2002]. This means that serum cystatin C is superior to serum creatinine in detecting impaired GFR.

### 4.4 IL-18

IL-18 is a proinflammatory cytokine and powerful mediator of ischemia induced AKI in animal models [Melnikov, Ecder, Fantuzzi et al. 2001]. Il-18 is induced and cleaved in the proximal tubules and is detected in urine following experimental AKI [Melnikov, Faubel, Siggmund et al. 2002]. In a cross-sectional study, IL-18 levels were significantly higher in patients with established AKI but not in those with urinary tract infections. The AUC for diagnosis of established AKI is 0.95 [Parikh, Jani, Melnikov et al. 2004]. In general, it is considered that IL-18 is specific for ischemic AKI but may also be a non-specific marker of inflammation and has shown inconsistent results [Moore, Bellomo, Nichol 2010].

### 4.5 L-FABP

L-FABP is expressed in various organs including the liver and kidneys. The function of L-FABP is cellular uptake of fatty acids from plasma and promotion of intracellular fatty acid metabolism. Since free fatty acids can be easily oxidized, they can lead to oxidative stress and cellular injury. L-FABP inhibits the accumulation of intracellular fatty acids and prevents oxidation of free fatty acids. L-FABP is an important cellular antioxidant during oxidative stress [Noiri, Doi, Negishi et al. 2009].

L-FABP is filtered by glomeruli and reabsorbed in the proximal tubules. This partly explains the increase of L-FABP in injury of the proximal tubules. Renal L-FABP expression is up-regulated and urinary L-FABP excretion is accelerated by accumulation of free fatty acids in proximal tubule injury [Kamijo, Sugaya, Hikawa et al. 2004, ].

In a clinical study, urine L-FABP appeared to to be a more sensitive predictor of AKI than serum creatinine, and differentiated patients with septic shock from those with severe sepsis [Nakamura, Sugaya, Koide 2009]. Urine L-FABP can predict AKI in pediatric cardiopulmonary bypass surgery with AUC of 0.81 at 4-hours post-surgery [Portilla, Dent, Sugaya et al. 2008]. Although urine L-FABP is an early, accurate biomarker of AKI, it appears later than NGAL [Moore E, Bellomo R, Nichol. 2010].

## 5. Treatment

People who have risk factors of AKI (eg, past history of AKI, CKD or diabetes mellitus) should be treated as carefully as possible [Lamaire, Adam, Becker et al. 1999]. The best method for preventing contrast media induced AKI is to avoid use of contrast media. If contrast media must be used, the most effective prevention is to avoid volume depletion and to assure adequate volume [Davidson, Hlatky, Morris et al. 1989, Cigarroa, Lange, Williams et al. 1989]. The effect of administration of *N*-acetylcysteine (NAC) is controversial [Fishbane 2008] and there is no convincing evidence of benefits in periprocedual blood purification [Frank H, Werner D, Lorusso V et al. (2003), Vogt B, Ferrari P, Schonholzer C et al. (2001)]. Since renal autoregulatory capacity maintains renal blood flow, several vasopressors including dopamine, norepinephrine, vasopressin and terlipressin, have been used or tested for prevention of renal ischemia. There is no clear convincing evidence on the beneficial effects of these agents for treating AKI [Rudnik MR, Kesselheim A, Goldfarb S (2006)].
There are currently no specific pharmacological interventions for patients with established AKI but renal replacement therapy (RRT) is a key component of supportive care. AKI associated with cancer shows substantial morbidity and mortality. Among critically ill cancer patients, 12-49% experience AKI and 9-32% need RRT [Lanore JJ, Brunet F, Pchard st al. 1991, Benoit, Hoste, Depuydt et al. 2005, Azoulay, Recher, Alberti C et al. 1999, Azoulay, Moreau, Alberti et al. 2000, Darmon, Thiery, Ciroldi et al. 2005]. These figures are much higher than those for critically ill patients without cancer. Most of the studies on AKI in cancer patients focus on patients with hematological malignancies whose mortality is over 80% when RRT is necessary [Zager, O'Quigley, Zager et al. 1989]. Studies focusing on AKI in renal tumor patients have not been reported. In a cohort study, the benefits of early organ support including RRT was shown in the patients with non-hematological cancers associated with AKI [Darmon, Thiery, Ciroldi et al. 2007]. AKI, which has multiple causes and shows higher mortality in cancer patients, allows physicians to perform reluctant RRT, but there are no adequate treatment guidelines for AKI in patients with malignancies.

### 5.1 Dosage in renal replacement therapy (RRT)

The effectiveness of RRT can be adjusted by the rate of solute clearance (duration of the session) and/or the frequency of RRT sessions. The assessment of RRT dose is traditionally performed by single-pooled Kt/V urea. This refers to fractional clearance of urea (K), which takes into consideration therapy duration (t) and volume of distribution of urea in the body (V). In contrast to end stage kidney disease (ESKD) patients, critically ill patients with AKI have an unstable metabolic status (eg. hypercatabolism and fluid expansion). When continuous RRT (CRRT) is performed, ultrafiltration volume acts as a surrogate for clearance, based on with sieving coefficient of most small solutes such as urea. Therefore, application of Kt/V urea in critically ill patients has its limitations [Schiffl, Lang, Fischer 2002]. The RRT adequacy is more complex than small-solute removal. Fluid overload has been independently associated with increased mortality of AKI [Payen, de Pont, Sakr et al. 2008, Bouchard J, Soroko S Chertow G et al. 2009].

### 5.2 Intensity of RRT and outcome

Renal replacement therapy (RRT) is usually performed in critically ill patients by intermittent hemodialysis or continuous RRT (CRRT). CRRT is performed together with hemofiltration, dialysis or a combination of them. The efficacy of CRRT for critically ill patients is not superior to that of intermittent hemodialysis [Himmelfarb 2007]. Studies on the dose of intermittent hemodialysis (IHD) or CRRT and their outcomes have shown conflicting results although some clinical trials suggested an improvement in survival with higher doses of RRT [Ronco, Bellomo, Homel et al. 2000, Palvesky, Zhang, O'Connor et al. 2008, Bellomo, Cass, Cole et al. 2009, Tolwani, Cruz, Fumagalli et al. 2008, Boumann, Oudemans-Van Straaten, Tijssen et al. 2002, Saudan, Niederberger, Seigneux et al. 2006]. One of the reasons for this phenomenon is that there is considered to be an inflection point separating the dose-response portion and dose-independent portion between RRT dose and survival. Recent multicenter randomized trials showed that higher intensity of CRRT or IHD did not reduce mortality of critically ill patients with AKI [Palvesky, Zhang, O'Connor et al. 2008, Bellomo, Cass, Cole et al]. If a critically ill patient with AKI is given RRT, the mortality is expected to be over 90%. Under-dialysis for critically ill patients with AKI results in higher mortality because of uremic complications. The correct dose is around the infection point, at which the RRT dose is not too small but not excessive.

### 5.3 Recommendation of RRT for critically ill patients with AKI

The balance of current evidence suggests that CRRT should be performed with an effluent flow rate higher than 20-25ml/kg/h in hemodynamicaly unstable patients with AKI. Alternative-day IHD is acceptable in more stable patients and minimum single pool Kt/V urea of 1.2-1.4 is recommended [Schiffl 2010]. Clinicians should check whether patients actually receive the current optimal doses of RRT. Higher doses and more intensive therapy can be considered if patients become extremely hypercatabolic or have a volume overload.

## 6. Conclusion

Although a large number of studies have been performed on AKI, little is known about its pathophysiology, appropriate diagnosis or treatment. It is hoped that further studies will improve the prognosis of patients with AKI. It appears that suitable treatments should be selected for AKI especially in patients with malignancies.

## 7. Acknowledgement

This work is partly supported by grants by Ministry of Education, Culture, Sports, Science and Technology of Japan and Ministry of Health, Labor and Welfare of Japan.

## 8. References

Arany I, Safirstein RL (2003). "Cisplatin nephrotoxicity." *Semin Nephrol* 23: 460-64.

Azoulay E, Moreau D, Alberti C et al. (2000). "Predictors of short-term mortality in critically ill patients with solid malignancies." *Intensive Care Med* 26: 1817-23.

Azoulay E, Recher C, Alberti C et al. (1999). "Changing use of intensive care for hematological patients: the example of multiple myeloma." *Intensive Care Med* 25: 1395-1401.

Baeksgaard L, Sorensen JB (2003). "Acute tumor lysis syndrome in solid tumors- a case report and review of the literature." *Cancer Chemother Pharmacol* 51: 187-92.

Baker RJ, Pusey CD (2004). The changing profile of acute tubulointerstitial nephritis. *Nephrol Dial Transplant* 19(1): 8-11.

Bellomo R, Cass A, Cole L et al. (2009). 'Intensity of continuous renal replacement therapy in critically ill patients." *N Engl J Med* 361: 1627-38.

Bellomo R, Ronco C, Kellum JA et al. (2004). "Acute renal failure - definition, outcome, measures, animal models, fluid therapy and information technology needs: The Second International Consensus Conference of the Acute Dialysis Quality Initiative (ADQI) Group." *Crit Care* 8: R204-R210.

Benoit DD, Hoste EA, Depuydt PO et al. (2005). "Outcome in critically ill medical patients treated with renal replacement therapy for acute renal failure: comparison between patients with and those without haematological malignancies." *Nephrol Dial Transplant* 20: 552-8.

Bouchard J, Soroko S, Cherow G et al. (2009). "Fluid accumulation, survival and recovery of kidney function in critically ill patients with acute kidney injury." *Kideny Int* 76: 422-7.

Bouman C, Oudemans-Van Straaten H, Tijssen J et al. (2002). 'Effects of early high-volume continuous venovenous hemofiltration on survival and recovery of renal function in intensive care patients with acute renal failure: a prospective, randomized trial." *Crit Care Med* 30: 2205-11.

Briguori C, Quintavalle C, De Micco F et al. (2011) "Nephrotoxicity of contrast media and protective of acetylcysteine." *Arch Toxicol* 85: 165-73.

Briguori C, Tavano D, Colombo A (2003). "Contrast agent-associated nephrotoxicity" *Prog Cardiovasc Dis* 45(6): 493-503.

Chertow GM, Burdick E, Honour M et al. (2005). "Acute kidney injury, mortality, length of stay, and costs in hospitalized patients." *J Am Soc Nephrol* 16: 3365-70.

Choudhury D (2010). "Acute kidney injury: current perspectives." *Postgrad Med* 122(6): 29-40.

Cigarroa RG, Lange RA, Williams RH et al. (1989). "Dosing contrast material to prevent contrast nephropathy in patients with renal disease." *Am J Med* 86: 649-52.

Cowland JB, Borregaad N (1997). "Molecular characterization and pattern of tissue expression of gene for neutrophil gelatinase associated lipocalin from humans." *Genomics* 45: 17-23.

Darmon M, Thiery G, Ciroldi M et al. (2005). "Intensive care in patients with newly diagnosed malignancies and a need for cancer chemotherapy." *Crit Care Med* 33: 2488-93.

Darmon M, Thiery G, Ciroldi M et al. (2007). "Should dialysis be offered to cancer patients with acute kidney injury?" *Intensive Care Med* 33:765-72.

Davidson CJ, Hlatky M, Morris KG et al. (1989). "Cardiovascular and renal toxicity of a nonionic radiographic contrast agent after cardiac catheterization: a prospective trial." *Ann Intern Med* 110: 119-24.

Denker B, Robles-Osorio ML, Sabath E (2011). "Recent advances in diagnosis and treatment of acute kidney injury in patients with cancer." *Eur J Intern Med* 22(4): 348-54.

Dent CL, Ma Q, Dastrala S et al. (2007). "Plasma NGAL predicts acute kidney injury, morbidity and mortality after pediatric cardiac surgery: a prospective uncontrolled cohort study." *Crit Care* 11: R127.

Fishbane S (2008). "N-acetylcysteine in the prevention of contrast-induced nephropathy." *Clin Am Soc Nephrol* 3: 281-7.

Frank H, Werner D, Lorusso V et al. (2003). "Simultaneous hemodialysis during coronary angiography fails to prevent radiocontrast-induced nephropathy in chronic renal failure." *Clin Nephro*l 60: 176-82.

Goetz DH, Holmes MA, Borregaad N et al. (2002). 'The neutrophil lipocalin NGAL is a bacteriostatic agent that interferes with siderophore mediated iron aquisition. *Mol Cell* 10: 1045-56.

Goncalves GM, Zamboni DS, Camara OS (2010). "The role of innate immunity in septic kidney injuries." *Shock* 34 Suppl 1: 22-6.

Gordon LI, Kwaan HC (1997). "Cancer- and drug-associated thrombotic thrombocytopenic purpura and hemolytic uremic syndrome." *Semin Hemotol* 34: 140-7.

Gurevich F, Parazella MA (2009). "Renal effects of anti-angiogenesis therapy: Update for the internist." *Am J Med* 122(4): 322-8.

Han WK, Bailly V, Abichandani R et al. (2002). "Kidney Injury Molecule-1 (KIM-1): a novel biomarker for human renal proximal tubule injury." *Kidney Int* 62: 237-44.

Han WK, Waikar SS, Johnson A et al. (2008). "Urinary biomarkers in the early diagnosis of acute kidney injury." *Kidney Int* 73(7): 863-9.

Himmelfarb J 2007. 'Continuous renal replacement therapy in the treatment of acute renal failure: critical assessment is required." *Clin J Am Soc Nephrol* 2: 385-9.

Himmelfaub J, Ikizler TA (2007). "Acute kidney injury: changing lexicography, definitions, and epidemiology." *Kidney Int* 71(10): 971-6.

Ichimura T, Bonventre JV, Bailly V et al. (1998). "Kidney injury molecule-1 (KIM-1), a putative epitherial adhesion molecule containing a novel immunoglobulin domain, is up-regulated in renal cell after injury." *J Biol Chem* 273: 4135-42.

Jasek AM, Day HJ (1994). "Acute spontaneous tumor lysis syndrome." *Am J Hematol* 47: 129-31.

John R, Herzenberg AM (2009). "Renal toxity of therapeutic drugs." *J Clin Pathol* 62: 505-15.

Kalantarinia K (2009). "Novel imaging techniques in acute kidney injury." *Curr Drug Targets* 10(12): 1184-9.

Kamijo A, Sugaya T, Hikawa A et al. (2004). "Urinary excretion of fatty acid-binding protein reflects stress overload on the proximal tubules." *Am J Pathol* 165: 1243-55.

Kapoor M, Chan GZ (2001). "Malignancy and renal disease." *Crit Care Clin* 17: 571-98.

Kwaan HC, Gordon LI (2001). "Thrombotic microangiopathy in the cancer patient." *Acta Haematol* 106: 52-6.

Kwitkowski VE, Prowell TM, Ibrahim A (2010). "FDA approval summary: temsirolimus as treatment for advanced renal cell carcinoma" *Oncologist* 15(4): 428-35.

Lamaire N, Adam A, Becker CR et al. (2006). 'CIN Consensus Working Panel. Baseline renal function screening. *Am J Cardiol* 98: 21K-26K.

Lameire N, Van Biesen W, Vanholder R (2010). "Electrolyte disturbances and acute kidney injury in patients with cancer." *Semin Nephrol* 30(6): 534-47.

Lanore JJ, Brunet E, Pochard F et al. (1991). "Hemodialysis for acute renal failure in patients with hematological malignancies." *Crit Care Med* 19: 346-51.

Li M, Khan AM, Maderdrut JL et al. (2010). "The effect of PACAP38 on MyD88-mediated signal transduction in ischemia/hypoxia-induced acute kidney injury." *Am J Nephrol* 32(6): 522-32.

Lin CJ, Lim KH, Cheng YC et al. (2007). "Tumor lysis syndrome after treatment with gemcitabine for metastatic transitional cell carcinoma." *Med Oncol* 24(4): 455-7.

Malyszko J (2010). "Biomarkers of acute kidney injury in different clinical settings: A time to change the paradigm?" *Kidney Blood Res* 33: 368-82.

Mehta RL, Kellum JA, Shah SV et al. (2007). "Acute Kidney Injury Network: report on an initiative to improve outcomes in acute kidney injury." *Crit Care* 11: R31.

Melnikov VY, Ecder T, Fantuzzi G et al. (2001). "Impaired IL-18 processing protects caspase-1 deficient mice from ischemic acute renal failure." *J Clin Invest* 107: 1145-52.

Melnikov VY, Faubel S, Siegmund B et al. (2002). "Neutrophil-independent mechanisms of caspase-1 and IL-18-mediated ischemic acute tubular necrosis in mice." *J Clin Invest* 110: 1083-91.

Mishra J, Dent C, Tarabishi R et al. (2005). "Neutrophil gelatinase-associated lipocalin (NGAL) as a biomarker for acute kidney injury after cardiac surgery." *Lancet* 365: 1231-8.

Moore E, Bellomo R, Nichol A (2010). "Biomarkers of acute kidney injury in anesthesia, intensive care and major surgery: from the bench to clinical research to clinical practice." *Minerva Anestesiologica* 76(6): 425-40.

Mori K, Lee HT, Rapoport D et al. (2005). "Endocytic delivery of lipocalin-siderophore-ion complex rescues the kidney from ischemia-perfusion injury." *J Clin Invest* 115: 610-21.

Nakamura T, Sugaya T, Koide H. (2009). "Urinary liver-type fatty acid binding protein in septic shock: effect on polymyxin B-immobilized fiber hemoperfusion." *Shock* 31: 454-9.

Noiri E, Doi K, Negishi K et al. (2009). " Urinary fatty acid-binding protein-1: An early predictive biomarker of kidney injury." *Am J Physiol Renal Physiol* 296: F669-79.

Nolan CR 3rd., Anger MS, Kelleher SP (1986). "Eosinophiluria - a new method of detection and definition of the clinical spectrum." *N Engl J Med* 315: 1516-9.

Oleksowicz L, Bhagwati N, DeLeon-Fernandez M (1999). "Deficient activity on von Willebrand's factor-cleaving protease in patients with disseminated malignancies." *Cancer Res* 59: 2244-50.

Palevsky P, Zhang J, O'Connor T, Chertw G et al. (2008). "Intensity of renal support in critically ill patients with acute kidney injury." *N Engl J Med* 359: 7-20.

Parikh CR, Jani A, Melnikov VY et al. (2004). "Urinary interleukin-18 is a marker of human acute tubular necrosis." *Am J Kidney Dis* 43: 405-14.

Payen D, de Pont A, Sakr Y et al. (2008). "A positive fluid balance is associated with worse outcome in patients with acute renal failure." *Crit Care* 12: R74.

Penne F, Vignau C, Auburtin M et al. (2005). "Outcome of severe adult thrombotic microangiopathies in the intensive care unit." *Intensive Care Med* 31: 71-8.

Persons DA, Garst J, Vollmer R et al. (1998). "Tumor lysis syndrome and acute renal failure after treatment of non-small cell lung carcinoma with combination irinotecan and cisplatin." *Am J Clin Oncol* 21(4): 426-9.

Portilla D, Dent C, Sugaya T et al. (2008). "Liver fatty acid-binding protein as a biomarker of acute kidney injury after cardiac surgery." *Kidney Int* 73: 465-72.

Rock GA, Shumak KH, Buskard NA et al (1991). "Comparison of plasma exchange with plasma infusion in the treatment of thrombotic thrombocytopenic purpura. Canadian Apheresis Group." *N Engl J Med* 325: 393-7.

Ronco C, Bellomo R, Homel P et al. (2000). "Effects of different doses in continuous veno-venous hemofiltration on outcomes of acute renal failure: a prospective randomized trial." *Lancet* 356: 26-30.

Rossert J (2000). "Drug-induced acute interstitial nephritis." *Kidney Int* 60: 804-17.

Rudnik MR, Kesselheim A, Goldfarb S (2006). "Contrast-induced nephropathy: how it develops, how to prevent it." *Cleve Clin Med* 73: 75-7.

Saudan P, Niederberger M, De Seigneux et al. (2006). "Adding a dialysis dose to continuous hemofiltration increases survival in patients with acute renal failure." *Kidney Int* 70: 1312-7.

Schiffl H, Lang S, Fischer R (2002). "Daily hemodialysis and outcome of acute renal failure." *Nephron Clin Pract* 107: c163-9.

Schmidt-Ott KM, Mori K, Kalandadze A (2006). "Neutrophil gelatinase associated lipocalin-mediated iron traffic kidney epithelia." *Curr Opin Nephrol Hypertens* 15: 442-9.

Schuchter LM, Hensley ML, Meropol NJ et al. (2002). "2002 update of recommendations for the use of chemotherapy and radiotherapy protectants: clinical practice guidelines of American Society of Clinical Oncology." *J Clin Oncol* 20: 2895-2903.

Shimizu-Tokiwa A, Kobata M, Io H et al. (2002). "Serum cystatin C is a more sensitive marker of glomerular function than serum creatinine." *Nephron* 92(1): 224-6.

Srisawat N, Hoste EEA, Kellum JA (2010). "Modern classification of acute kidney injury" *Blood Purif* 29: 300-7.

Sternberg CN, Yagoda A, Scher HI et al. (1989) "Methotrexate, vinblastine, doxorubicin, and cisplatin for advanced transitional cell carcinoma of the urothelium. Efficacy and patterns of response and relapse." *Cancer* 64: 2448-58.

Tanji N, Ozawa A, Miura N et al. (2010). 'Long-term results of combined chemotherapy with gemcitabine and cisplatin for metastatic urothelial carcinomas. *Int J Clin Oncol* 15: 369-75.

Tanji N, Yokoyama M (2011). "Treatment of metastatic renal cell carcinoma and renal pelvic cancer." *Clin Exp Nephrol* 15: 331-8.

Tannock I, Gospodarowicz M, Connolly J et al. (1989) 'M-VAC (methotrexate, vinblastine, doxorubicin and cisplatin) chemotherapy for transitional cell carcinoma: the Princess Margaret Hospital experience. *J Urol*: 142: 289-92.

Tolwani A, Campbell R, Stofan B et al. (2008). "Standard versus high-dose CVVHDF for ICU related acute renal failure." *J Am Soc Nephrol* 19: 1233-8.

Villa P, Jimenez M, Soriano MC et al. (2005). "Serum cystatin C concentration as a marker of acute renal dysfunction in critically ill patients." *Crit Care* 9: R139-43.

Vogt B, Ferrari P, Schonholzer C et al. (2001). "Prophylactic hemodialysis after radiocontrast media in patients with renal insufficiency is potentially harmful." *Am J Med* 111: 629-38.

Zager RA, O'Quigley J, Zager BK et al. (1989). ''Acute renal failure following bone marrow transplantation: a retrospective study of 272 patients.'' *Am J Kidney Dis* 13: 210-6.

von der Maase H, Hansen SW, Roberts SW et al. (2000). 'Gemcitabine and cisplatin versus methotrexate, vinblastine, doxorubicin, and cisplatin in advanced or metastatic bladder cancer: results of large, randomized, multinational, multicenter, phase III study. *J Clin Oncol* 18: 3068-77.

# 12

# Chronic Kidney Disease Update

Waqar H. Kazmi and Khurram Danial
*Karachi Medical & Dental College, Abbasi Shaheed Hospital, Karachi*
*Pakistan*

## 1. Introduction

Chronic kidney disease (CKD) is a worldwide public health issue. In the United States there is a rising incidence and prevalence of kidney failure with poor outcomes and high cost. Most chronic nephropathies are characterized by a progressive course that leads, at a variable rate, to loss of kidney function and the need for renal replacement therapy. The progression of CKD typically moves through phases from initial diminution of renal reserve to mild, moderate and severe reductions in glomerular filtration rate (GFR), to end-stage renal disease (ESRD). There is growing evidence that some of the adverse outcomes of CKD can be prevented or delayed by preventive measures, early detection and treatment.

## 2. Definitions and classification

The definition and classification of CKD may help identify affected patients, possibly resulting in the early institution of effective therapy. To achieve this goal, guidelines were proposed from the National Kidney Foundation of the United States through its Kidney Disease Outcomes Quality Initiative (K/DOQI) program (National kidney Foundation [NKF], 2002). These guidelines have been reviewed and accepted internationally (Levey et al., 2005; Uhlig et al., 2005; Levin et al., 2008).
The K/DOQI working group defined CKD in adults as:

- Evidence of structural or functional kidney abnormalities (abnormal urinalysis, imaging studies, or histology) that persist for at least three months, with or without a decreased GFR. The most common manifestation of kidney damage is persistent albuminuria, including microalbuminuria.
  OR
- Decreased GFR (as defined by a GFR of less than 60 ml/min per 1.73 $m^2$), with or without evidence of kidney damage.

Based upon these definitions, the following is the recommended classification of CKD by stage and the estimated prevalence within the United States of each stage, as determined by a National Health and Nutrition Examination Survey (NHANES) performed in 1999 to 2004 (KDOQI, 2002; Coresh et al., 2003; Levey et al., 2003; Coresh et al., 2005; MMWR, 2007; Coresh et al, 2007).

- Stage 1 disease is defined by a normal GFR (greater than 90 ml/min per 1.73 $m^2$) and persistent albuminuria (1.8 percent of the total United States population)
- Stage 2 disease is a GFR between 60 to 89 ml/min per 1.73 $m^2$ and persistent albuminuria (3.2 percent)

- Stage 3 disease is a GFR between 30 and 59 ml/min per 1.73 $m^2$ (7.7 percent)
- Stage 4 disease is a GFR between 15 and 29 ml/min per 1.73 $m^2$ (0.21 percent)
- Stage 5 disease is a GFR of less than 15 ml/min per 1.73 $m^2$ or ESRD (2.4 percent for stages.)

### 2.1 Estimation of glomerular filtration rate (GFR)

Patients with kidney disease may have a variety of different clinical presentations. Some have symptoms that are directly referable to the kidney (gross hematuria,or flank pain), or to extrarenal symptoms (edema, hypertension, signs of uremia). Many patients, however, are asymptomatic and are noted during routine examination to have an elevated serum creatinine concentration, or an abnormal urinalysis.

Once kidney disease is discovered, the presence or degree of kidney dysfunction and rapidity of progression are assessed, and the underlying disorder is diagnosed. Although the history and physical examination can be helpful, the most useful information is initially obtained from estimation of the GFR and examination of the urinary sediment.

Estimation of the GFR is used clinically to assess the degree of kidney impairment and to follow the course of the disease. However, the GFR provides no information on the cause of the kidney disease. This is achieved by the urinalysis, measurement of urinary protein excretion, and, if necessary, radiologic studies and/or kidney biopsy.

### 2.2 Laboratory measurement for diagnosis of CKD

#### 2.2.1 For all patients at increased risk for CKD

- Serum creatinine to estimate GFR;
- Albumin-to-creatinine or protein-to-creatinine ratio in a first-morning or random untimed 'spot' urine specimen;
- Examination of the urine sediment or dipstick for red bloodcells and white blood cells.

#### 2.2.2 For patients found to have CKD

- Imaging of the kidneys, usually by ultrasound;
- Serum electrolytes (sodium, potassium, chloride and bicarbonate)

#### 2.2.3 Estimation of GFR

Once kidney disease is discovered, the presence or degree of kidney dysfunction and rapidity of progression are assessed, and the underlying disorder is diagnosed. Early identification of patients with CKD would allow treatment that could slow the progression to ESRD, improve clinical outcomes, and constrain the growth of costs in the ESRD program. Although the history and physical examination can be helpful, the most useful information is initially obtained from estimation of the GFR and examination of the urinary sediment.

Estimation of the GFR is used clinically to assess the degree of kidney impairment and to follow the course of the disease. However, the GFR provides no information on the cause of the kidney disease. This is achieved by the urinalysis, measurement of urinary protein excretion, and, if necessary, radiologic studies and/or kidney biopsy.

The GFR is equal to the sum of the filtration rates in all of the functioning nephrons, thus, estimation of the GFR gives an approximate measure of the number of functioning nephrons. GFR cannot be measured directly. Instead it is measured as the urinary clearance of an ideal filtration marker.

The most reliable assessment of GFR is based on the measurement of kidney clearance of a filtration marker such as Inulin which is a physiologically inert substance that is freely filtered at the glomerulus, and is neither secreted, reabsorbed, synthesized, nor metabolized by the kidney (Rahn et al., 1999). Thus, the amount of inulin filtered at the glomerulus is equal to the amount excreted in the urine, which can be measured. Inulin, however, is in short supply, expensive, and difficult to assay and is not suitable for routine clinical practice, and is cumbersome even for clinical research. Furthermore, the classic protocol for measuring inulin clearance requires a continuous intravenous infusion, multiple blood samples, and bladder catheterization.

Various less cumbersome methods for measuring clearance are available: using alternative filtration markers (such as radioactive or non-radioactive iothalamate, iohexol, DTPA, or EDTA), bolus administration of the marker (subcutaneous or intravenous), spontaneous bladder emptying, and plasma clearance (Rahn et al., 1999; Levey, 1990; Brandstrom et al., 1998). While these methods are simpler, all have disadvantages that limit their application in clinical practice and affect the interpretation of research studies.

In the United States, the most common methods utilized to estimate the GFR are the serum creatinine concentration, the creatinine clearance, or estimation equations based upon the serum creatinine: such as the Cockcroft-Gault equation and Modification of Diet in Renal Disease (MDRD) Study equations.

The K/DOQI guidelines classified patients by CKD stage, which is defined in part by the estimated GFR (table 1). The GFR should be estimated from the MDRD and Cockcroft-Gault equations, which take into account the serum creatinine concentration, and some or all of the following variables: age, gender, race, and body size.

The Cockcroft-Gault formula estimates creatinine clearance in milliliters per minute, and the MDRD equation estimates GFR in milliliters per minute per 1.73 $m^2$, and this difference should be kept in mind when comparing their outputs. However, the estimation equations have not been validated, and may be less accurate, in some populations. These include individuals with high, normal, or near-normal renal function, children, certain ethnic groups, pregnant women, and those with unusual muscle mass, body habitus, and weight (eg, morbid obesity or malnourished). Some, therefore, recommend measuring the creatinine clearance to estimate the GFR in these patients with stable renal function. Most patients with CKD stages 3 to 5 progress relentlessly to ESRD. A straight-line relationship is often found between the reciprocal of serum creatinine (1/SCr) values or the estimated GFR and time. The rate of progression of CKD varies according to the underlying nephropathy and how the kidney responds to injury.

Because of the problems with changes in creatinine production and secretion, other endogenous compounds have been evaluated in an effort to provide a more accurate estimation of GFR including symmetric dimethylarginine (Kielstein et al., 2006) and cystatin C. Perhaps the best studied and most promising is cystatin C, a low molecular weight protein, that is a member of the cystatin superfamily of cysteine protease inhibitors. Cystatin C is filtered at the glomerulus and not reabsorbed. However, it is metabolized in the tubules, which prevents use of cystatin C to directly measure clearance.

Cystatin C is thought to be produced by all nucleated cells; its rate of production has been thought to be relatively constant, and not affected by changes in diet, although this is not proven. Cystatin C has been purported to be unaffected by gender, age or muscle mass. However, higher cystatin C levels have now been associated with male gender, greater height and weight, and higher lean body mass (Knight et al., 2004; Groesbeck et al., 2008;

Macdonald et al., 2006). Cystatin C levels increase sharply with age (Knight et al., 2004). Analysis of a sub-sample of 7596 participants drawn from National Health and Nutrition Examination Survey III (NHANES III) revealed that more than 50 percent of individuals over age 80 have an elevated cystatin C level, and non-Hispanic whites and males have higher levels of cystatin C (Kottgen et al., 2008). These data were not adjusted for GFR; therefore, it is unclear whether they are related to different levels of kidney function among the populations, or difference in the non-GFR determinants of cystatin C. In addition, cystatin is affected by hyper- and hypothyroidism, and has been correlated with markers of inflammation (C-reactive protein), body size (in particular fat mass), and diabetes (Manetti et al., 2005; Stevens et al., 2009). Together, these data suggest that levels of cystatin C are affected by factors other than GFR.

Although reference ranges have been reported, there is no current standard for serum cystatin C measurements (Shlipak et al., 2005; Mussap & Plebani, 2004). In addition, testing for cystatin C is only available in a limited number of laboratories.

The serum cystatin C concentration may correlate more closely with the GFR than the serum creatinine concentration (Newman et al., 1995; Coll et al., 2000; Fliser & Ritz, 2001; Mussap et al., 2002; Ahlstrom et al., 2004; Hoek et al., 2003; Dharnidharka et al., 2002; Poge et al., 2006; Stevens et al., 2008). In multiple studies, serum cystatin C was more sensitive in identifying mild reductions in kidney function than serum creatinine (Coll et al., 2000; Hoek et al., 2003; Dharnidharka et al., 2002). Using the clearance of radioactive iothalamate as the gold standard, serum cystatin C levels began increasing at GFR levels of approximately 90 mL/min per 1.73 $m^2$, while the serum creatinine only increased when the GFR was approximately 70 mL/min per 1.73 $m^2$. Whether cystatin C correlates better with GFR than serum creatinine in patients with diabetic nephropathy is unclear (Oddoze et al., 2001; Perkins et al., 2005).

Estimation equations based on serum cystatin C have also been formulated (Grubb et al., 2005; Sjostrom et al., 2005; Grubb et al., 2005). It has been proposed that cystatin C-based equations would be more accurate in populations with lower creatinine production, such as the elderly, children, renal transplant recipients, or patients with cirrhosis (White et al., 2005; Poge et al., 2006). In one study of over 3000 patients with known CKD, an equation for the estimated GFR based upon cystatin C was nearly as accurate as GFR estimated from the serum creatinine adjusted for age, sex, and race when compared to GFR measured by iothalamate clearance (Stevens et al., 2008). The addition of age, sex and race to cystatin C reduced bias in some subgroups defined by these variables, and an equation that uses both serum creatinine and cystatin C with age, sex and race was better than equations that used only one of these markers.

Steroid use may affect cystatin C levels, therefore, limiting its use in transplant recipients. As an example, for the same level of cystatin C, measured GFR was 19 percent higher in transplant recipients than in patients with native kidney disease.

Although cystatin C appears to be more accurate for the assessment of GFR than serum creatinine in certain populations, whether measurement of cystatin C levels will improve patient care is at present unknown [Deinum & Derkx, 2000).

### 2.3 Markers of kidney damage

Markers of kidney damage include proteinuria, hematuria, and other abnormalities of the urinary sediment, and radiologic evidence of damage. The most common cause of CKD in adults are diabetes and hypertension, and, therefore, the most common marker for kidney damage is increased excretion of protein, and specifically of albumin. Measurement of protein excretion is useful in a variety of clinical settings, particularly to establish the diagnosis and to follow the course of glomerular disease.

In normal subjects, low molecular weight proteins and small amounts of albumin are filtered. The actual amount of albumin filtered each day in humans is controversial. The majority view is that no more than about 2 to 4 g of albumin per day are filtered normally, but some investigators claim that as much as 200 g of albumin are filtered each day (with the bulk of this filtered albumin "reclaimed" in the early proximal tubule) (Russo et al., 2007). The filtered proteins enter the proximal tubule where they are almost completely reabsorbed and then catabolized by the proximal tubular cells. Some of the catabolized proteins (including albumin) are excreted as peptides in the urine. These are not detected by dipstick or the immuno-nephelometric albumin-specific assays, but are detected by chromatographic assays. The net result is the normal daily protein excretion of less than 150 mg (usually 40 to 80 mg), of which approximately about 4 to 7 mg is intact, immuno-reactive albumin.

Previously, abnormal proteinuria was generally defined as the excretion of more than 150 mg of protein per day. However, it is now clear that early renal disease is reflected by lesser degrees of proteinuria, particularly increased amounts of albuminuria.

The normal rate of albumin excretion is less than 20 mg/day (15 µg/min); the rate is about 4 to 7 mg/day in healthy young adults and increases with age and with an increase in body weight. Persistent albumin excretion between 30 and 300 mg/day (20 to 200 µg/min) is called microalbuminuria. In patients with diabetes, this is usually indicative of incipient diabetic nephropathy (unless there is some co-existent renal disease). In non-diabetics, the presence of microalbuminuria is associated with cardiovascular disease.Values above 300 mg/day (200 µg/min) are considered to represent overt proteinuria or macroalbuminuria, the level at which the standard dipstick becomes positive. At this level, practically all protein in the urine consists of albumin.

The standard urinary dipstick measures albumin concentration via a colorimetric reaction between albumin and tetrabromophenol blue producing different shades of green according to the concentration of albumin in the sample

- Negative
- Trace — between 15 and 30 mg/dl
- 1+ — between 30 and 100 mg/dl
- 2+ — between 100 and 300 mg/dl
- 3+ — between 300 and 1000 mg/dl
- 4+ — >1000 mg/dl

The urine dipstick is, therefore, not very accurate in assessing the severity of proteinuria since the protein concentration is a function of urine volume as well as the quantity of protein present. As an example, suppose a patient excretes 500 mg of protein per day. If the urine volume is two liters, the protein concentration will be 25 mg/dl, resulting in a trace to 1+ findings on the dipstick. However, if the urine volume is only 500 ml, the protein concentration will be 100 mg/dl and the dipstick will read 2+.

The urine dipstick is also a relatively insensitive marker for initial increases in protein excretion, not generally becoming positive until protein excretion exceeds 300 to 500 mg/day. Limited data suggest that the combination of specific gravity plus dipstick proteinuria may significantly improve the ability to detect proteinuria (Constantiner et al., 2005).

The dipstick may also be insufficiently sensitive in multiple myeloma. Given that the dipstick primarily detects urinary albumin, it may be negative in patients with multiple myeloma who may excrete relatively large amounts of monoclonal immunoglobulin light chains. In contrast, testing the urine with sulfosalicylic acid will detect all proteins, as evidenced by the degree of turbidity (Rose, 1987). As a result, any patient with unexplained renal failure, a benign urine sediment, and a negative dipstick for protein should have the urine tested with sulfosalicylic acid. A positive finding suggests the presence of non-albumin proteins in the urine, which in adults usually represents immunoglobulin light chains.

The accurate measurement of protein excretion in the urine can be performed by several different techniques. The gold standard for measurement of protein excretion is a 24 hour urine collection, with the normal value being less than 150 mg/day. However, an adequate collection must be ensured. This is cumbersome for patients and physicians; thus, measurement on random specimens has become an accepted alternative method.

The preferred method of measuring urinary protein excretion in patients with proteinuria is either the total protein-to-creatinine ratio or albumin-to-creatinine ratio for microalbuminuria on a random urine specimen (Eknoyan et al., 2003; KDOQI, 2002).

These ratios on a random urine specimen correlate fairly closely with daily protein excretion in g/1.73 $m^2$ of body surface area (Ginsberg et al., 1983; Schwab et al., 1987; Abitbol et al., 1990; Steinhauslin & Wauters, 1995; Chitalia et al., 2001; Zelmanovitz et al., 1997; Bakker, 1999). Thus, a ratio of 4.9 (as with respective urinary protein and creatinine concentrations of 210 and 43 mg/dl) represents daily protein excretion of approximately 4.9 g/1.73 $m^2$.

The accuracy of the ratio is diminished when creatinine excretion is either markedly increased in a muscular man (the ratio will underestimate proteinuria) or markedly reduced in a cachectic patient (the ratio will overestimate proteinuria).

Because of this markedly increased convenience, the total protein-to-creatinine ratio or albumin-to-creatinine ratio are preferred to the 24 hour urine collection for quantitative measurement of significant urinary protein. First morning specimens are preferred, but random daytime specimens are acceptable if first morning specimens are not available (Witte et al., 2009). Specimens obtained in the evening or overnight appear to be least accurate.

The range of the urinary albumin-to-creatinine ratio with microalbuminuria varies by gender, being 20 to 200 mg/g and 30 to 300 mg/g for males and females, respectively. This is a result of the higher muscle mass observed in males.

Hematuria or pyuria originating in the renal parenchyma, glycosuria in the absence of hyperglycemia, and abnormal radiologic or pathologic studies are others diagnostic criteria for CKD.

## 3. Natural history of CKD

The kidney is able to adapt to damage by increasing the filtration rate in the remaining normal nephrons, a process called adaptive hyperfiltration. As a result, the patient with mild renal insufficiency often has a normal or near-normal serum creatinine concentration. Additional homeostatic mechanisms (most frequently occurring within the renal tubules) permit the serum concentrations of sodium, potassium, calcium, and phosphorous and the total body water to also remain within the normal range, particularly among those with mild to moderate renal failure. Adaptive hyperfiltration, although initially beneficial, appears to result in long-term damage to the glomeruli of the remaining nephrons, which is manifested by proteinuria and progressive renal insufficiency. This process appears to be responsible for the development of renal failure among those in whom the original illness is either inactive or cured (Abboud & Henrich, 2010). The institution of measures to help prevent this process, such as antihypertensive therapy with an angiotensin converting enzyme inhibitor or an angiotensin II receptor blocker, may slow progressive disease and even preserve renal function. If these modalities are effective, the benefit is likely to be greatest if begun before a great deal of irreversible scarring has occurred.

Not all individuals have progressive loss of kidney function. Some studies show a high rate of progression, while others report relatively stable disease (Sarnak et al., 2005; Eriksen & Ingebretsen, 2006; Hallan et al., 2006). The rate of progression of CKD from one major stage to another varies based upon the underlying disease, presence or absence of comorbid conditions, treatments, socioeconomic status, individual genetics, ethnicity, and other factors.

Using epidemiologic data, general estimates for the rate of transition from a GFR between 15 to 60 ml/min per 1.73 $m^2$ to end stage disease may be approximately 1.5 percent per year, while the rate of transition from a GFR above 60 to below 60 ml/min per 1.73 $m^2$ may be approximately 0.5 percent per year (Hsu et al., 2004; Fox et al., 2004).

Historically, rate of decline in GFR of patients with diabetic nephropathy (DN) has been among the fastest, averaging about 10 ml/min/year. Control of systemic hypertension slows the rate of GFR decline to 5ml/min/year. In non-diabetic nephropathy, the rate of progression of CKD was 2.5 times faster in patients with chronic glumerulonephritis than in those with chronic interstitial nephritis, and 1.5 times faster than in those with hypertensive nephrosclerosis. Polycystic kidney disease (PKD) and impaired renal function may also have a faster rate of progression compared to those with other nephropathies.

## 4. Prevalence of chronic kidney disease

The prevalence of CKD has been evaluated based on serum creatinine concentrations and microalbuminuria in the following population studies from the United States, as well as some other countries.

In the Third National Health and Nutrition Examination Survey (NHANES III), serum creatinine concentration was obtained in a sample of 18,723 individuals aged 12 years and older between 1988 and 1994 (Jones et al., 1998). The prevalence of a serum creatinine level at or above 1.5, 1.7, and 2.0 mg/dl was 5.0, 1.9, and 0.6 percent for men, respectively, and 1.6, 0.7, and 0.3 percent for women.

By extrapolating the results of the NHANES III to the 1990 US Census population, it was estimated that the number of people with serum creatinine at or above 1.5, 1.7, and 2.0 mg/dl is 6.2, 2.5, and 0.8 million, respectively. It should be noted, however, that only a single creatinine measurement per patient was used to estimate the prevalence of CKD, and that serum creatinine was available in only 31 percent of the potentially eligible sample.

In a study of nearly 200,000 patients enrolled in a large health maintenance organization (HMO) in the southwestern US in 1997, the prevalence of at least one gender specific elevated serum creatinine (>1.2 mg/dl in women and >1.4 mg/dl in men) was 3.7 percent, and of at least two elevated serum creatinine levels separated by at least 90 days was 1.7 percent (Nissenson et al., 2001).

The prevalence estimates from this HMO study, as applied to United States Census data, led to the estimate of 9.1 million Americans in 1990 who had at least one elevated serum creatinine concentration, and 4.2 million Americans who had at least two elevated creatinine values separated by 90 days or greater.

The prevalence of CKD in Norway was estimated from a population-based health survey of Nord-Trondelag County (HUNT II), which included 65,181 adults in 1995 through 1997 (participation rate 70.4%) (Erikson & Ingebretsen, 2006). The primary analysis used gender-specific cutoffs in estimating persistent albuminuria for CKD stages 1 and 2. Total CKD prevalence in Norway was 10.2% (SE 0.5): CKD stage 1 (GFR>90 ml/min per 1.73 $m^2$ and albuminuria), 2.7% (SE 0.3); stage 2 (GFR 60 89 ml/min per 1.73 $m^2$ and albuminuria), 3.2% (SE 0.4); stage 3 (GFR 30 to 59 ml/min per 1.73 $m^2$, 4.2% (SE 0.1); and stage 4 (GFR 15 to 29 ml/min per 1.73 $m^2$, 0.2% (SE 0.01).

Forty two percent of men and 44 percent of women over the age of 85 had an MDRD-estimated GFR less than 60 ml/min per 1.73 $m^2$ in the Nijmegen Biomedical Study, a population-based cross-sectional study conducted in the eastern part of the Netherlands. In a report from Taiwan, the prevalence of an estimated GFR <60 ml/min per 1.73 $m^2$ was 7 % (Hsu et al., 2006).

In a population-based survey from Pakistan, Kazmi et al have reported the prevalence of CKD stages 3 and 4 to be about 21 million (Kazmi et al., 2007).

| Stage | Description | GFR (ml/min/1.73$m^2$) |
|---|---|---|
| 1 | Kidney damage with normal GFR | 90 or more |
| 2 | Mildly deceased GFR | 60 - 89 |
| 3 | Moderately decreased GFR | 30 - 59 |
| 4 | Severely decreased GFR | 15 - 29 |
| 5 | Advanced kidney failure requiring dialysis/kidney transplant | < 15 |

Table 1. National Kidney Foundation K/DOQI Classification of Chronic Kidney Disease based on GFR levels.

## 5. Screening for chronic kidney disease

The NKF-K/DOQI guidelines for CKD, which have been reviewed and endorsed by the 2006 Kidney Disease Improving Global Outcomes (KDIGO) Controversies Conference, recommend that all individuals should be assessed as part of routine health examinations to determine whether they are at increased risk for developing CKD (KDOQI, 2002).

Some data suggest, however, that screening the general population may decrease the incidence of ESRD resulting from glomerulonephritis. However, screening the general population is unlikely to be cost-effective. Screening for CKD among select patients who are at risk for development of CKD is justified because therapeutic interventions may slow or prevent the progression toward ESRD. Such patients include those with a history of diabetes, cardiovascular disease, hypertension, hyperlipidemia, obesity, metabolic syndrome, smoking, HIV or hepatitis C virus infection, and malignancy. A family history of CKD, age >60 years and treatment with potentially nephrotoxic drugs should also prompt screening for CKD. Testing for CKD can be done with a urinalysis, a first morning or a random "spot" urine sample for albumin or protein and creatinine assessment, and a serum creatinine level. Depending upon the presence of particular risk factors, additional testing such as renal ultrasonography may be required, such as in patients with a family history of polycystic kidney disease. Once the diagnosis is established and the cause and/or potentially reversible factors are identified and treated, CKD should be staged according to the classification proposed by the NKF-K/DOQI.

## 6. Mechanisms of progression of chronic kidney disease

Regardless of the nature of the underlying nephropathy, the progression of CKD is associated with the progressive sclerosis of glomeruli, tubulointerstitial fibrosis, and vascular sclerosis which can be initiated by endothelial, mesangial, or epithelial cell injury or damage. The kidney responds to injury by adaptive changes that lead to remodeling evolving towards either healing and functional recovery or scarring with loss of kidney function and progressive CKD. Healing is characterized by recovery of kidney function and structure. It occurs primarily in AKI when acutely damaged tubules recover from the initial insult and replace lost tubular cells to reconstitute the integrity of the tubules and to restore kidney function.

On the other hand, most forms of chronic kidney damage, such as those induced by diabetes, hypertension, chronic glomerulonephritis, or chronic exposure to infections, evolve to progressive scarring with loss of function and CKD. Scarring is characterized by progressive loss of intrinsic renal cells and their replacement by fibrous tissue made of collagenous extracellular matrix.

Within glomerular capillaries, endothelial cells are the first to be exposed to damage induced by hemodynamic, immunologic, or metabolic insults. Glomerular endothelial injury is associated with reduction or loss of their physiologic anticoagulant and anti-inflammatory properties and the acquisition of procoagulant and inflammatory characteristics.

Glomerular endothelial injury can induce proliferation, phenotype change (expression of adhesion molecules), release of vasoactive agents (endothelin, nitric oxide), infiltration of glomerular tufts by inflammatory cells and conversion to a prothrombotic state. Glomerular endothelial injury is characterized by proliferation, apoptosis, detachment, and (particularly) thrombosis.

Mesangial cells are the glomerular capillary equivalent to the smooth muscle cells and in that capacity respond to injury in a similar fashion; death, transformation, proliferation, and migration as well as synthesis and deposition of extracellular matrix.

The mesangial response to injury is characterized by alterations in cell cycle proteins that favor cell proliferation, phenotype change (to an actin positive myofibroblast), extracellular matrix production, and apoptosis. Many of these effects involve agonist interaction with specific receptors on the mesangial cell, including receptors for IgA, toll-like receptors, and transferrin receptors. Platelet derived growth factor (PDGF) appears to be the principal mediator of mesangial cell migration and proliferation in glomerular disease, an effect possibly magnified in hypoxic conditions. Receptors for PDGF are also upregulated. Further support for a role for PDGF is provided by a study that demonstrated prevention of renal scarring by antagonism of PDGF in an animal model of glomerulonephritis.

Mesangial cell proliferation is associated with the increased expression of cyclin-dependent kinases and reduced expression of cyclin kinase inhibitors, such as P21 and P27. Mesangial cell proliferation is an essential precursor to subsequent mesangial matrix expansion and sclerosis, due primarily to the actions of TGF and CTGF. Increased prostanoid synthesis, possibly modulated by TGF, may also have a role in this process. Therapeutic interventions, which target mesangial cell proliferation or matrix production, can therefore greatly ameliorate both acute and chronic forms of glomerular injury in those disorders in which glomerular cell proliferation is prominent.

The relative inability of podocytes to replicate in response to injury may lead to their stretching along the GBM, expressing areas of denuded Glomerular basement membrane (GBM) that would attract and interact with parietal epithelial cells leading to the formation of capsular adhesions and subsequent segmental glomerulosclerosis. This may lead to the accumulation of amorphous material in the paraglomerular space and the subsequent disruption of glomerular-tubular junction resulting in atubular glomeruli.

### 6.1 Extrinsic cells

**Neutrophils:** Neutrophils are present in the early biopsies of patients with post-streptococcal glomerulonephritis (GN), membranoproliferative GN, Henoch-Schönlein purpura (HSP), systemic lupus erythematosus (SLE), and some forms of rapidly progressive glomerulonephritis (RPGN) [Ishida-Okawara et al., 2004; Tipping & Holdsworth, 2003).

Neutrophil localization in glomerular capillaries is dependent upon the generation of chemotactic factors within and around an inflammatory focus; the most prominent chemo-attractants in glomerular disease are C5a (derived from activation of complement) and several chemokines, such as interleukin-8, which can be bound to endothelial cells via heparan sulfate proteoglycans (Segerer et al., 2000; De Vriese et al., 1999; Kitching et al., 2002; Rops et al., 2004; Johnson et al., 2001; Segerer & Schlondorff, 2007).

Once attracted, neutrophil localization involves the interaction between adhesion molecules expressed on glomerular endothelial cells, such as selectins, integrins (CD11/CD18), and Ig-like molecules (ICAM-1), and their corresponding ligands on the neutrophil (Segerer et al., 2000; De Vriese et al., 1999; Johnson et al., 2001; Ito et al., 2001).

At the site of immune deposit formation, neutrophils phagocytose the immune complex aggregates, become activated and undergo a respiratory burst that generates reactive oxygen species (Johnson et al., 1987). Several studies have shown hydrogen peroxide to be the principal neutrophil-derived oxidant that mediates glomerular injury. Hydrogen peroxide is nephritogenic because of interactions with another neutrophil-derived cationic enzyme myeloperoxidase (MPO) (which also localizes in glomeruli because of charge) and a halide to form hypohalous acids, which halogenate the glomerular capillary wall (Johnson et al., 1987; Johnson et al., 2001).

Neutrophils also store cationic serine proteases, such as elastase and cathepsin G, within azurophilic granules. The activation of neutrophils within glomeruli causes the extracellular release of these proteins, thereby resulting in the degradation of elements of the glomerular capillary wall. MPO and PR3, both cationic proteases localized in the primary granules of neutrophils, are also involved in the pathogenesis of ANCA-positive crescentic glomerulonephritis; they are localized in primary granules and displayed on the cell surface in response to certain cytokines. There they are accessible to ANCA antibody and become activated, resulting in capillary localization and release of oxidants and proteases (Xiao et al., 2005). Evidence in animal models suggests that ANCA-neutrophil interaction also induces release of a complement-activating factor that contributes to the mediation of injury (Huugen et al., 2007; Jennete & Falk, 2008).

**Macrophages:** Macrophages are also prominent constituents of several glomerular lesions, particularly ones that exhibit crescent formation such as RPGN, SLE, and cryoglobulinemic nephropathy (Hooke et al., 1987; Rastaldi et al., 2000; Kurts et al., 2007). The importance of monocytes/macrophages in mediating glomerular injury is well-documented by studies, such as macrophage depletion and inhibition of macrophage inhibitory factor (MIF) (Kurts et al., 2007). The protective effect of absent granulocyte macrophage colony stimulating factor is illustrated in GM-CSF -/- mice, which exhibited less infiltration of monocytes compared to wild type and were protected from crescentic glomerular injury (Timoshanko et al., 2005).

Macrophages localize to glomeruli via interactions with both deposited immunoglobulins (through Fc receptors) and several chemokines, such as macrophage chemo-attractant protein-1 (MCP-1) and macrophage inflammatory protein-1-alpha (MIP-1alpha) and RANTES (Timoshanko et al., 2005; Shimizu et al., 2003). Unlike neutrophils, macrophages are also readily recruited by lymphocyte-derived molecules, such as MIF, that result from the interaction between specifically sensitized T-cells and intraglomerular antigens (Chitalia et al., 2001). In addition, monocytes also localize through interaction with leukocyte adhesion molecules, such as ICAM-1 and VCAM-1, as well as osteopontin (Kurts et al., 2007; Okada et al., 2000).

Thus, macrophages may serve as effector cells in both humoral and cell-mediated forms of immune injury and are presumed to be the principal effector cells in inflammatory glomerular lesions induced by sensitized T-cells in the absence of antibody (Kurts et al., 2007). As with neutrophils, macrophages may generate oxidants and proteases. However, unlike neutrophils, they release tissue factor (which initiates fibrin deposition and crescent formation) and TGF beta (which contributes to the synthesis of extracellular matrix and eventual development of sclerosis).

**T cells:** T cells are rarely conspicuous in glomerular lesions, but can be detected, particularly in diseases primarily mediated by macrophages such as crescentic GN (Tipping & Holdsworth, 2003; Hooke et al., 1987; Kurts et al., 2007). Although there is experimental evidence that glomerular injury can be induced by systemic T-cells in the absence of antibody deposition, little evidence exists that glomerular T-cells alone are nephritogenic, with the exception of permeability factors (Renneke et al., 1994). Instead, T-cell mediated injury occurs primarily via the release of chemokines and recruitment of macrophages, which subsequently function as effector cells. In addition, T cells may be the source of permeability factors that contribute to non-inflammatory glomerular injury (Kurts et al., 2007).

**Platelets:** Platelets are prominent in several glomerular lesions, usually ones that involve intraglomerular thrombosis such as SLE, anti-phospholipid antibody syndromes, and thrombotic microangiopathies. In addition to their role in thrombotic processes involving endothelial cell injury, platelets also release a number of products that participate in and augment glomerular injury, more broadly including vasoactive, mitogenic, and chemotactic substances (Barnes, 2001). For example, platelet-derived factors such as PAF and platelet factor 4 enhance glomerular permeability to proteins and immune complex deposition, and PDGF and TGF contribute to mesangial cell proliferation and sclerosis, respectively. Platelets have also been shown to contribute to neutrophil-mediated glomerular injury through non-chemotactic mechanisms.

### 6.2 Tubulo-interstitial disease (fibrosis)

All forms of CKD are associated with marked tubulointerstitial injury (tubular dilatation, interstitial fibrosis), even if the primary process is a glomerulopathy (Ong & Fine, 1994;

Nath, 1982). Furthermore, the degree of tubulo-interstitial disease is a better predictor of the GFR and long-term prognosis than is the severity of glomerular damage in almost all chronic progressive glomerular diseases, including IgA nephropathy, membranous nephropathy, membranoproliferative glomerulonephritis, and lupus nephritis (Nath, 1982; D'Amico, 1992; Alexopoulos et al., 1990; Bajema et al., 1999; Bazzi et al., 2002; Meyer, 2003). It is possible in these settings that tubulointerstitial disease causes tubular atrophy and/or obstruction, eventually leading to nephron loss.

The mechanism by which tubulointerstitial fibrosis develops is incompletely understood [Alexopoulos et al., 1990; Lan et al., 1991; Eddy, 1994; Nath, 1998). Infiltration of the kidney by macrophage and T lymphocytes (and perhaps bone marrow derived fibroblast-like cells), resulting in the subsequent production of transforming growth factor beta (TGF-beta) and other profibrotic factors, may be central to the development of this process (Lan et al., 1991).

Other possible contributors include calcium phosphate deposition, and metabolic acidosis with secondary interstitial ammonia accumulation.

### 6.3 Angiotensin II

Non-hemodynamic effects of angiotensin II also appear to contribute to the development of tubulointerstitial fibrosis, mediated via one of the angiotensin II type 1 receptors that are present in the glomerulus (Ruiz-Ortega et al., 2006). Animal studies have suggested that activation of angiotensin II receptor type 1B, which is largely limited to the glomerulus, but not type 1A, may accelerate renal injury (Crowly et al., 2009). This effect is likely due to the generation of profibrotic factors such as TGF-beta, connective tissue growth factor, epidermal growth factor, and other chemokines (Aros & Remuzzi, 2002). Further support for this role is provided by the finding that the expression of angiotensin II type 1 receptors in podocytes is associated with focal segmental glomerulosclerosis (Hoffmann et al., 2004). It also appears that renin may lead to a receptor-mediated increase in TGF-beta that is independent of angiotensin II (Huang et al., 2006).

Actions of angiotensin II may also be mediated via epidermal growth factor (EGF) receptors, which are present throughout the nephron, and when stimulated, promote cell proliferation and collagen production via transforming growth factor-alpha (TGF-alpha), EGF, and other growth factors (Lautrette et al., 2005; Chen et al., 2006). In experimental models, infusion of angiotensin II induces glomerulosclerosis and tubular atrophy. This effect is not seen in mice lacking EGF receptors or TGF-alpha, and pharmacologic inhibition of angiotensin II prevented these renal lesions. Angiotensin II also participates in cytokine- and chemokine-mediated recruitment of inflammatory cells into the kidney.

### 6.4 Vascular sclerosis

Vascular sclerosis is an integral feature of the renal scarring process. Renal arteriolar hyalinosis is present in CKD at an early stage, even in the absence of severe hypertension. Vascular sclerosis is associated with progressive renal failure in glomerulonephritis. Hyalinosis of afferent arterioles has been implicated in the pathogenesis of diabetic glomerulosclerosis. Changes in postglomerular arterioles and damage to peritubular capillaries may further exacerbate interstitial ischemia and fibrosis. Ischemia and the ensuing hypoxia are fibrogenic influences that stimulate tubular cells and renal fibroblast to produce ECM components and reduce their collagenolytic activity.

## 7. Factors affecting progression of chronic kidney disease

A variety of chronic kidney diseases progress to ESRD, including chronic glomerulonephritis, diabetic nephropathy, and polycystic kidney disease. Although the underlying problem often cannot be treated, extensive studies in experimental animals and humans suggest that progression in CKD may be largely due to secondary factors that are sometimes unrelated to the activity of the initial disease. These include systemic and intraglomerular hypertension, glomerular hypertrophy, the intrarenal precipitation of calcium phosphate, hyperlipidemia, and altered prostanoid metabolism (tables 2, 3). (Jacobson, 1991; Renneke et al., 1989; Loghman-Adham, 1993; Nagata & Kriz, 1942; Yu, 2003).

### 7.1 Genetic factors

A number of genetic factors (eg, single nucleotide polymorphisms and modifier genes) may influence the immune response, inflammation, fibrosis, and atherosclerosis, possibly contributing to accelerated progression of CKD (Nordfors et al., 2005; Hsu et al., 2006). Indirect evidence in support of such factors can be found in familial clustering of all-cause ESRD, with approximately one-quarter of dialysis patients having relatives with ESRD (Freedman et al., 2005). This is consistent with the hypothesis that common kidney diseases and progression to ESRD are influenced by the inheritance of specific genes. Genetic studies have suggested possible links between CKD and a variety of alterations or polymorphisms of genes coding for putative mediators including the renin angiotensin system, nitric oxide synthase, kallikrein, growth factors including platelet-derived growth factors and cytokines.

With respect to specific genes, apolipoprotein E (ApoE) polymorphisms may alter the risk of atherosclerotic disease, and, therefore, progression of CKD. The ApoE epsilon-2 allele is associated with elevated lipoprotein and triglyceride levels, whereas the ApoE epsilon-4 allele is associated with elevated levels of high density lipoprotein and lower triglycerides. In a secondary analysis of the Atherosclerosis Risk in Communities Study of 14, 520 patients with a median follow-up of 14 years, individuals with an ApoE epsilon-4 allele (present in 30 percent) had a 15 percent reduction in risk of progression of CKD compared to individuals with ApoE epsilon-3 allele (present in 90 percent) (Hsu et al., 2005). The risk with the ApoE epsilon-2 allele was not significantly different compared with ApoE epsilon-3.

| Risk factors | Definition |
|---|---|
| Susceptibility factors | Factors predisposing to CKD include genetic and familial predisposition, race, maternal-fetal factors (low birth weight, malnutrition in utero), age (elderly), gender (male) |
| Initiation factors | Factors directly trigger kidney damage include diabetes, hypertension, cardiovascular disease, dyslipidemia, obesity, hyperuricemia and nephrotoxin exposure |
| Progression factors | Factors associated with worsening of already established kidney damage include poor glycemia control, poor blood pressure control, cardiovascular disease, proteinuria, alcohol consumption, nephrotoxin exposure, and acute kidney injury |

Table 2. Types of risk factors for chronic kidney disease and its outcomes.

| |
|---|
| Intraglomerular hypertension and hypertrophy |
| Phosphate retention, with interstitial CaPO4 deposition |
| Increased prostaglandin synthesis |
| Hyperlipidemia, especially in the nephrotic syndrome |
| Metabolic acidosis |
| Obesity |
| Smoking |
| Type of underlying kidney disease |
| Proteinuria |
| Tubulointerstitial disease |
| Retained "uremic" toxins |
| Filtered iron in nephrotic syndrome |

Table 3. Secondary factors and progression of CKD.

### 7.2 Hypertension

Systemic hypertension is both a cause and consequence of CKD. The incidence of hypertension increases as CKD advances. The prevalence of hypertension requiring treatment in patients with stage 4 CKD is greater than 80%. There is strong evidence that high blood pressure is a risk factor for the progression of CKD in humans. It is believed that the transmission of systemic hypersion into the glomerular capillary beds and the resulting glomerular hypertension contribute to the initiation of glomerulosclerosis and, there is clear evidence that strict control of the blood pressure is beneficial in slowing the rate of progression of CKD.

### 7.3 Proteinuria

Proteinuria alone may contribute to disease progression (Burton & Harris, 1996; Eddy et al., 1991; Benigini et al., 2004; Hirschberg & Wang, 2005). Proposed mechanisms include mesangial toxicity, tubular overload and hyperplasia, toxicity from specific filtered compounds such as transferrin/iron and albumin-bound fatty acids, and induction of proinflammatory molecules such as MCP-1 and inflammatory cytokines (Wang et al., 1997).
It is possible, for example, that a marked increase in protein filtration and subsequent proximal reabsorption leads to tubular cell injury and the release of lysozymes into the interstitium. To the degree that proteinuria alone might be important, reversing intraglomerular hypertension with protein restriction or antihypertensive therapy may be beneficial both by diminishing hemodynamic injury to the glomeruli and by reducing protein filtration (which is in part dependent upon the intraglomerular pressure), thereby lowering proteinuria.

### 7.4 Hyperlipidemia

Hyperlipidemia is common in patients with CKD, particularly those with the nephrotic syndrome. In addition to accelerating the development of systemic atherosclerosis, experimental studies suggest that high lipid levels also may promote progression of the renal disease (Keane, 1994; Grone & Grone, 2008). The major experimental evidence in support of this hypothesis are the observations in experimental animals that cholesterol loading enhances glomerular injury and that reducing lipid levels with a drug such as lovastatin slows the rate of progressive injury (Keane, 1994; Diamond & Karnovsky, 1987;

Rubin et al., 1994; Michel et al., 1997). Furthermore, the beneficial effect of lipid lowering may be additive to that of lowering the blood pressure in at least some models of CKD (Rubin et al., 1994).

The factors responsible for the lipid effects are incompletely understood. In different animal models, a high cholesterol intake may be deleterious in association with a rise in intraglomerular pressure (Diamond & Karnovsky, 1987), while lipid-lowering agents may be beneficial without affecting glomerular hemodynamics. These disparate observations suggest that mechanisms other than intraglomerular pressure alone may play a contributory role. It has been shown experimentally, for example, that hyperlipidemia activates the mesangial cells (which have LDL receptors), leading to stimulation of mesangial cell proliferation and to increased production of macrophage chemotactic factors, fibronectin (a component of the extracellular matrix), type IV collagen, plasminogen activator-1 and reactive oxygen species.

Each of these changes could contribute to glomerular injury. In addition, statins may act independent of plasma lipid levels by directly inhibiting mesangial cell proliferation and production of monocyte chemo-attractants.

The applicability of these findings to human disease is uncertain. There are numerous secondary analyses of data from lipid trials suggesting that high lipid levels are associated with a faster rate of progression, and that statins slow the rate of progression of kidney failure.

### 7.5 Hyperuricemia

Hyperuricemia can develop in patients with CKD due to decreased urinary excretion. It has been proposed that hyperuricemia may contribute to progression, in part by decreasing renal perfusion via stimulation of afferent arteriolar vascular smooth muscle cell proliferation (Ohno et al., 2001; Iseki et al., 2004; Sanchez-Lozada et al., 2005; Schwarz et al., 2006).

Combined data from two community-based cohorts comprising 13,388 individuals were examined for an association between baseline uric acid and the development of CKD during 9 years of follow-up. Baseline uric acid was associated with increased risk for CKD with odds ratios of 1.07 (95% CI 1.01 to 1.14) and 1.11 (95% CI 1.02 to 1.21) per 1 mg/dl increase in uric acid, in both GFR and serum creatinine based models.

In a Japanese study, hyperuricemic patients with IgA nephropathy had a worse prognosis than those with normal uric acid level, and a serum uric acid greater than 6mg/dl was an independent predictor of ESRD in women.

### 7.6 Phosphate retention

A tendency to phosphate retention is an early problem in kidney disease, beginning as soon as the GFR starts to fall. In addition to promoting bone disease, the excess phosphate also may contribute to progression of CKD. Higher serum phosphorus concentrations have been associated with a greater risk of progression. In an observational study of 985 patients followed for a median of two years, the adjusted hazard ratio for doubling of the serum creatinine was 1.3 for every 1.0 mg/dl [0.33 mmol/l] increase in serum phosphorus (Schwarz et al., 2006).

A similar relationship was noted for the calcium-phosphorus product.

A potential causative mechanism could be calcium phosphate precipitation in the renal interstitium (Gimenez et al., 1987), which might initiate an inflammatory reaction, resulting in interstitial fibrosis and tubular atrophy.

These observations do not prove a cause-and-effect relationship and there are no data addressing the possible role of improved calcium and phosphorus control in slowing the progression of CKD. However, there are other compelling reasons for optimizing phosphorus control in patients with CKD.

### 7.7 Type of underlying kidney disease

The type of kidney disease appears to be a risk factor. Glomerulonephritis, diabetic and hypertensive nephropathies, and polycystic kidney disease tend to progress faster than tubulointerstitial disease.

### 7.8 Metabolic acidosis and increased ammonium production

As the number of functioning nephrons declines, each remaining nephron excretes more acid (primarily as ammonium). The local accumulation of ammonia can directly activate complement, leading to secondary tubulointerstitial damage (at least in experimental animals) (Nath et al., 1985). On the other hand, buffering the acid with alkali therapy prevents the increase in ammonium production and minimizes the renal injury. Although the renal protective effect of alkali therapy is unproven in humans, there are other reasons (prevention of osteopenia and muscle wasting) why correction of the acidemia might be desirable.

### 7.9 Smoking

Cigarette smoking increases systemic blood pressure and affects renal hemodynamics. In diabetic and non-diabetic patients, smoking is associated with a faster rate of decline of CKD. In one study of men with CKD, smoking increased the risk for ESRD threefold in patients treated with ACE inhibitors; with the odds ratio increasing to 10 in those taking other antihypertensive agents.

## 8. Clinical manifestations of chronic kidney disease

A wide range of disorders may develop as a consequence of the loss of renal function. In the early phase, stage 1 and 2, the patient is asymptomatic, blood urea nitrogen (BUN) and serum creatinine (SCr) are normal or near-normal, and acid base, fluid, and electrolyte balances are maintained through an adaptive increase of function in the remaining nephrons. A reduction of GFR to 30 to 59 ml/min/1.73 $m^2$ define stage 3, moderate impairment of GFR. The patient usually has no symptoms, although SCr and BUN are increased, and serum levels of hormones such as erythropoietin, calcitriol, and parathyroid hormones (PTH) are usually abnormal. Stage 4, severe impairment of GFR, involves a further loss of kidney function. Finding, if present, are mild; patients may have anemia, acidosis, hypocalcemia, hyperphosphatemia and hyperkalemia. The final stage of kidney disease, stage 5 is defined by a GFR of less than 15ml/min/1.73 $m^2$, is usually characterized by worsening of all the aforementioned findings, and symptoms including fatigue, dysgeusia, anorexia, nausea, and pruritis may develop.

### 8.1 Hypertension

Hypertension is present in approximately 80 to 85 percent of patients with CKD [MMWR, 2007]. The prevalence of hypertension increases linearly as the GFR falls and, as in patients without renal disease, is increased in patients with higher body weight and in blacks. Data from the Modification of Diet in Renal Disease Study, for example, showed that the prevalence of hypertension rose progressively from 65 to 95 percent as the GFR fell from 85 to 15 ml/min per 1.73 $m^2$ (Buckalew et al., 1996).

One or more of the following factors may contribute in the individual patient:

- Sodium retention is generally of primary importance, even though the degree of extracellular volume expansion may be insufficient to induce edema.
- Increased activity of the renin-angiotensin system (probably due to regional ischemia induced by scarring) is often responsible for at least part of the hypertension that persists after the restoration of normovolemia.
- Enhanced activity of the sympathetic nervous system has been demonstrated in patients with CKD. The afferent signal may arise in part within the failing kidneys, since it is not seen in patients who have undergone bilateral nephrectomy (Ligtenberg et al., 1999; Neumann et al., 2004).

Secondary hyperparathyroidism raises the intracellular calcium concentration, which can lead to vasoconstriction and hypertension (Raine et al., 1993). Lowering parathyroid hormone secretion by the chronic administration of an active vitamin D analog can reduce both intracellular calcium and the systemic blood pressure.

- Hypertension may occur or be exacerbated in patients with advanced CKD treated with erythropoietin; this effect is in part related to the degree of elevation in the hematocrit.
- Impaired nitric oxide synthesis and endothelium-mediated vasodilatation has been demonstrated in patients with uremia (Passauer et al., 2005; Passauer et al., 2005). Although the mechanisms are unclear, potential explanations include reduced nitric oxide availability due to a state of increased oxidative stress, or cofactor deficiency-induced uncoupling of nitric oxide synthase.

In addition to these factors that can raise the mean arterial pressure, two other factors may be important:

- Patients with end-stage renal disease are more likely to have an increase in pulse pressure and isolated systolic hypertension (London et al., 1992). Why this occurs is incompletely understood but increased aortic stiffness appears to play an important role.
- Patients with CKD may not demonstrate the normal nocturnal decline in blood pressure (called "nondippers"), a possible risk factor for hypertensive complications.

The optimal blood pressure in hypertensive patients with CKD is uncertain. The rate of loss of GFR appears to be more rapid when the mean arterial pressure remains at or above 100 mmHg (which reflects a diastolic pressure of 80 to 85 mmHg in the absence of systolic hypertension). To slow progression of CKD, the optimal blood pressure depends in part on the degree of proteinuria.

We recommend a blood pressure goal of less than 130/80 mmHg, which is consistent with JNC 7 and the K/DOQI Clinical Practice Guidelines on hypertension and antihypertensive agents in CKD. However, evidence from the Modification of Diet in Renal Disease study, the AASK trial, and a meta-analysis from the ACE inhibition and Progressive Renal Disease (AIPRD) study group suggest that an even lower systolic pressure may be more effective in slowing progressive renal disease in patients with a spot urine total protein-to-creatinine ratio =1000 mg/g (which represents protein excretion of greater than 1000 mg/day). Caution is advised about lowering the systolic blood pressure below 110 mmHg.

The desired degree of blood pressure control typically requires combination therapy in patients with CKD. The regimen should include an ACE inhibitor or angiotensin II receptor blocker, which are the preferred drugs to prevent progressive proteinuric CKD, and a diuretic for fluid control

A loop diuretic is recommended for the treatment of hypertension and edema in patients with CKD. The thiazide diuretics in conventional dosage become less effective as monotherapy when the GFR falls below 20 ml/min. They do, however, produce an additive effect when administered with a loop diuretic for refractory edema.

Calcium channel blockers are also effective in the hypertension of CKD. These agents are relatively unique in that they seem to be more effective in patients who are volume expanded.

### 8.2 Volume overload

Sodium and intravascular volume balance are usually maintained via homeostatic mechanisms until the GFR falls below 10 to 15 ml/min. However, the patient with mild to moderate CKD, despite being in relative volume balance, is less able to respond to rapid infusions of sodium and is therefore prone to fluid overload. As kidney function declines, most patients develop sodium retention and extracellular volume expansion. They may complain of ankle swelling or shortness of breath as a result of pulmonary edema.

Patients with CKD and volume overload generally respond to the combination of dietary sodium restriction and diuretic therapy, usually with a loop diuretic given daily.

### 8.3 Anemia

Anemia has been defined by the World Health Organization (WHO) as a hemoglobin (Hgb) concentration below 13.0 g/dl for adult males and post-menopausal women, and a Hgb below 12.0 g/dl for pre-menopausal women . Based upon these criteria, nearly 90 percent of patients with a GFR less than 25 to 30 ml/min have anemia, many with Hgb levels below 10 g/dl.

Anemia is an almost universal complication of CKD. It contributes considerably to reduced quality of life of patients with CKD and has been increasingly recognized as an adverse risk factor. Renal anemia is typically an isolated normochromic, normocytic anemia with no leukopenia or thrombocytopenia.

It is principally due to reduced renal erythropoietin production and, to a lesser degree, to shortened red cell survival and decreased responsiveness to the hormone.

Anemia can develop well before the onset of uremic symptoms due to ESRD and is a common feature in many patients with CKD who do not require dialysis, with decreasing hemoglobin levels as GFRs decline below 60 ml/min per 1.73 $m^2$. As an example, based upon over 15,000 participants in the NHANES survey, the prevalence of anemia (Hbg <12 g/dL in men and <11 g/dL in women) increased from one percent at an estimated GFR of 60 ml/min per 1.73 $m^2$ to 9 percent at an estimated GFR of 30 ml/min per 1.73 $m^2$ and to 33 to 67 percent at an estimated GFR of 15 ml/min per 1.73 $m^2$. Kazmi et al. (2001) in a study on anemia in pre-dialysis patients have demonstrated that even among CKD patients in the serum creatinine <2mg/dl category, 24% of the patients had hemoglobin levels <11g/dl (Figure 1). Anemia has also been implicated as a contributing factor in many of the symptoms associated with reduced kidney function. These include fatigue, depression, reduced exercise tolerance, dyspnea, and cardiovascular consequences, such as left ventricular hypertrophy (LVH) and left ventricular systolic dysfunction. It is also associated with an increased risk of morbidity and mortality principally due to cardiac disease and stroke, and with an increased risk of hospitalization, hospital length of stay, and mortality in patients with predialysis CKD.

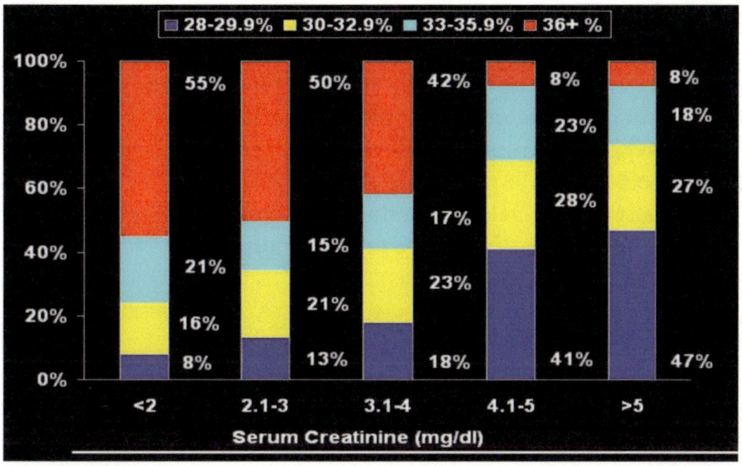


Fig. 1. Prevalence of anemia in patients with different stages of CKD (Kazmi et al., Am J Kidney Dis, 2001).

### 8.4 Hyperkalemia

The ability to maintain potassium excretion at near normal levels is generally maintained in patients with renal disease as long as both aldosterone secretion and distal flow are maintained (Gonik et al., 1971; Hsu & Chertow, 2002). Thus, hyperkalemia generally develops in the patient who is oliguric, or who has an additional problem such as a high potassium diet, increased tissue breakdown, or hypoaldosteronism (due in some cases to the administration of an ACE inhibitor or ARB) (Gennari & Segal, 1995). Impaired cell uptake of potassium also may contribute to the development of hyperkalemia in advanced CKD. Unlike patients with acute kidney failure, those with CKD may tolerate high plasma potassium concentrations without electrocardiographic changes or arrhythmias.

Hyperkalemia due to ACE inhibitor or ARB therapy is most likely to occur in patients in whom the serum potassium concentration is elevated or in the high normal range prior to therapy. In this setting, institution of a low-potassium diet or concurrent use of a loop diuretic (to increase urinary potassium losses) often ameliorates the degree of hyperkalemia. In selected patients, low dose Kayexalate (5 grams with each meal) can be used to lower the serum potassium concentration without the side effects associated with larger doses. In addition to treating hyperkalemia, there are several measures that can help prevent hyperkalemia in patients with CKD. These include ingestion of a low potassium diet (eg, less than 40 to 70 meq/day [1500 to 2700 mg/day]) and avoiding, if possible, the use of drugs that raise the serum potassium concentration such as nonsteroidal antiinflammatory drugs (Allon, 1995). Nonselective beta-blockers make the postprandial rise in the serum potassium concentration but do not produce persistent hyperkalemia.

Spontaneous hypokalemia is uncommon in CKD, but it can be seen in salt wasting nephropathy, Fanconi's syndrome, hereditary or acquired tubulointerstitial disease, and renal tubular acidosis .in patients with CKD, hypokalemia is usually caused by low dietary potassium intake combined with high doses of diuretics or by gastrointestinal loss.

### 8.5 Metabolic acidosis

There is an increasing tendency to retain hydrogen ions among patients with CKD. (Uribarri et al., 1995; Warnock, 1988; Widmer et al., 1979). This can lead to a progressive metabolic acidosis with the serum bicarbonate concentration tending to stabilize between 12 and 20 meq/l, and rarely falling below 10 meq/l (Warnock, 1988; Walia et al., 1986).

Previously, exogenous alkali was not usually given to treat the generally mild metabolic acidosis (arterial pH generally above 7.25) in asymptomatic adults with CKD. This was primarily due to concerns related to the exacerbation of volume expansion and hypertension. However, these concerns appear to be overstated. The treatment of acidosis is desirable to prevent osteopenia and muscle catabolism. In fact, bone buffering of some of the excess hydrogen ions is associated with the release of calcium and phosphate from bone, which can worsen the bone disease. Uremic acidosis can increase skeletal muscle breakdown and diminish albumin synthesis, leading to loss of lean body mass and muscle weakness. The administration of bicarbonate increases serum albumin and the lean body mass (de Brito-Ashurst et al., 2009).

It is now recommended to start alkali therapy to maintain the serum bicarbonate concentration above 23 meq /l (de Brito-Ashurst et al., 2009). If alkali is given, sodium bicarbonate (in a daily dose of 0.5 to 1 meq/kg per day) is the agent of choice. Sodium citrate (citrate is rapidly metabolized to bicarbonate) may be used in patients who are unable to tolerate sodium bicarbonate, since it does not produce the bloating associated with bicarbonate therapy. Sodium citrate should be avoided in the rare patient who may be taking aluminum-containing antacids since it markedly enhances intestinal aluminum absorption.

An alternative method to correct the metabolic acidosis in patients on maintenance dialysis is to increase the bicarbonate concentration in the dialysate. Levels as high as 42 meq/l may be required with hemodialysis to prevent predialysis acidosis. This regimen is generally well tolerated and does not induce significant postdialysis alkalosis.

### 8.6 Renal osteodystrophy

Four main types of renal bone disease can be seen in patients with CKD. These are osteitis fibrosa cystica, adynamic bone disease, osteomalacia, and mixed renal osteodystrophy, with the last disorder being a mixture of the first three. The prevalence of the different types of bone disease has changed over the last several decades. At present, the most common disorder is adynamic bone disease, with osteitis fibrosa, osteomalacia, and mixed disease less frequently observed.

A tendency toward phosphate retention begins early in renal disease, due to the reduction in the filtered phosphate load. Although this problem is initially mild with hyperphosphatemia being a relatively late event, phosphate retention is intimately related to the common development of secondary hyperparathyroidism that play an important role in the pathogenesis of bone disease and in other uremic complications.

Dietary phosphate restriction may limit the development of secondary hyperparathyroidism in patients with CKD. An intake of about 800 mg/day may be desirable and is recommended by the K/DOQI guidelines in patients with elevated phosphate and/or PTH levels.

Once the GFR falls below 25 to 30 ml/min, the addition of oral phosphate binders are usually required to prevent hyperphosphatemia (Abboud & Henrich, 2010; Sarnak et al., 2005). The K/DOQI guidelines recommend that serum phosphorus levels should be between 2.7 and 4.6 mg/dl (0.87 and 1.49 mmol/l) among patients with stage 3 and 4 CKD, and between 3.5 and

5.5 mg/dl (1.13 and 1.78 mmol/l) among those with ESRD (or stage 5 disease) (Sarnak et al., 2005). Patients are also prescribed biologically active vitamin D e.g calcitriol or vitamin D prohormones that are converted to active dihydroxylated compounds in the liver.

### 8.7 Malnutrition

Malnutrition is common in patients with advanced chronic renal disease because of a lower food intake (principally due to anorexia), decreased intestinal absorption and digestion, and metabolic acidosis (Kopple et al., 2000; Garg et al., 2001; Bammens et al., 2003). Among participants =60 years of age in the United States NHANES III, a GFR <30 ml/min was independently associated with malnutrition (odds ratio of 3.6) (Garg et al., 2001).

It is, therefore, desirable to monitor the nutritional status of patients with CKD. Biochemical indicators include a fall in serum albumin, transferrin, and cholesterol. Weight should be carefully monitored in patients who progress to CKD stages 4 to 5 ,these should be measured approximately every one to three months for those with estimated GFRs <20 ml/min, and more frequently if necessary for those with GFRs =15 ml/min.

### 8.8 The uremic syndrome

The uremic syndrome can be defined as deterioration of multiple biochemical and physiological function in parallel with progressive renal failure, thereby resulting in complex but variable symtomatology. A myriad of uremic retention solutes accumulates in the uremic patients with ESRD which are directly or indirectly attributable to deficient renal clearance that impair cell regulatory mechanisms involving the cardiovascular, gastrointestinal, hematopoietic, immune, nervous and endocrine systems.

These retained solutes are called uremic toxins when they contribute to the uremic syndrome. The uremic syndrome is characterized not only by solute accumulation but also by hormonal alterations such as decreased production of erythropoietin and calcitriol, decreased clearance of insulin, end-organ resistance to insulin and PTH. The signs and symptoms vary from one patient to another, depending partly on the rate and severity of the loss of kidney function.

Uremic toxins can be subdivided into three major groups based upon their chemical and physical characteristics:

- Small, water-soluble, non-protein-bound compounds, such as urea
- Small, lipid-soluble and/or protein-bound compounds, such as the phenols
- Larger so-called middle-molecules, such as beta2-microglobulin

### 8.9 Dyslipidemia

Abnormal lipid metabolism is common in patients with renal disease. Patients with CKD stage 3 develop a disturbance of lipoprotein metabolism characterized by accumulation of partially metabolized very-low-density lipoprotein particle and a disturbance in the maturation of high-density-lipoprotein .The primary finding in CKD is hypertriglyceridemia with the total cholesterol concentration usually being normal (perhaps due in part to malnutrition in some patients). Patients with CKD should be assessed for dyslipidemia, including a total cholesterol, LDL, HDL, and triglycerides.

Among patients with CKD, the degree of hypertriglyceridemia that occurs may not be sufficient to significantly increase coronary risk, but other changes have been found that might contribute to the accelerated atherosclerosis commonly seen in ESRD. First, dietary modification may be helpful for the hypertriglyceridemia. Drug therapy in patients without

renal failure may be beneficial in selected patients with isolated marked hypertriglyceridemia (serum triglycerides =500 mg/dl [=5.65 mmol/l]) who have proven coronary disease, a strong family history of Coronary heart disease (CHD), or multiple coexisting cardiac risk factors. Whether this approach is beneficial in patients with renal failure is not known, but it should be considered. Fibrate dose should be reduced in any patient with CKD stage 3 to 4, and these agents are best avoided in those with stage 5 disease.
In the patient with hypercholesterolemia, a statin can effectively and safely lower the plasma cholesterol concentration to or near acceptable levels, although low starting doses are recommended because of drug accumulation. The goal LDL-cholesterol is similar to that in patients with CHD, which has been less than 100 mg/dl (2.6 mmol/l).
Limited data suggest that lipid lowering may have an additional benefit in patients with CKD, which is slowing the rate of progression of the underlying renal disease.

### 8.10 Sexual dysfunction in females

Disturbances in menstruation, fertility, and sexual dysfunction are commonly encountered in women with CKD, usually leading to amenorrhea by the time the patient reaches ESRD. The menstrual cycle typically remains irregular with scanty flow after the initiation of maintenance dialysis, although normal menses are restored in some women (Holley et al., 1997; Peng et al., 2005). In others, menorrhagia develops, sometimes leading to significant blood loss and increased transfusion requirements.
The major menstrual cycle abnormality in uremic women is anovulation, resulting in infertility. Women receiving chronic dialysis also tend to experience decreased libido and reduced ability to reach orgasm (Hou, 1999; Finkelstein et al., 2007).
Although rare, pregnancy can occur in women with advanced kidney failure, but fetal wastage is markedly increased (Hou, 1999). Some residual renal function is usually present in the infrequent pregnancy that can be carried to term. Although luteinizing hormone levels are high, there is absence of the preovulatory peak in LH and estradiol concentrations. The failure of LH to rise in part reflects a disturbance in the positive estradiol feedback pathway, since the administration of exogenous estrogen to mimic the preovulatory surge in estradiol fails to stimulate LH release. In contrast, feedback inhibition of gonadotropin release by low doses of estradiol remains intact. This can be illustrated by the ability of the antiestrogen clomiphene to enhance luteinizing hormone (LH) and follicle stimulating hormone (FSH) secretion.
Women with CKD commonly have elevated circulating prolactin concentrations and galactorrhea due to increased secretion and decreased metabolic clearance. The hypersecretion of prolactin in this setting appears to be relatively autonomous, as it is resistant to maneuvers designed to stimulate or inhibit its release. Similar observations have been made in uremic males.
The elevated prolactin levels may impair hypothalamic-pituitary function and contribute to sexual dysfunction and galactorrhea in these patients. Bromocriptine treatment corrects the hyperprolactinemia in these patients but does not restore normal menses, thereby suggesting that other mechanisms are involved.

### 8.11 Sexual dysfunction in males

Disturbances in sexual function are a common feature of chronic kidney disease (Palmer, 2003; Holdsworth et al., 1978). Over 50 percent of uremic men complain of symptoms that include erectile dysfunction, decreased libido, and marked decline in the frequency of intercourse (Diemont et al., 2000). Prolactin levels are elevated in CKD stage 5 and may contribute to gynecomastia and sexual dysfunction. Testosterone levels are often low-normal, and gonadotropins may be raised, implying testicular failure. This is accompanied by poor spermatogenesis, leading to low sperm counts and reduced fertility. These problems may improve, but rarely normalize with the institution of maintenance dialysis, commonly resulting in a decreased quality of life (Rosas et al., 2003). By comparison, a well-functioning renal transplant is much more likely to restore sexual activity; however, some features of reproductive function may remain impaired, particularly reduced libido and erectile dysfunction.

It is presumed that the uremic milieu plays an important role in the genesis of this problem. Other organic (and not necessarily uremic) factors that may contribute to erectile dysfunction include peripheral neuropathy, autonomic dysfunction, peripheral vascular disease, and pharmacologic therapy.

### 8.12 Thyroid dysfunction

The kidney normally plays an important role in the metabolism, degradation, and excretion of several thyroid hormones. It is not surprising, therefore, that impairment in kidney function leads to disturbed thyroid physiology. All levels of the hypothalamic-pituitary-thyroid axis may be involved, including alterations in hormone production, distribution, and excretion.

As a result, abnormalities in thyroid function tests are frequently encountered in uremia. However, the overlap in symptomatology between the uremic syndrome and hypothyroidism requires a cautious interpretation of these tests. Nevertheless, it is ordinarily possible in the individual uremic patient to assess thyroid status accurately by physical diagnosis and thyroid function testing.

Epidemiologic data suggests that predialysis patients with CKD have an increased risk of hypothyroidism (Lo et al., 2005; Chonchol et al., 2008). Many cases are subclinical. Free thyroxin [T4] and serum thyroid stimulating hormone [TSH] are usually normal but most patients with ESRD have decreased plasma levels of free triiodothyronine (T3), which reflect diminished conversion of T4 (thyroxine) to T3 in the periphery (Kaptein et al., 1988). This abnormality is not associated with increased conversion of T4 to the metabolically inactive reverse T3 (rT3), since plasma rT3 levels are typically normal. This finding differentiates the uremic patient from patients with chronic illness. In the latter setting, the conversion of T4 to T3 is similarly reduced, but the generation of rT3 from T4 is enhanced.

### 8.13 Insulin metabolism

Impaired tissue sensitivity to insulin occurs in almost all uremic subjects and is largely responsible for the abnormal glucose metabolism seen in this setting (Mak & DeFronzo, 1992). Both experimental and clinical studies suggest that hepatic glucose production and uptake are normal in uremia and that skeletal muscle is the primary site of insulin resistance (Androgue, 1992). How this occurs is not clear, but a post-receptor defect is of primary importance (Smith & DeFronzo, 1982). Furthermore, the abnormality appears to specifically involve glycogen synthesis, as the rate of glucose oxidation is relatively normal. It is of interest in this regard that other actions of insulin such as promoting potassium uptake by the cells, and inhibiting proteolysis are also maintained in renal failure.

Accumulation of a uremic toxin or toxins and excess parathyroid hormone (PTH), resulting from abnormalities in phosphate and vitamin D metabolism are thought to be responsible for the insulin resistance (McCaleb et al., 1985). As an example, the observation that tissue sensitivity to insulin can be substantially improved by dialysis is consistent with a role for uremic toxins. The expected response to impaired tissue sensitivity would be an augmentation in insulin secretion in an attempt to normalize glucose metabolism. In many cases, however, insulin secretion tends to be blunted; these patients tend to have the greatest impairment in glucose tolerance.

One factor that can suppress insulin release in CKD is the associated metabolic acidosis. In addition, deficiency of calcitriol (1,25-dihydroxyvitamin D) and excess PTH may interfere with the ability of the beta cells to augment insulin secretion in response to hyperglycemia or amino acids. A PTH-induced elevation in the intracellular calcium concentration may be responsible for the impairment in insulin release by decreasing both the cellular content of ATP and Na-K-ATPase pump activity in the pancreatic beta cells.

There is little change in the metabolic clearance rate of insulin in renal disease until the GFR has fallen to less than 15 to 20 ml/min. At this point, there is a dramatic reduction in insulin clearance which is also mediated by a concomitant decline in hepatic insulin metabolism. The hepatic defect may be induced by a uremic toxin, since it is largely reversed with adequate dialysis.

Insulin requirements show a biphasic course in diabetic patients with renal disease. It is not uncommon for glucose control to deteriorate as renal function deteriorates, as increasing insulin resistance can affect both insulin-dependent and non-insulin-dependent diabetics. Thus, insulin requirements may increase in the former, while the institution of insulin therapy may be necessary in the latter.

In comparison, the marked fall in insulin clearance in advanced renal failure often leads to an improvement in glucose tolerance. This may allow a lower dose of insulin to be given or even the cessation of insulin therapy. Decreased caloric intake, due to uremia-induced anorexia, also may contribute to the decrease in insulin requirements.

### 8.14 Hypoglycemia

An unusual manifestation of disturbed glucose metabolism in CKD is the development of spontaneous hypoglycemia. This complication can be seen in both diabetic and nondiabetic subjects. As an example, in a retrospective analysis of 243,222 patients, the incidence of hypoglycemia was significantly higher among patients with CKD (defined as estimated GFR <60 ml/min per 1.73 $m^2$) compared with patients without chronic kidney disease, both among those with diabetes (10.72 versus 5.33 per 100 patient-months, respectively) and without diabetes (3.46 versus 2.23 per 100 patient-months, respectively) (Moen et al., 2009).

Multiple factors may play a contributory role. These include decreased caloric intake, reduced renal gluconeogenesis due to the reduction in functioning renal mass, impaired release of the counter-regulatory hormone epinephrine due to the autonomic neuropathy of renal failure, concurrent hepatic disease, and decreased metabolism of drugs that might promote a reduction in the plasma glucose concentration such as alcohol, propranolol and other nonselective -blockers, and disopyramide.

### 8.15 Psychological manifestations

Psychiatric illness is common among patients with chronic disorders, particularly in those with ESRD. In a review based upon United States Renal Disease Systems (USRDS) data (Kimmel et al., 1998) the psychological problems associated with CKD included affective disorders, particularly depression, organic brain diseases eg, dementia and delirium drug-related disorders (such as alcoholism), schizophrenia and other psychoses and personality disorders.

These disorders account for a 1.5 to 3.0 times higher rate of hospitalization among dialysis patients compared to those with other chronic illnesses, thereby resulting in significant morbidity. In the previous study of approximately 175,000 dialysis patients, 9 percent were hospitalized with a mental disorder during a one-year period. A subsequent study from Japan reported a one-year 10.6 percent incidence of psychiatric disorders in dialysis patients (Fukunishi et al., 2002). Dementia, delirium, and major depression were the most common disorders in this four-year follow-up study.

Patients maintained on hemodialysis are more likely to be hospitalized for a psychiatric disorder than are those treated with peritoneal dialysis. This difference may be due to patient selection for a particular dialysis modality or the increased incidence among hemodialysis patients of disruptive behaviors that may lead to hospitalization. Overall, the type of dialysis modality does not appear to have a significant impact upon symptoms related to depression, sexual function, and life satisfaction.

### 8.16 Gastrointestinal manifestations

Gastrointestinal complications are common in advanced CKD and in some cases may be the first or only complaint on presentation. Anorexia, nausea, vomiting, and uremic fetor are common manifestations of uremia. Vomiting may occur without nausea and is often prominent in the early morning. Stomatitis, gastritis and enteritis can develop with ESRD in patients not treated with dialysis or transplantation. In one study of 60 patients with ESRD, panendoscopy revealed esophagitis, gastritis, and duodenitis in 13, 22, and 60 percent of patients, respectively, while biopsies showed histologic evidence of gastritis and duodenitis in 46 and 43 percent, respectively (Margolis et al., 1978). The incidence of gastritis appears to decline with increasing duration of dialysis. The pathogenesis of mucosal inflammation in these patients is unclear.

In general, there is an increased risk of bleeding in hemodialysis patients because of uremia-induced platelet dysfunction as well as the intermittent use of heparin with dialysis treatments. These systemic abnormalities may in part help explain the perceived higher incidence of upper gastrointestinal (UGI) bleeding in patients with ESRD. The causes of UGI bleeding among patients with ESRD may be somewhat different and a larger study found that angiodysplasia was a more frequent cause of upper GI bleeding in patients with renal failure compared to those without renal dysfunction. In this report, 727 patients with upper GI bleeding underwent diagnostic endoscopy. Among the 60 patients with CKD, the most common causes of bleeding were gastric ulcer (37 percent), duodenal ulcer (23 percent), and angiodysplasia (13 percent). Compared to patients without renal disease, angiodysplasia as a cause of UGI bleeding was significantly more common in those with renal failure (13 versus 1.3 percent, $P<0.01$).

Rarely, pancreatitis is a significant clinical problem and additional reported risk factors in this patient population may include vascular disease, polycystic kidney disease, drug ingestion (possibly including valproic acid and iodixanol), and hyperparathyroidism.

Lower gastrointestinal disorders of importance in CKD patients include uremic colitis (principally of historic interest), ischemic bowel disease, spontaneous colonic perforation, fecal impaction, diverticular disease, and angiodysplasia. A positive fecal occult blood test appears to be more informative as kidney function declines. One study of 531 patients with a positive test, for example, found that clinical significant findings increased from 24 to 33 to 43 percent in patients with normal/stage 1 CKD, stage 2/3 CKD, and stage 4/5 CKD, respectively (Bini et al., 2006). Similar findings were observed with adenomas, carcinomas, and vascular ectasias.

## 9. Prevention of progression of chronic kidney disease

A kidney disease that progresses to ESRD usually does so by two mechanisms; those of primary kidney disease and those of natural progression. For most CKD patients, the first evidence of natural progression is proteinuria increasing from low to heavy levels. Only later does decreasing GFR appear. However, for certain diseases such as polycystic kidney disease, a decrease in GFR or the presence of hypertension may be the heralding features.

### 9.1 Monitoring proteinuria

Proteinuria magnitude generally is the strongest single predictor of GFR decline. Therapy-induced proteinuria reduction slows GFR decline.The most detailed analysis of proteinuria and progression are from the Modification in Diet in Renal Disease and Ramipril Efficacy in nephropathy trials which show that for each 1.0gm reduction in proteinuria by 4 to 6 months of the antiproteinuric intervention, GFR decline is slowed by about 1 to 2 ml/min/yr. With regard to frequency of proteinuria testing, every 2 to 3 months for those with nephrotic range proteinuria and every 4 to 6 months for those with non-nephrotic proteinuria are usually sufficient to assess proteinuria trends.

### 9.2 Monitoring GFR trends

The GFR is equal to the sum of the filtration rates in all of the functioning nephrons; thus, estimation of the GFR gives an approximate measure of the number of functioning nephrons. A reduction in GFR implies either progression of the underlying disease or the development of a superimposed and often reversible problem, such as decreased renal perfusion due to volume depletion. An increase in GFR, on the other hand, is indicative of improvement in renal function, whereas a stable GFR in patients with renal disease implies stable disease.

The most common methods utilized to estimate the GFR in adults are the serum creatinine concentration, the creatinine clearance, and estimation equations based upon the serum creatinine concentration: the Cockcroft-Gault equation and Modification of Diet in Renal Disease (MDRD) study equation.

The K/DOQI working groups have published guidelines recommending that patients with CKD should be classified by disease stage, with each stage being defined in part by GFR estimation. In adults, the GFR should be estimated from the MDRD Study and Cockcroft-Gault equations, which take into account the serum creatinine concentration and some or all of the following variables: age, gender, race, and body size. Since the MDRD Study equation was derived from patients (largely white) with nondiabetic renal disease (mean GFR of 40 ml/min per 1.73 $m^2$) in the United States, it can be reliably used in such patients with significant kidney disease. It also appears to be accurate in African-Americans and those with diabetic kidney disease.

However, the estimation equations have not been validated, and may be less accurate, in some populations. These include individuals with high, normal, or near-normal renal function, children, certain ethnic groups, pregnant woman, and those with unusual muscle mass, body habitus, and weight (eg, morbid obesity or malnourished). Some therefore recommend measuring the creatinine clearance to estimate the GFR in these patients with stable renal function.

Serum creatinine and GFR estimation equations can only be used in patients with stable kidney function. With acute renal failure, for example, the GFR is initially markedly reduced but there has not yet been time for creatinine to accumulate and for the SCr to reflect the degree of renal dysfunction.
What is important to know in the patient with kidney disease is whether the GFR (and therefore disease severity) is changing or is stable. This can usually be determined by monitoring changes in the serum creatinine or the estimated GFR in patients with a relatively constant body mass and diet.

### 9.3 Angiotensin-converting enzyme inhibitors

The degree of proteinuria in glomerular disease tends to vary directly with the intraglomerular pressure. It was, therefore, proposed that a treatment-induced reduction in protein excretion (in the absence of a large fall in GFR) reflected a desirable decline in intraglomerular pressure, and would result in improved renal outcomes. Although both angiogenesis-converting enzyme [ACE] inhibitors and angiotensin receptor blockers [ARBs] are kidney protective; an ACE inhibitor is the first choice because it is not clear whether ARBs are cardioprotective to the level of ACE inhibitors. ACE inhibitor should be used even if the patient is not hypertensive and regardless of the level of proteinuria. ACE inhibitors slow progression even in those with a low grade of proteinuria. Although the greatest benefit is in those with heavy proteinuria. Measures that may increase ACE inhibitor kidney protection include a low salt, reduced-protein diet, diuretic therapy, the low BP goal and statin therapy. ACE inhibitors are antiproteinuric, even in inflammatory glomerulonephritis. ACE inhibitor should be continued even if GFR decline to stage 4 CKD [15 to 29 ml/min 1.73 $m^2$]. To prevent hyperkalemia, dietary potassium restriction, and the concomitant use of a loop diuretic and sodium bicarbonate may be needed. Advancing the ACE inhibitor dose to tolerance may increase its antiproteinuric effect and decrease the likeihood of aldosterone escape (increasing plasma aldosterone levels during stable ACE inhibitor therapy), which may diminish the ACE inhibitor reno-protection. In addition to lowering the intraglomerular pressure, experimental studies suggest that the beneficial effect of ACE inhibitors may also be related to a number of other factors:

- Angiotensin II is a growth factor; therefore, diminishing its production may minimize glomerular hypertrophy which, by decreasing the capillary radius, can reduce the tension on the glomerular capillary wall (Fogo, 2000).
- Angiotensin II, either directly or via increased glomerular pressure, can enhance the release of extracellular matrix and collagen from mesangial and tubular cells, thereby promoting both glomerular and tubulointerstitial fibrosis (Boffa et al., 2003). This effect is mediated at least in part by enhanced release of transforming growth factor-beta, matrix proteins, platelet-derived growth factors, and plasminogen activator inhibitor-I. Administration of an ACE inhibitor and/or angiotensin II receptor blocker decreases cytokine release, due most likely to a fall in glomerular pressure and/or reversal of the direct action of angiotensin II.

The ability of ACE inhibitors and/or angiotensin II receptor blockers to block the profibrotic effect of angiotensin II may be particularly due to their effect to decrease transforming growth factor-beta and plasminogen activator inhibitor-I levels (among others), and/or increase hepatocyte growth factor concentrations. Due to these effects, ACE inhibitors and angiotensin II receptor blockers may help reverse renal sclerosis, as observed in multiple animal models of progressive kidney dysfunction (Remuzzi et al., 2002).

- An ACE inhibitor may directly improve the size selective properties of the glomerulus, thereby preventing the accumulation of macromolecules in the mesangium and a secondary increase in mesangial matrix production (Remuzzi et al., 1990). Whether this effect is related to or is independent of the associated reduction in intraglomerular pressure is not clear.
- Inhibition of angiotensin II production via ACE inhibition also lowers the release of aldosterone.
- Due to decreased degradation, ACE inhibitors increase bradykinin concentrations, which may ameliorate renal tubulointerstitial fibrosis. Support for this was provided by an animal model in which unilateral ureteral obstruction-induced interstitial fibrosis was significantly increased in bradykinin B2 receptor knockout mice (Schanstra et al., 2002). Bradykinin may dampen fibrosis by increasing extracellular matrix degradation via enhanced metalloproteinase-2 and other enzymatic activity. A similar benefit by this mechanism would not be expected with an angiotensin II receptor blocker, which does not increase bradykinin levels.

### 9.4 Angiotensin II receptor blockers

The renoprotective effectiveness of angiotensin II receptor blockers (ARBs) has been best described in type 2 diabetic nephropathy. It seems likely that they will have a similar renoprotective effect as ACE inhibitors in nondiabetic CKD, but supportive data are limited (Lee et al., 2006). Studies in humans have found that ARBs are as effective as ACE inhibitors in reducing protein excretion in patients with CKD (Hilgers & Mann, 2002). In a 2008 meta-analysis of randomized trials (mostly small), the reduction in proteinuria at 5 to 12 months was similar with ARBs and ACE inhibitors (ratio of means 1.08, 95% CI 0.96-1.22). In addition, the reduction in proteinuria with ARBs was significantly greater than that with amlodipine (ratio of means 0.62, 95% CI 0.55-0.70). As with ACE inhibition, there appears to be a dose effect, with greater reduction of proteinuria at higher (even supramaximal) doses in both nondiabetic and diabetic patients. In the SMART trial, for example, 269 patients with proteinuria greater than 1 g/day, despite seven weeks of the maximum approved dose of candesartan (16 mg/day) were randomly assigned to candesartan at a dose of 16, 64, or 128 mg/day. Patients who received 128 mg/day had a significantly greater reduction in proteinuria at 30 weeks compared to those who received 16 mg/day (mean difference in percent change of proteinuria of 33 percent). The blood pressure was not different between groups. Although hyperkalemia required the withdrawal of 11 patients from the trial, there was no difference in the incidence of hyperkalemia between groups. Further studies of the efficacy, safety, and cost are required before such high dose therapy can be recommended.

#### 9.4.1 ACE inhibitors plus ARBs

The reduction in proteinuria appears to be greater when ACE inhibitors are used in combination with ARBs than with either drug alone. However, it has not been proven that combination therapy improves renal outcomes, and adverse effects are more common.

#### 9.4.2 ARB plus aliskiren

The first effective oral direct renin inhibitor, aliskiren, was approved by the United States Food and Drug Administration in March 2007. Aliskiren lowers blood pressure to a degree comparable to most other agents. In the AVOID trial, aliskiren plus losartan was associated with a significant 20 percent greater reduction in proteinuria compared to losartan alone, in the absence of a significantly greater effect on blood pressure (Parving et al., 2008). The role of aliskiren in preventing progression of CKD is not yet known (Ingelfinger, 2008).

### 9.5 Control protein intake

In a variety of animal models (such as subtotal nephrectomy and diabetic nephropathy), lowering protein intake protects against the development of glomerular scarring (called glomerulosclerosis). This effect is mediated, in part, by changes in glomerular arteriolar resistance, leading to a reduction in intraglomerular pressure and decreased glomerular hypertrophy.

Studies in humans indicate that an increase in the GFR can be induced by animal protein and by amino acid mixtures; in comparison, vegetable protein and egg whites alone produce little or no effect. Why the latter sources of protein have little hemodynamic activity is not clear, but lower concentrations of the amino acids that cause renal vasodilatation (such as glycine and alanine) and lesser stimulation of vasodilator prostaglandins may be involved. Enhanced secretion of glucagons, a direct renal vasodilator, may be a mediator of protein-induced hyper filtration (King & Levey, 1993). A high protein diet also increases the release of at least two other hormones that can raise the GFR, including insulin-like growth factor I (IGF-I) and kinins. IGF-1 is a direct renal vasodilator that can increase both renal blood flow and the GFR. In addition to a possible role in protein-induced hyperfiltration, IGF-1 may play an important role in the hyperfiltration and glomerular hypertrophy observed in type 1 diabetes mellitus. The renin-angiotensin system may also modulate the effect of protein on glomerular filtration. Angiotensin II leads to a preferential increase in efferent arteriolar resistance, causing an increase in intraglomerular pressure and hyperfiltration. Lowering angiotensin II production induces efferent dilatation, which decreases intraglomerular pressure and perhaps the GFR. However, there are conflicting data on the effect of a low protein diet on renal renin release. Both a reduction in renin gene expression (which could contribute to the protective effect of a low protein diet in renal disease) and an increase in gene expression have been described.

Intrarenal mechanisms, including tubuloglomerular feedback, may contribute to protein-induced hyper filtration (Woods, 1993). An increase in the filtered load of amino acids may enhance proximal sodium reabsorption via sodium-amino acid cotransporters in the proximal tubule. The ensuing decrease in sodium chloride delivery to the macula densa may then activate tubuloglomerular feedback, leading to an elevation in GFR in an appropriate attempt to restore macula densa delivery to normal.

Multiple well-designed randomized controlled human trials have evaluated both the efficacy and safety of protein restriction in patients with progressive CKD and reducing dietary protein intake from the usual level of about 1 to 1.5g/kg ideal weight per day, to about 0.6 to 0.8 g/kg per day slows GFR decline in those with proteinuria of more than 1gm. It is generally well tolerated and does not lead to malnutrition in patients with CKD provided caloric goals are met, dietary protein is of high biologic value, and metabolic acidosis is avoided. Dietary protein intake should be monitored periodically by urine urea excretion in 24 hour urine collections. In nutrient balance, urine urea nitrogen of 8.0g/day represents a protein intake of 50g/day, which is the target for a 70kg person. If the dietary goals are generally being met, 24-hour urine testing every 4 to 6 months is sufficient, otherwise, testing at 2- to 3-month intervals is recommended.

Therefore, we suggest the use a low protein diet (0.6 to 0.8 g/kg per day) in select predialysis patients who are highly motivated to follow such a diet. However, the adoption of this diet should NOT preclude the initiation of dialysis in patients with severe CKD, if indicated.

### 9.6 Restrict salt intake

High salt intake e.g NaCl 200mmol/day, sodium 4.6g/day, NaCl 11.7g/day, can completely override the antiproteinuric effects of ACE inhibitors, ARBs, or NDHCCBs. Also, a high salt diet can activate the tissue renin angiogenesis aldosterone system, inducing renal and myocardial fibrosis, even though the circulating RAS is suppressed. The recommended NaCl intake in CKD is about 80 to 120mmol/day [2 to 3g Na, 4.6 to 6.9g NaCl]. Salt intake should be monitored periodically by 24-hour urine collection. Those achieving their NaCl goal have 80 to 120mmol Na in their 24-hour urine collection because dietary NaCl is excreted almost entirely in urine, unless there are abnormal non-renal NaCl losses.

### 9.7 Diuretic therapy

Diuretic therapy improves BP control and proteinuria in those treated with ACE inhibitors, or ARBs. Nevertheless, the ideal is to avoid a diuretic, if possible, because of its multiple metabolic dysfunctions, especially induction of diabetes mellitus and stimulation of the RAS.

### 9.8 Control blood lipids

There is indirect evidence of beneficial effects of statins on vessel stiffening and endothelial function in patients with CKD. Once renal injury has occurred, the yearly decline in GFR may be accelerated and perpetuated by dyslipidemia. However, this effect has been derived from post-hoc analyses, which are limited by unmeasured confounders that are closely correlated to dyslipidemia. If real, this effect is fairly modest.

Although statins have demonstrated cardiovascular benefits and result in improved cardiovascular outcomes in patients without CKD, the effect of statins on primary cardiovascular outcomes in patients with ESRD or less severe renal insufficiency is uncertain. Among dialysis patients, both the 4-D and AURORA trials found NO difference between statin therapy and placebo with respect to cardiovascular death, nonfatal myocardial infarction, and stroke despite significant lipid-lowering. However, the results from 4-D and AURORA should NOT be extrapolated to patients with CKD not on dialysis. There are meta-analyses and post-hoc analyses of randomized trials that have reported decreased all-cause and cardiovascularity mortality with statins.

If administered, patients with CKD should be treated with the lowest dose of statin that reduces the LDL-C to less than 100 mg/dl (2.6 mmol/l). However, more aggressive LDL-lowering to less than 70 mg/dl (1.8 mmol/l) is a reasonable option, if the additional therapy does not impose undue burdens from side effects or cost.

With respect to adverse effects, good side effect profiles with statins have been reported patients with CKD, dialysis patients, renal transplant recipients. However, accurate estimates of the risk of adverse events (especially myopathy) are not available in patients with ESRD or moderate to severe chronic renal insufficiency, since the existing clinical trials with statins in these patients have been quite small.

### 9.9 Smoking cessation

Smoking cessation should be encouraged, with smoking stoppage being associated with a reduced rate of progression of CKD. In an increasing number of studies, smoking also appears to correlate with an enhanced risk of developing kidney disease (primarily nephrosclerosis) as well as increasing the rate of progression among those with existing CKD.

### 9.10 Avoidance of administration of nephrotoxic drugs

The administration of drugs or diagnostic agents that adversely affect renal function are a frequent cause of worsening renal function. Among patients with CKD, common offenders include aminoglycoside antibiotics (particularly with unadjusted doses), nonsteroidal antiinflammatory drugs, and radiographic contrast material, particularly in diabetics. The administration of such drugs should, therefore, be avoided or used with caution in patients with underlying CKD.

Certain drugs also interfere with either creatinine secretion or the assay used to measure the serum creatinine. These include cimetidine, trimethoprim, cefoxitin, and flucytosine. In these settings, there will be no change in GFR; the clinical clue that this has occurred is the absence of a concurrent elevation in the blood urea nitrogen (BUN).

### 9.11 Reduce obesity

Obesity is associated with multiple other conditions that are known to cause compromised renal function, including hypertension, diabetes, and the metabolic syndrome. However, data from the Framingham Offspring Study, the Hypertension Detection and Follow-Up Program, and the Multiphasic Health Testing Services Program suggest that obesity may be independently associated with the risk of developing CKD. Focal glomerulosclerosis and obesity-related glomerulopathy (glomerular enlargement and mesangial expansion) with associated proteinuria have been described in patients with severe obesity. Obesity-related glomerulopathy may be reversible with weight loss.

### 9.12 Correction of anemia

The anemia of CKD is, in most patients, normocytic and normochromic, and is due primarily to reduced production of erythropoietin by the kidney (a presumed reflection of the reduction in functioning renal mass), and to shortened red cell survival. Anemia is a common feature in many patients with CKD who do not yet require dialysis, with anemia becoming increasingly common as GFRs decline below 60 ml/min per 1.73 $m^2$, particularly among diabetics. As an example, based upon over 15,000 participants in the NHANES survey, the prevalence of anemia (Hbg <12 g/dl in men and <11 g/dl in women) increased from 1 percent at an eGFR of 60 ml/min per 1.73 $m^2$ to 9 percent at an eGFR of 30 ml/min per 1.73 $m^2$ and to 33 to 67 percent at an eGFR of 15 ml/min per 1.73 $m^2$ (Astor et al., 2002).

As stated in the 2006 K/DOQI Guidelines, the evaluation of anemia in those with CKD should begin when the Hgb level is less than 12 g/dl in females, and Hgb levels of less than 13.5 g/dl in adult males . These levels are based on the Hgb levels below the fifth percentile for the adult general population as noted in the NHANES database.

The anemia observed with CKD is largely diagnosed by excluding non-renal causes of anemia in the patient with a suitably decreased GFR. The evaluation of patients should, therefore, include red blood cell indices, absolute reticulocyte count, serum iron, total iron binding capacity, percent transferrin saturation, serum ferritin, white blood cell count and differential, platelet count, and testing for blood in stool. The content of hemoglobin in reticulocytes can also be assessed. This work-up should be performed prior to administering epoietin alfa (EPO) or darbepoietin alfa therapy. The dialysis patient is in a state of continuous iron loss from gastrointestinal bleeding, blood drawing, and/or, most important with hemodialysis, the dialysis treatment itself. Hemodialysis patients lose an average of 2 g of iron per year. Thus, iron deficiency will develop in virtually all dialysis patients receiving EPO or darbepoetin alfa unless supplemental iron therapy is given orally or intravenously. An important issue in the diagnosis of iron deficiency in the patient with CKD or ESRD is that the laboratory criteria are markedly different from those in patients with relatively normal renal function.

Absolute iron deficiency is likely to be present in patients with ESRD when:

- The percent transferrin saturation (plasma iron divided by total iron binding capacity x 100, TSAT) falls below 20 percent
- The serum ferritin concentration is less than 100 ng/ml among predialysis and peritoneal dialysis patients or is less than 200 ng/ml among hemodialysis patients. This difference in the serum ferritin level is based upon accumulating evidence in hemodialysis patients that the maintenance of ferritin levels above 200 ng/ml is associated with decreased erythropoietin requirements.

In addition to absolute iron deficiency, it is now recognized that dialysis patients may have functional iron deficiency. This is characterized by the presence of adequate iron stores as defined by conventional criteria, but an inability to sufficiently mobilize this iron from the liver and other storage sites to adequately support erythropoiesis with the administration of erythrocyte stimulating agents (ESA).

Functional iron deficiency, which usually responds somewhat to iron therapy, must be distinguished from inflammatory iron block, which usually does not. Inflammatory iron block occurs among patients with refractory anemia due largely to an underlying inflammatory state. Both functional deficiency and inflammatory block are associated with transferrin saturation =20 percent and elevated ferritin level (between 100 to 800 ng/ml or even higher). The response to EPO and/or parenteral iron may help distinguish between functional iron deficiency and inflammatory block.

With increasing doses of ESA, ferritin levels may decrease in patients with functional deficiency but not with inflammatory iron block.

Inflammatory block is most likely present if the weekly administration of intravenous iron (50 to 125 mg) for up to 8 to 10 doses fails to result in increased erythropoiesis; instead, this course of iron therapy typically results in a progressive increase in ferritin concentration. Among patients with inflammatory block, further intravenous iron should not be given until the inflammatory condition has resolved. This is thought to be particularly important in patients with active, ongoing infections.

By comparison, among patients with functional iron deficiency, additional intravenous iron (in association with an increase in EPO dose) can be effective in increasing Hgb levels, at least over the short-term.

Serial evaluation of iron indices is necessary for the early detection of iron deficiency on dialysis once therapy with EPO or darbepoetin alfa is initiated. Serum ferritin levels and the percent transferrin saturation should be measured at baseline and then periodically thereafter.

In patients with adequate iron stores who are on maintenance oral or intravenous iron, monitoring every three months is probably adequate, especially after the first few months when iron stores are most likely to become depleted. By comparison, monitoring every one to two months is recommended in patients just starting EPO therapy or in whom the dose has been increased, in those with marginal iron status, or in those with declining serum ferritin or TSAT levels. A reduction in serum ferritin can be expected during the first few months after the initiation of EPO as iron is mobilized from iron stores and used for red cell production.

Prior to initiation of treatment with erythropoietic stimulating agents (ESA), we recommend the administration of iron therapy among hemodialysis patients with absolute iron deficiency and anemia. This is principally because ESA therapy requires significant amounts of supplemental iron for effective erythropoiesis. Although normal body stores of iron are 800 to 1000 mg, approximately 1000 mg is required among hemodialysis patients to raise hemoglobin levels from approximately 8 g/dl to 11 to 12 g/dl with the initiation of ESA therapy. After target hemoglobin levels are achieved, approximately 500 mg of iron is required every three months to maintain target levels with ESA therapy.

Among those with percent transferrin saturation =20 percent and ferritin between 200 and 500 ng/ml, we administer iron therapy prior to the use of ESAs if an underlying infection has been excluded. We do not routinely administer intravenous iron without an ESA to patients with ferritin levels above 500 ng/ml and anemia, although each patient should be individually assessed.

The most common cause of resistance to ESA is iron deficiency, which can be present at the time of initiation of ESA treatment or can develop as the result of exhaustion of iron stores due to the increase in erythropoiesis caused by ESA treatment. As shown in numerous observational and prospective studies, the administration of iron to obtain adequate iron stores increases hemoglobin levels in patients who are not on ESA treatment, as well as those who are, and lowers ESA doses.

If iron indices indicate absolute (transferrin saturation <20 percent and serum ferritin <200 ng/mL) or functional iron deficiency (transferrin saturation <20 percent and serum ferritin >200 ng/ml in the setting of ESA therapy), a sufficient amount of iron to correct the iron deficiency should be administered to raise the transferrin saturation above at least 20 to 25 percent and serum ferritin level above 200 ng/ml, we suggest administering one of the following regimens:

- 125 mg of sodium ferric gluconate complex in sucrose can be given at each consecutive hemodialysis treatment for a total of eight doses (1000 mg in total).

  OR

- 100 mg iron sucrose can be given at each consecutive hemodialysis treatment for a total of 10 doses (1000 mg in total).

Repeat the initial loading regimen if the transferrin saturation remains below 20 percent, the hemoglobin level does not increase to the target level, or the serum ferritin level remains below 200 ng/ml.

Our goal with any loading regimen is to increase hemoglobin levels and raise the transferrin saturation above at least 20 to 25 percent and serum ferritin level above 200 ng/mL, while not increasing the transferrin saturation above 50 percent or the serum ferritin level above 500 ng/ml.

Among hemodialysis patients, use of parenteral iron rather than oral iron therapy is recommended . The different parenteral preparations of iron available in the United States are iron dextran, sodium ferric gluconate complex in sucrose, and iron sucrose. These preparations are largely equivalent in efficacy. However, sodium ferric gluconate complex in sucrose and iron sucrose are much safer than iron dextran, which is associated with a significant risk of anaphylaxis. Iron replete patients are characterized by transferrin saturation levels between 20 to 50 percent and serum ferritin levels between 200 to 500 mg/l. Among such patients receiving erythropoietin stimulating agents, weekly administration of parenteral iron is sufficient to maintain Hgb.

As previously mentioned, the anemia of CKD, if left untreated, can result in deterioration in cardiac function, and decreased cognition and mental acuity. It can also be accompanied by debilitating symptoms, such as fatigue, weakness, lethargy, anorexia, and sleep disturbances. In addition, anemic patients commonly lack the stamina needed to perform normal daily activities or to work.

Furthermore, anemia in patients with CKD is also associated with an increased risk of morbidity and mortality principally due to cardiac disease and stroke, and with an increased risk of hospitalization, hospital length of stay, and mortality in patients with predialysis CKD.

### 9.12.1 Administration of erythropoiesis-stimulating agents

Correction of anemia with erythropoiesis-stimulating agents is associated with some clinical benefits. These include improvements in quality of life, increased energy levels, greater capacity for work and exercise, restored sexual function, improved appetite and participation in social activities, as well as reduced depression and fatigue.

The erythropoietin deficiency evident in patients with CKD can be corrected by the exogenous administration of erythropoiesis-stimulating agents. Two such agents are currently available in the United States:

- Epoetin alfa (recombinant human erythropoietin)
- Darbepoetin alfa, a unique molecule that stimulates erythropoiesis with a longer half-life than rHuEPO

### 9.12.2 Epoetin alfa (recombinant human erythropoietin [rHuEPO]

Several general principles govern the administration of recombinant human EPO

- The response to EPO is dose-dependent, but varies greatly among patients.
- The response is dependent on the route of administration (intravenous versus subcutaneous) and the frequency of administration. With subcutaneous administration, frequency is not as important as with the intravenous route. Response is less dependent on route of administration for darbepoetin alfa than for epoetin.
- The response may be limited by low iron stores, bone marrow fibrosis, infection, inflammation, inadequate dialysis, and other conditions.
- Hypertension may complicate therapy, particularly if the hemoglobin is raised quickly. This is primarily limited to patients undergoing dialysis. We recommend that target hemoglobin levels in dialysis patients treated with EPO or darbepoetin alfa should be maintained between 10 and 12 g/dl. In addition, the Hgb target should NOT exceed 13 g/dl.

The vast majority of cases of recombinant human erythropoietin (EPO) - related acquired pure red cell aplasia (PRCA) have occurred in patients treated with a particular epoetin alfa product. The underlying cause may be organic compounds (leached by polysorbate from uncoated rubber stoppers in prefilled syringes) that are acting as adjuvants, resulting in anti-EPO antibody development. Virtually all reported cases of anti-EPO antibody mediated PRCA have occurred in patients with chronic kidney disease who have received the drug subcutaneously. EPO-induced PRCA should be considered in the patient with significant anemia who has been treated with EPO for at least three to four weeks, and has previously responded to treatment with EPO. The condition is characterized by a sudden decline in hemoglobin level despite continued use of EPO, markedly reduced reticulocyte count, and normal white blood cell (WBC) and platelet counts. To definitively diagnose

EPO-induced PRCA, a bone marrow aspirate and evaluation for the presence of neutralizing anti-EPO antibodies should be performed. The bone marrow reveals severe erythroid hypoplasia, with less than five percent red blood cell precursors, and there may be evidence of a block in the maturation of erythroid precursors. Platelet and white cell precursors are entirely normal. Anti-EPO antibodies are detected by radioimmunoprecipitation assay (RIPA), enzyme linked immunosorbent assays (ELISA), or other assay, as available. Cessation of all erythropoietic stimulating agents with NOT switching to an alternative EPO product or to darbepoetin alfa in patients with PRCA is recommended. Patients should be transfused for symptomatic anemia.

Given that spontaneous remissions after cessation of EPO therapy are rare, the administration of immunosuppressive therapy in most patients is recommended. Initial therapy consisting of prednisone (1.0 mg/kg per day) plus oral cyclophosphamide (50 to 100 mg per day) for a maximum of three to four months. A reasonable alternative for first-line therapy is cyclosporine alone at a dose of 200 mg daily (or 100 mg twice daily) for a maximum of three to four months. Patients who do not respond to initial treatment with either oral cyclophosphamide plus prednisone or with cyclosporine alone may be subsequently treated with the other regimen.

### 9.12.3 Dose of EPO

The initial dose of EPO should vary based upon the baseline hemoglobin level, overall clinical setting, mode of administration, and the target hemoglobin level. A large number of studies have found that there is wide interpatient variability, as the dose of EPO required to reach hemoglobin levels above 11 g/dl among hemodialysis patients ranges from less than 50 to more than 300 U/kg three times per week.

In general, at a starting dose of 100 U/kg given intravenously three times per week, 90 percent of patients will attain a hemoglobin level of 11 to 12 g/dl, compared to 70 percent who will reach this level with 50 U/kg given intravenously three times per week. The logic of starting with the higher dose and then titrating down is that a month of therapy may be wasted on the nonresponders if the lower dose is used initially. In addition, titrating up from a smaller initial dose allows the hematocrit to rise more smoothly and more economically than with the titrate down approach.

In addition, numerous studies have found that intravenous therapy may also require, on average, approximately 30 percent more EPO than with the subcutaneous route. Thus, if subcutaneous doses are given, an initial dose for adults is 80 to 120 U/kg per week (typically 6000 U/week) given in one to three doses.

### 9.12.4 Dosage adjustments

In general, to attain hemoglobin levels of 11 g/dl or higher, a dose increase of 25 percent would be appropriate after four weeks if initial dosing levels do not result in a rate of increase in the hemoglobin of approximately 0.3 to 0.5 g/dl per week. Patients with hemoglobin levels that are increasing at this rate generally do not need adjustments in the EPO dose. Once the desired hemoglobin level is reached, smaller changes in the EPO dose, either titrating up or down, are usually satisfactory to maintain desired levels. Changing the dose of EPO more than once over a two- to four-week period is unnecessary in most instances.

Some patients respond to the administration of EPO with a marked acceleration in hemoglobin values. Among those with increases in hemoglobin of greater than 2.5 to 3 g/dl per month, the EPO dose should be reduced by at least 25 percent. Some clinicians recommend holding EPO for a short period of time (i.e., one week) before resuming treatment at the reduced dosing level if the hemoglobin exceeds the target value, while others recommend that EPO doses not be held but instead be reduced in dose. For hemodialysis patients in whom EPO administration has been initiated or the dose has recently changed, the hemoglobin should be measured once per week to adequately assess the response; by comparison, the hemoglobin of patients with stable hemoglobin levels and EPO dose can be assessed every two to four weeks, although in many dialysis facilities weekly hemoglobin levels are commonly obtained.

### 9.12.5 Hyporesponsivess to EPO

Some patients are relatively resistant to EPO and require large doses. This may be an important clinical observation since a poor response to EPO therapy may be associated with increased mortality. Higher doses of EPO have also been associated with an increased mortality, an effect that persists after adjustment for the usually lower hematocrit in such patients A large EPO requirement is defined as either the requirement of excessive doses during initiation of therapy, or inability to achieve or maintain target Hgb levels despite the large dose in the iron-replete patient. Different guidelines have suggested different definitions:

- 450 U/kg per week intravenous EPO or 300 U/kg per week subcutaneous EPO, per K/DOQI (NKF-DOQI, 2001).
- 300 U/kg per week of EPO (approximately 20,000 U/week) and 1.5 mcg/kg per week of darbepoetin alfa (approximately 100 mcg/week), per the revised European Guidelines (Locatelli et al., 2004).

The most common cause of resistance to EPO is absolute iron deficiency which may be due to external blood losses and/or exhaustion of iron stores due to an increase in erythropoiesis caused by EPO treatment. Additional causes include the following:

- Bone disease due to secondary hyperparathyroidism;
- Occult malignancy and unsuspected hematologic disorders
- Multiple myeloma/myelofibrosis/myelodysplastic syndrome.
- Chronic inflammation (with inhibition possibly due to enhanced cytokine production)
- Although now rare, the accumulation of aluminum in bone.
- Hemoglobinopathies, as patients with sickle cell disease or trait may have an inadequate response to the administration of EPO.
- The administration of angiotensin converting enzyme inhibitors and/or angiotensin II receptor antagonists.
- Development of pure red cell aplasia associated with the presence of neutralizing anti-erythropoietin antibodies in patients treated with particular brands of EPO by the subcutaneous route.
- Presence of HIV infection.

### 9.12.6 Darbepoetin alfa

Darbepoetin alfa is biochemically distinct from rHuEPO. It contains up to 22 sialic acid molecules (compared with a maximum of 14 for rHuEPO), giving it higher potency and an approximately three times longer half life than that of rHuEPO (25.3 versus 8.5 hours) following intravenous administration, and.approximately twofold longer than that of subcutaneously administered rHuEPO (Macdougall et al., 1999).

Clinical studies performed in rHuEPO-naive patients (defined as patients who had not received rHuEPO within 12 weeks) confirmed that darbepoetin alfa corrects anemia in patients with CKD who have not previously been exposed to hematopoietic stimulators. Darbepoetin alfa, compared with rHuEPO, controls hemoglobin (Hb) with an extended dosing interval. In patients with CKD who are not on dialysis, subcutaneous darbepoetin alfa administered once weekly at an initial dose of 0.45 µg/kg or once every two weeks at a median dose of 60 µg achieved target Hb concentrations in 93 to 97 percent of patients in a median time of five to seven weeks (Locatelli et al., 2001). As with rHuEPO, darbepoetin alfa has beneficial effects on quality of life via its ability to correct renal anemia. Interim data from a United States study performed in 48 evaluable rHuEPO-naive patients with CKD revealed improvements in 20 of the 22 different measures of health-related quality of life after 16 weeks of treatment with darbepoetin alfa (Bahman et al., 2002). Over the same period, there was a mean increase in Hb levels of 3.3 g/dl. Several large trials have confirmed that patients stabilized on either subcutaneous or intravenous rHuEPO can be successfully switched to darbepoetin alfa given at extended dosing intervals of once weekly or once every two weeks, with maintenance of a constant Hgb (mean change of -0.08 to 0.16 g/dl) after 28 to 36 weeks of treatment.

### 9.12.7 Continuous Erythropoiesis Receptor Activator (C.E.R.A)

Alternative bioengineering techniques to prolong the half life of EPO further resulted in the development of C.E.R.A., which is a pegylated derivative of epoetin beta with an elimination half-life of around 130 hours when it is administered either intravenously or subcutaneously. Phase III studies suggested that many patients are able to maintain with once-monthly administration of C.E.R.A., and a superiority [PATRONUS] suggested greater efficacy with this frequency of administration compared with once monthly dosing of darbepoetin alfa when it is administered intravenously to hemodialysis patients.

### 9.12.8 Epomimetics

The discovery of a drug that can mimic the action of erythropoietin is another method for eliminating the need for recombinant EPO in renal failure (Vadas et al., 2008). Evidence in support of this possibility was provided by a study in which a number of short peptides were evaluated as possible agonists of the EPO receptor. Peptides whose sequence matched a minimum consensus sequence of only 14 amino acids bound to and activated the EPO receptor. This observation provides strong experimental evidence that the EPO-EPO receptor complex requires only a small number of contact points for full effect.

Hematide is a synthetic peptide-based ESA with an amino acid sequence that is unrelated to erythropoietin. It is currently undergoing evaluation in clinical trials.

## 9.13 Management of hyperparathyroidism

The treatment of secondary hyperparathyroidism in CKD has evolved based upon new insights into the pathogenesis and clinical features of this disorder, the recognition that abnormal calcium and phosphate homeostasis may impact upon morbidity and mortality as well as mineral homeostasis, and the development of new therapeutic agents that can suppress parathyroid hormone (PTH) without exacerbating hyperphosphatemia and causing hypercalcemia.

Because of the interdependence of calcium, phosphate, vitamin D and PTH, it is difficult to elucidate the primary and proximate causes of parathyroid gland dysfunction in patients with CKD. In addition, no single pharmacological intervention is sufficient to completely restore disordered calcium and phosphate homeostasis. The medical management of secondary hyperparathyroidism in patients with CKD principally involves the use of the combination of phosphate binders, active vitamin D analogs, and/or calcimimetics (which increase the sensitivity of the CaSR to calcium), with differences in management based in part upon the degree of renal dysfunction and whether the patient is on dialysis.

Kidney failure disrupts systemic calcium and phosphate homeostasis and affects the bone, gut, and parathyroid glands. This occurs because of decreased renal excretion of phosphate and diminished renal hydroxylation of 25-hydroxyvitamin D to calcitriol (1,25-dihydroxyvitamin D).

Circulating calcitriol levels begin to fall when the GFR is less than 40 ml/min (occasionally even less than 80 ml/min and are typically markedly reduced in subjects with end-stage renal failure. The loss of functioning renal tissue and physiologic suppression by hyperphosphatemia participate in the decline in calcitriol synthesis. Thus, progressive kidney dysfunction results in hyperphosphatemia and calcitriol deficiency. These ultimately result in hypocalcemia. These abnormalities directly increase PTH levels via different mechanisms.

The CaSR [calcium-sensing receptor] which is highly expressed in the parathyroid glands, permits variations in the serum calcium concentration to be sensed by the parathyroid gland, leading to the desired changes in PTH secretion. The fall in serum calcium concentration with renal failure, as sensed by the CaSR, is a potent stimulus to the release of PTH.

There are reductions in calcitriol-regulated calcium absorption in the gut and calcium release from bone, both of which promote the development of hypocalcemia; this is a potent stimulus to the release of parathyroid hormone (PTH), as previously mentioned.

Calcitriol acts on the vitamin D receptor (VDR) in the parathyroid gland to suppress PTH transcription, but not PTH secretion. The absence of vitamin D also decreases calcium and phosphorus absorption in the gastrointestinal tract. The net effect of low vitamin D levels is to directly increase PTH production due to removal of the normal suppressive effect of calcitriol on the parathyroid glands, and indirectly increase secretion through the gastrointestinal mediated hypocalcemic stimulus.

A decrease in calcitriol levels also lowers the number of vitamin D receptors in the parathyroid cells. The lack of calcitriol and the decreased number of receptors may both directly promote parathyroid chief cell hyperplasia and nodule formation through potential non-genomic effects.

If the physiologic abnormalities are not corrected, renal bone disease, referred to as renal osteodystrophy, will develop. Although frequently asymptomatic, this disorder can result in weakness, fractures, bone and muscle pain, and avascular necrosis. These symptoms and signs do not generally occur until the patient is undergoing maintenance dialysis.

There are several forms of renal osteodystrophy, including osteitis fibrosa cystica, adynamic bone disease, and osteomalacia. In some patients, there is evidence of more than one type, which is called mixed osteodystrophy. Osteitis fibrosa cystica and mixed osteodystrophy are largely the direct result of increased PTH levels, while adynamic bone disease is a consequence of excessive suppression of the parathyroid gland with current therapies.

### 9.14 Chronic kidney disease - mineral and bone disorder (CKD-MBD)

The 2009 KDIGO practice guidelines were developed to provide recommendations for the evaluation and management of chronic kidney disease-mineral and bone disorder (CKD-MBD) (KDIGO, 2009). The term CKD-MBD was created to describe the syndrome associated with mineral, bone, and calcific cardiovascular abnormalities. The guidelines were formulated in an attempt to minimize the morbidity and mortality associated with abnormal mineral metabolism, abnormal bone process, and extraskeletal calcification.

**Stepped treatment approach in patients with CKD grades 3 through 5 not yet on dialysis with PTH levels higher than target level:**

**Step 1.** Among patients with serum phosphate levels greater than target levels, first restricting dietary phosphate intake. Although the optimal limit is unclear, we usually limit phosphate intake to 900 mg per day.

**Step 2.** Among patients with serum phosphate levels greater than target levels despite dietary phosphorus restriction after two to four months, the administration of phosphate binders is recommended. The two principal options are calcium and non-calcium based phosphate binders:

- For patients with an initial serum calcium levels less than 9.5 mg/dl (<2.37 mmol/l), a calcium containing phosphate binder may be administered as long as hypercalcemia does not develop.
- For patients with an initial serum calcium level greater than than 9.5 mg/dl (<2.37 mmol/l), we recommend a non-calcium based phosphate binder rather than a calcium-containing phosphate binder. Either sevelamer or lanthanum carbonate can be given in this setting.

Among predialysis patients with stage 3 to 5 CKD and elevated plasma intact PTH, treatment with ergocalciferol be initiated if nutritional vitamin D deficiency exists, as demonstrated by a 25(OH)-vitamin D (calcidiol) level of less than 30 ng/ml. After initiating treatment, serum calcium and phosphorus should be monitored quarterly, and continued need for supplementation with ergocalciferol can be re-evaluated annually. If the serum level of corrected total calcium exceeds 10.2 mg/dl (2.54 mmol/l), ergocalciferol therapy should be discontinued.

**Step 3.** If elevated PTH levels remain despite optimal ergocalciferol and phosphate binder therapy over a six-month period, administration of low dose active oral vitamin D analog is recommended. Any one of the available active oral agents (calcitriol, alfacalcidol, doxercalciferol, or paricalcitol) may be administered using cost and formulary availability as guides. The optimal regimen is not clear. Treatment with a vitamin D analog should not be given to predialysis patients with stage 3 to 5 CKD with elevated serum phosphate levels. A vitamin D analog should also not be given unless the corrected serum total calcium concentration is less than 9.5 mg/dL (<2.37 mmol/L). In addition, initiation of vitamin D supplementation requires close outpatient follow-up to avert severe hypercalcemia, with serum calcium and phosphate being measured at least every three months. If the serum level of corrected total calcium exceeds 10.2 mg/dl (2.54 mmol/l), ergocalciferol therapy and all forms of vitamin D therapy should be discontinued.

**Step 4.** Among predialysis patients with secondary hyperparathyroidism that is refractory to therapy with vitamin D analogues, calcium supplements, and phosphate binders, cinacalcet may be useful. However, the use of cinacalcet in early stages of CKD is highly controversial. Some experts and the KDIGO working group recommend NOT giving cinacalcet given the paucity of data concerning efficacy and safety in predialysis patients with CKD (Levin et al., 2008). Alternatively, parathyroidectomy could be considered for patients with refractory hyperparathyroidism and hypercalcemia not responsive to medical therapy.

If cinacalcet is administered, however, laboratory values should be monitored closely (weekly after starting therapy or change in dose) because of the risk of hypocalcemia and elevations of serum phosphate. The initial dose of 30 mg/day should be cautiously titrated upwards every two weeks only if the serum calcium level is greater than 8.4 mg/dL (2.1 mmol/liter) and PTH is higher than the target range.

**Stepped approach to the management of hyperparathyroidism and bone mineral abnormalities in dialysis patients:**

**Steps 1 and 2** Serum calcium, albumin, phosphate, 25(OH) vitamin D and intact PTH levels are measured initially and then on an ongoing basis. The initial focus in managing secondary hyperparathyroidism should be the prevention and management of hyperphosphatemia.

As a first step, a dietary restriction of 900 mg/day of phosphorus is appropriate. There should be an emphasis on high biologic sources of phosphorus (meats, eggs) and avoidance of lower nutritional sources (certain vegetables, colas).

Serum phosphate and calcium levels are next optimized, which involves treating hyperphosphatemia without causing hypercalcemia. This is difficult to achieve with thrice weekly hemodialysis.

We suggest the following interventions based upon serum phosphate and calcium levels.

- Phosphate <5.5 mg/dl (<1.78 mmol/l) and calcium <9.5 mg/dL (<2.37 mmol/l) – Calcium-based phosphate binders should be administered. Daily elemental calcium intake from binders to less than 1,500 mg, and total elemental calcium from diet and binders to less than 2,000 mg (in the presence of concurrent therapy with active vitamin D analogues) is recommended. Either calcium carbonate or calcium acetate can be administered.
- Phosphate <5.5 mg/dl (<1.78 mmol/l) and calcium >9.5 mg/dl (>2.37 mmol/l) – No phosphate binder is necessary in most patients.
- Phosphate >5.5 mg/dl (>1.78 mmol/l) and calcium >9.5 mg/dl (>2.37 mmol/L) – We recommend the administration of a non-calcium containing phosphate binder rather than calcium containing binders. Either sevelamer or lanthanum can be given.
- Phosphate >5.5 mg/dl (>1.78 mmol/l) and calcium <9.5 mg/dl (<2.37 mmol/l) – First titrating a calcium-based phosphate binder (up to 1,500 mg of elemental calcium from binders alone if there is concurrent use of active vitamin D analogues). If phosphate remains above 5.5 mg/dl (>1.78 mmol/l), then add a non-calcium containing phosphate binder.

**Step 3.** The next step is to decide whether phosphate binder therapy is sufficient or whether a calcimimetic or vitamin D analogue should be added. This is based upon calcium, phosphate, and PTH levels that are measured when administering optimal phosphate binder therapy (as defined in step 2).

If calcium supplementation and phosphate binders are effective in controlling PTH (ie, level between 150 and 300 pg/ml), no additional therapy may be needed. Serial follow up of PTH levels should be performed at three month intervals to assess the continued control of disease.

If PTH levels remain greater than 300 pg/ml with optimal binder therapy, the choice is either cinacalcet or vitamin D analogues. The decision to use vitamin D or cinacalcet as the next step, without additional data on outcomes, should be based upon the calcium and phosphate levels that are measured when administering optimal phosphate binders:

If the calcium and phosphate levels are both toward the upper limit of target levels, we suggest administering cinacalcet. This is because cinacalcet lowers both these parameters, while vitamin D therapy has the potential to further increase calcium and phosphorus levels.

If the calcium level is near or below the lower limit of normal and the phosphate is well within the normal range, we suggest the administration of vitamin D, given that cinacalcet would further lower the serum calcium. There are no compelling data to use intravenous versus oral therapy or one form of vitamin D analogue over the other. Cost and patient compliance would be two considerations.

Based upon this rationale, we initiate cinacalcet in patients with PTH >300 pg/ml and the following measured levels of phosphate and calcium when administering optimal phosphate binder therapy:

- Phosphate >5.5 mg/dl (>1.78 mmol/l) and Calcium >8.4 mg/dl (>2.1 mmol/l)
- Phosphate <5.5 mg/dl (<1.78 mmol/l) and Calcium >9.5 mg/dl (>2.37 mmol/l)

Since cinacalcet lowers serum calcium levels, it should not be initiated if the serum calcium level is less than 8.4 mg/dl (less than 2.1 mmol/l).

We suggest that a vitamin D analogue would be the initial choice in patients with PTH >300 pg/ml, and the following measured levels of phosphate and calcium when administering optimal phosphate binder therapy:

- Phosphate <5.5 mg/dl (<1.78 mmol/l) and Calcium <9.5 mg/dl (<2.37 mmol/l)

Since vitamin D analogues raise serum calcium and phosphate levels, we recommend NOT initiating these agents if the serum calcium level is greater than 9.5 mg/dl (>2.37 mmol/l), serum phosphate is greater than 5.5 mg/dl (>1.78 mmol/l), or the Ca X P product is greater than 55 $mg^2/dl^2$.

**Step 4.** The final step is to adjust the doses of phosphate binders, active vitamin D, and cinacalcet to attempt to attain target values:

Among patients with inadequate reduction of PTH with initial therapies, serum phosphate <5.5 mg/dl (<1.78 mmol/l), and serum calcium <9.5 mg/dL (<2.37 mmol/l), we suggest adding active vitamin D among those already receiving cenacle

Among patients with inadequate reduction of PTH with initial therapies and serum calcium >8.4 mg/dl (>2.1 mmol/l), we suggest adding cinacalcet among those already receiving a vitamin D analogue.

## 10. Preparation for and initiation of renal replacement therapy

It is important to identify patients who may eventually require renal replacement therapy since adequate preparation can decrease morbidity and perhaps mortality. Early identification enables dialysis to be initiated at the optimal time with a functioning chronic access and may also permit the recruitment and evaluation of family members for the placement of a renal allograft prior to the need for dialysis. In addition, the ability of the individual to psychologically accept the requirement of life-long renal replacement therapy is often diminished if inadequate time has elapsed between the time of recognition of ESRD and the initiation of dialysis.

CKD progresses at a variable rate due to differences in the clinical course of the underlying diseases (particularly between individuals) and the recognition that the natural history of progressive renal disease can be altered by various therapeutic interventions, particularly strict blood pressure control with an ACE inhibitor or ARB. As a result, exactly if and when a patient may require dialysis or renal transplantation is unclear. In addition, some patients refuse renal replacement therapy until the onset of absolute indications, while others desire early initiation to avoid the complications of severe chronic kidney disease, such as malnutrition.

### 10.1 Referral to nephrologists

Patients with CKD should be referred to a nephrologist early in the course of their disease, preferably before the plasma creatinine concentration exceeds 1.2 (106 micromol/l) and 1.5 mg/dl (133 micromol/l) in women and men, respectively, or the eGFR is less than 60 ml/min per 1.73 $m^2$. These subspecialists are trained to help counsel the patient in choosing the optimal renal replacement therapy and to manage the many issues associated with CKD. Lower costs and/or decreased morbidity and mortality may be associated with early referral and care by subspecialists. Reasons for later referral may include disease specific factors, patient and physician dependent causes, and health care system related factors. Late referral to a nephrologist has been associated with higher mortality after the initiation of dialysis (Kazmi et al., 2004).

An equally important component of early identification is institution of renoprotective therapy (eg, ACE inhibitor, angiotensin II receptor blocker, and rigorous blood pressure control) as early as possible after identifying the presence of progressive chronic kidney disease. Protective therapy has the greatest impact if it is initiated before the plasma creatinine concentration exceeds 1.2 (106 micromol/l) and 1.5 mg/dl (133 micromol/l) in women and men, respectively, or the eGFR is less than 60 ml/min per 1.73$m^2$. At this point, most patients have already lost more than one-half of their GFR. Waiting until the disease progresses further diminishes the likelihood of a successful response but still should be attempted.

### 10.2 Choice of renal replacement therapy

Once it is determined that renal replacement therapy will eventually be required, the patient should be counseled to consider the advantages and disadvantages of hemodialysis (in-center or at home), peritoneal dialysis (continuous or intermittent modalities), and renal transplantation (living or deceased donor). The 2006 K/DOQI guidelines recommend that patients with a GFR less than 30 ml/min per 1.73 $m^2$ should be educated concerning these issues.

Kidney transplantation is the treatment of choice for ESRD. A successful kidney transplant improves the quality of life and reduces the mortality risk for most patients, when compared with maintenance dialysis. To facilitate early transplantation, a 2008 NKF/KDOQI conference suggested early education and referral to a transplantation center plus the identification of potential living donors.

However, not all patients are appropriate candidates for a kidney allograft because of absolute and/or relative contraindications to this procedure or the subsequent required medications. Referral to a transplant program should occur once renal replacement therapy is thought to be required within the next year.

For these individuals and for those who are suitable transplant recipients but must wait for an available kidney, the choice between hemodialysis or peritoneal dialysis is influenced by a number of considerations such as availability, convenience, comorbid conditions, home situation, age, gender, and the ability to tolerate volume shifts.

In the United States, the universal availability of renal replacement therapy forces the nephrologist to consider its application in every patient in whom it might be indicated. However, the patient, particularly the elderly and terminally ill, may refuse dialysis, a choice which is assuming more prominence as patients and physicians grapple with the increasing use of advance directives, and the laudable goals of death with dignity and life with quality. Nevertheless, not all nephrologists are willing to recommend no treatment, especially when dialysis facilities are available with no need to ration therapy. These issues can be a source of conflict among physicians, patients, and their families.

### 10.3 Indications for renal replacement therapy

The decision to initiate dialysis in a patient with CKD involves the consideration of subjective and objective parameters by the physician and the patient. These parameters are often modulated by the patient's perception of his or her quality of life and by possible anxiety about starting new therapy that is technologically complex.

There are a number of clinical indications to initiate dialysis in patients with CKD. These include:

- Pericarditis or pleuritis (urgent indication)
- Progressive uremic encephalopathy or neuropathy, with signs such as confusion, asterixis, myoclonus, wrist or foot drop, or, in severe, cases, seizures (urgent indication)
- A clinically significant bleeding diathesis attributable to uremia (urgent indication)
- Fluid overload refractory to diuretics
- Hypertension poorly responsive to antihypertensive medications
- Persistent metabolic disturbances that are refractory to medical therapy. These include hyperkalemia, metabolic acidosis, hypercalcemia, hypocalcemia, and hyperphosphatemia.
- Persistent nausea and vomiting
- Weight loss or signs of malnutrition

However, these indications are potentially life-threatening. They occur when the patient has very advanced CKD, such as may be observed in those who present with severe uremia and have not had prior medical contact. For patients under medical care, delaying initiation of dialysis until one or more of these complications is present may put the patient at unnecessary jeopardy; dialysis should therefore be initiated well before these indications have developed. Patients with CKD should, therefore be closely followed and the GFR estimated.

## 11. Cardiovascular disease in patients with chronic kidney disease

### 11.1 Introduction

Cardiovascular disease (CVD) is common in the general population, affecting the majority of adults past the age of 60 years. The prevalence of coronary heart disease (CHD) is approximately one-third to one-half that of total CVD.

It is increasingly appreciated that chronic renal dysfunction alone is an independent risk factor for the development of CHD, and for more severe coronary heart disease (CHD)

(USRDS, 2010). Chronic kidney disease (CKD) is also associated with an adverse effect on prognosis from cardiovascular disease. This includes increased mortality after an acute coronary syndrome and after percutaneous coronary intervention (PCI) with or without stenting.

Patients on renal replacement therapy appears to be at extraordinary risk for premature death due to cardiovascular complications. Although accelerated atherosclerosis may be one important cause of the high cardiovascular mortality in this patient group, the CVD pattern is atypical in that volume overload and left ventricular hypertrophy (LVH) are very common. In addition, the incidence of sudden cardiac death, arrhythmias, hypertension, coronary artery disease (CAD), peripheral vascular disease (PVD), and pericarditis is markedly increased, and cardiac arrest or arrhythmia is the major cause of cardiovascular death in this patient population. CKD patients should therefore be considered in the "highest-risk" group for CVD, irrespective of levels of traditional CVD risk factor. The presence of cardiovascular disease is an important predictor of mortality in patients with ESRD, as it accounts for almost 50 percent of deaths. Of these, approximately 20 percent can be attributed to the consequences of CAD. Patients with varying stages of CKD but who are not yet dialysis-dependent also have a markedly increased risk of morbidity and mortality from CVD, including CHD.

### 11.2 Epidemiology

The incidence/prevalence of coronary disease in the dialysis population depends in part upon the definition that is used (Herzog, 2003). A confounding issue is that coronary disease often presents in atypical fashion in dialysis patients. As a result, the presence of CHD is frequently overlooked due to the absence of classic symptoms and/or signs of heart disease. Overall, the incidence is much higher than that observed in the general population.

Approximately 40 percent of incident dialysis patients have ischemic heart disease (Cheung et al., 2004), with an annual rate of myocardial infarction and/or angina of approximately 10 percent.

- Almost 40 percent of the 1846 patients enrolled in the HEMO report were noted to have ischemic heart disease at study initiation (Cheung et al., 2004). During the mean follow-up period of 2.8 years, angina and acute myocardial infarction were responsible for 43 percent of all cardiac hospitalizations, with ischemic heart disease causing 62 percent.
- Utilizing data from Wave II of the United States Renal Data System (USRDS) Dialysis Morbidity and Mortality study, the incidence of an acute coronary syndrome was 2.9 percent per year among 3374 incident dialysis patients followed for approximately two years (Trespalacios et al., 2002).
- In one Japanese study, the presence of significant occult coronary artery disease using coronary angiography (greater than 50 percent stenosis) was found in 16 of 30 asymptomatic patients (53 percent) initiating renal replacement therapy (Ohtake et al., 2005).

Cardiac disease, including coronary artery disease, left ventricular hypertrophy (LVH) and heart failure (HF), is common in patients with chronic kidney disease (CKD). LVH appears to be increasingly prevalent as the glomerular filtration rate (GFR) declines and with increased dialysis vintage.

- LVH has been found in as many as 30 to 45 percent of patients with chronic kidney disease (CKD) not yet on dialysis, with a higher prevalence and more severe LVH in those with increasingly lower degrees of renal function (Moran et al., 2008).

- Concentric LVH has been documented by echocardiography in 42 percent of patients at the start of dialysis and in as many as 75 percent of patients who have been on hemodialysis for 10 years (Parfrey & Foley, 1999).

### 11.3 Association with traditional and non-traditional risk factors

Although CKD alone is an independent risk factor for CHD, it is worthwhile to review the variety of abnormalities commonly observed in these patients that enhance the overall risk of cardiovascular disease (Table 4).

Traditional cardiovascular risk factors, such as hypertension (which may be accompanied by left ventricular hypertrophy), smoking history, diabetes, dyslipidemia and older age, are highly prevalent in CKD populations. The number of cardiovascular risk factors appears to correlate with the severity of kidney dysfunction.

Patients with CKD are also more likely to have the metabolic syndrome, which could contribute to the increase in cardiovascular risk (Chen et al., 2004). This syndrome is defined as some combination of insulin resistance, dyslipidemia, elevated serum glucose, abdominal obesity, and hypertension.

There are additional possible risk factors that are relatively unique to patients with moderate to severe CKD. These include retention of uremic toxins, anemia, increased calcium intake, abnormalities in bone mineral metabolism, proteinuria, and/or an "increased inflammatory-poor nutrition" state.

The purported link between some of these additional factors and an enhanced risk for CHD is uncertain. As an example, studies examining the relationship between coronary artery calcification and abnormalities in mineral metabolism (phosphorus, calcium, and parathyroid hormone) in patients with moderate to severe CKD have demonstrated increased coronary artery calcification, but conflicting data on independent risk factors (Dellegrottaglie et al., 2006).

| Traditional CVD Risk Factors | CKD Related "Nontraditional" CVD Risk Factors |
|---|---|
| Older age | Type (diagnosis) of CKD |
| Male gender | Decreased GFR |
| White Race | Proteinuria |
| Hypertension | Renin-angiotensin system activity |
| Elevated LDL cholesterol | Extra-cellular fluid volume overload |
| Decreased HDL cholesterol | Abnormal Calciam and Phosphorus |
| Diabetes mellitus | Metabolism |
| Tobacco use | Dyslipidemia |
| Physical inactivity | Anemia |
| Menopause | Malnutrition |
| Psychosocial stress | Inflammation |
| Family history of CVD | Infection |
| | Thrombogenic fectors |
| | Oxidative stress |
| | Elevated homocysteine |
| | Advanced glycation end-products (AGEs) |
| | Uremic toxins |

Table 4. Traditional vs. CKD- related factors associated with an increased risk for CVD.

Elevated levels of CRP and asymmetric dimethylarginine were both associated with increased risks of all cause and cardiovascular mortality in the Modification of Diet in Renal Disease study, after adjustment for known cardiovascular risk factors (Menon et al., 2005; Young et al., 2009), though a similar relationship for CRP was not seen in the Irbesartan for Diabetic Nephropathy trial. Hyperhomocysteinemia has also been inconsistently associated with increased cardiovascular risk.

Anemia has emerged as an important, independent risk factor for the development and progression of LVH and HF in CKD, and of adverse cardiovascular outcomes, including mortality. The presence of LVH is important clinically because it is associated with increases in the incidence of heart failure, ventricular arrhythmias, death following myocardial infarction, decreased LV ejection fraction, sudden cardiac death, aortic root dilation, and a cerebrovascular event.

### 11.3.1 Inflammation

The chronic inflammatory milieu of uremia may contribute to vascular calcification. A large number of proinflammatory or antiinflammatory substances have been evaluated as possible factors underlying this abnormal milieu. These include osteopontin, osteoprotegerin and fetuin. Osteopontin (a chemoattractant) concentrations in blood and in atherosclerotic plaques are increased in hemodialysis patients compared to age-matched healthy controls, and may correlate with aortic calcification score.

Inflammatory states and chronic kidney disease are also associated with altered levels of osteoprotegerin and alpha-2-Heremann Schmitt glycoprotein (AHSG, or human fetuin). Both of these factors are considered protective against extraosseous calcification.

Normal levels of fetuin help clear apoptotic cells, which act as potential niduses for crystal formation in medial arterial calcification, by augmenting phagocytosis. In vitro, fetuin appears to inhibit the precipitation of hydroxyapatite from supersaturated solutions of calcium and phosphate via the formation of a fetuin-mineral complex (FMC), which contains calcium phosphate, matrix Gla protein (MGP), fetuin, and other fetuin-like compounds.

Low fetuin levels, which are observed with CKD and other chronic inflammatory states, are associated with increased vascular calcification, cardiovascular mortality, and overall mortality in some studies of dialysis patients. The sera of dialysis patients with low fetuin concentrations also demonstrated impaired capacity to inhibit calcium/phosphate precipitation.

### 11.3.2 Oxidative and carbonyl stress

Increased production of cytokines due to oxidative stress is also observed among patients with renal failure. Oxidative stress, which occurs when there is an excessive free-radical production or low antioxidant level, could be an important condition for the development of endothelial dysfunction, inflammation, and atherogenesis. Lower plasmalogen levels, an indicator of such stress, have been reported in malnourished and inflamed patients with CKD.

With renal failure, molecules that are not cytokines may also accumulate and provoke an inflammatory response. As an example, advanced glycosylated end-products (AGE), which result from carbonyl stress, can clearly initiate inflammation in patients with renal failure.

### 11.3.3 Decreased antioxidants

The oral intake or the level of some antioxidants is lower than normal in both CRF and ESRD patients. An acute-phase response is also associated with decreased plasma levels of several antioxidants, such as serum vitamin C concentrations. Low serum vitamin C levels are in turn associated with increased cardiovascular morbidity and mortality.

### 11.3.4 Vascular calcification

Vascular calcification in patients with CKD, noted radiologically for decades, has been of increasing interest within the renal literature. The presence of calcium in the intimal layer may be a marker for plaque vulnerable to rupture and is associated with occlusive disease, while the presence of calcium in the vessel media may have direct adverse effect on vascular distensibility. The reduced vascular compliance may lead to increased pulse pressure, reduced coronary perfusion, and abnormal autonomic and endothelial vasomotor function. Such overall vascular stiffness may have a profound negative effect upon survival for dialysis patients. Risk factors to both types of calcification include excess calcium and phosphate, hyperparathyroidism/chronic inflammation and decreased circulating, or tissue-bound, inhibitors of the calcification process. Both appear to progress by a series of elaborate mechanisms similar to bony ossification and may involve genetic susceptibility or gene polymorphisms.

### 11.3.5 Chronic kidney disease alone as a risk factor for CHD

Based upon observational data in patients with CKD due to a variety of systemic and kidney-specific diseases, CKD is associated with an increased risk of adverse cardiovascular outcomes and is considered a CHD risk equivalent and the risk increases with increasing renal dysfunction and/or severity of proteinuria. The presence of both decreased renal function and increased proteinuria appears to further enhance the risk of cardiovascular disease versus that associated with either alone.

All patients with the same degree of renal dysfunction also do not have the same risk of cardiovascular disease. As an example, the overall risk for a 25 year old nonsmoking man with moderate CKD due to IgA nephropathy is not the same as that of a 65 year old man with a similar degree of CKD due to IgA but with a long history of smoking, hypertension, and elevated serum cholesterol levels. Thus, in addition to the evaluation for the presence of CKD, the proper assessment of overall cardiovascular risk requires an adequate assessment for the presence and severity of the other major risk factors for cardiovascular disease. Therefore, patients with either an estimated GFR that is less than 60 ml/min per 1.73 $m^2$ or with proteinuria greater than one gram/day to have sufficient increased cardiovascular risk to be considered a CHD risk equivalent.

## 11.4 Treatment and prevention of cardiovascular disease

### 11.4.1 Therapeutic lifestyle changes

Therapeutic lifestyle changes are a part of decreasing the risk of adverse cardiovascular outcomes in patients with CKD.

### 11.4.2 Smoking

In hemodialysis patients, smoking greatly increases the risk for cardiovascular morbidity and mortality. However, unlike that found in the general population, there are no studies showing beneficial cardiovascular outcomes with smoking cessation in dialysis patients. Despite this, we recommend that dialysis patients completely stop smoking, given the marked benefits of smoking cessation observed in the general population.

### 11.4.3 Weight reduction

In those with normal renal function, obesity is associated with an increased risk for cardiovascular disease. By comparison, the benefits of weight reduction in dialysis patients are unclear. In contrast, there appears to be a survival advantage in obese dialysis patients. The higher mortality risks in dialysis patients with lower body mass indices may be attributed to malnutrition. Limited data suggest that increased muscle mass confers greater survival advantage than increased fat in the dialysis population. In general, we do not currently recommend weight reduction for dialysis patients, although it is reasonable to recommend an increase in muscle rather than fat. Weight reduction may be attempted in morbidly obese patients.

### 11.4.4 Exercise

Regular exercise has a variety of possible cardiovascular benefits in those with normal renal function. By comparison, a paucity of data exists concerning the association between cardiovascular benefits, survival, and exercise in dialysis patients. This was examined using data for 2507 patients from the Dialysis Morbidity and Mortality Wave 2 study. Decreased mortality was associated with patients who exercised two to three and four to five times per week. However, for unclear reasons, daily exercise provided no survival benefit.

### 11.4.5 Oxidative stress

A number of studies have demonstrated that hemodialysis patients are, in general, at a state of increased oxidative stress, suggesting the possibility that antioxidant therapies may improve clinical outcomes. Limited evidence suggests that an attempt to lower oxidative stress may improve cardiovascular disease outcomes in ESRD.

### 11.4.6 Hyperhomocysteinemia

Hyperhomocysteinemia is common in patients with ESRD. As observed in those with normal kidney function, lowering homocysteine levels does not improve cardiovascular outcomes in dialysis patients. Folic acid and B vitamins decrease homocysteine levels in this population .Treatment with high doses of folic acid and B vitamins did not improve survival or reduce the incidence of vascular disease in patients with advanced CKD or ESRD. This was best shown in the double-blind randomized controlled trial Homocysteinemia in Kidney and End Stage Renal Disease (HOST), which compared the effect of folic acid (40 mg/day), pyridoxine (100 mg/day), and vitamin B12 (2 mg/day) versus placebo on vascular outcomes in 2056 patients with advanced CKD, including ESRD. At a median follow-up of 3.2 years, there was NO difference between the groups in terms of total mortality, myocardial infarction, stroke, and amputations.

### 11.4.7 Mineral metabolism issues

Cardiovascular disease in dialysis patients may be due in part to the presence of excess vascular calcification, particularly in the form of extensive coronary artery calcification. A key question is what drives the development and maintenance, or progression, of such abnormal calcification. Abnormalities of mineral metabolism and therapeutic maneuvers aimed at correcting these abnormalities have been implicated as primary underlying pathogenic factors. These include hyperphosphatemia, administration of calcium-containing oral phosphate binders, elevated parathyroid hormone levels, and (possibly) decreased serum vitamin D levels.

No prospective randomized studies have demonstrated a cardiovascular benefit and/or a survival advantage with any of the current therapeutic options, including limiting calcium intake, use of non-calcium or calcium-containing phosphate binders, active vitamin D therapy, and administration of calcimimetics. However, observational studies have shown improved survival in hemodialysis patients treated with active vitamin D analogues. Despite the absence of evidence from randomized trials, we generally aim for a calcium x phosphate product less than 55 $mg^2/dL^2$ using current therapeutic options. However, it is possible that even lower levels (<50 $mg^2/dl^2$) offer further survival advantage.

#### 11.4.8 Diabetes mellitus

Guidelines from the American Heart Association and the American Diabetes Association recommended optional glycemic control, reaching blood pressure target levels and lipids monitoring (with subsequent dysplipidemia treatment). In CKD patients with diabetes, CVD must be treated aggressively.

#### 11.4.9 Anemia

Because anemia is contributing to the development of LVH in ESRD and partial correction of severe anemia with epoetin results in regression of LVH , epoetin treatment is advocated . Treatment of severe anemia is also associated with less ischemic symptoms in patient with CAD. However, although life quality improves after anemia correction; the evidence that epoetin treatment reduces cardiovascular mortality in ESRD is based on data from observational studies only.

## 12. References


Abitbol C, Zilleruelo G, Freundlich M, & Strauss J. (1990). Quantitation of proteinuria with urine protein/creatinine ratios and random testing with dipsticks in children. *J Pediatr,* Vol. 116, No. 2, pp. 243-7.

Abboud H, & Henrich WL. (2010). Clinical practice. Stage IV chronic kidney disease. *N Engl J Med,* Vol. 362, No. 1, pp. 56-65.

Adrogué HJ. (1992). Glucose homeostasis and the kidney. *Kidney Int,* Vol. 42, No. 5, pp. 1266-82.

Ahlstrom A, Tallgren M, Peltonen S, & Pettila V. (2004). Evolution and predictive power of serum cystatin C in acute renal failure. *Clin Nephrol,* Vol. 62, No. 5, pp. 344-50.

Alexopoulos E, Seron D, Hartley RB, & Cameron JS. (1990). Lupus nephritis: Correlation of interstitial cells with glomerular function. *Kidney Int,* Vol. 37, No. 1, pp. 100-9.

Allon M. (1995). Hyperkalemia in end-stage renal disease: Mechanisms and management. *J Am Soc Nephrol,* Vol. 6, No. 4, pp. 1134-42.

Aros C, Remuzzi G. (2002). The renin-angiotensin system in progression, remission and regression of chronic nephropathies. *J Hypertens Suppl,* Vol. 20, No. 3, pp. S45-53.

Astor BC, Muntner P, Levin A, Eustace JA, & Coresh J. (2002). Association of kidney function with anemia: the Third National Health and Nutrition Examination Survey (1988-1994). *Arch Intern Med,* Vol. 162, No. 12, pp. 1401-8.

Bajema IM, Hagen EC, Hermans J, Noël LH, Waldherr R, Ferrario F, Van Der Woude FJ, & Bruijn JA. (1999). Kidney biopsy as a predictor for renal outcome in ANCA-associated necrotizing glomerulonephritis. *Kidney Int,* Vol. 56, No. 5, pp. 1751-8.

Bakker AJ. (1999). Detection of microalbuminuria. Receiver operating characteristic curve analysis favors albumin-to-creatinine ratio over albumin concentration. *Diabetes Care,* Vol. 22, No. 2, pp.307-13.

Bammens B, Verbeke K, Vanrenterghem Y, & Evenepoel P. (2003). Evidence for impaired assimilation of protein in chronic renal failure. *Kidney Int,* Vol. 64, No. 6, pp. 2196-203.

Barnes, JL. (2001). Platelets. In: Immunologic Renal Diseases, 2nd ed, Neilson, EG, Couser, WG (Eds), Lippincott Williams and Wilkins, Philadelphia, p 593.

Bazzi, C, Petrini, C, Rizza, V, Arrigo G, Napodano P, Paparella M, D'Amico G. Urinary N-acetyl-beta-glucosaminidase excretion is a marker of tubular cell dysfunction and a predictor of outcome in primary glomerulonephritis. Nephrol Dial Transplant 2002; 17, No. 11, pp. 1890-6.

Benigni A, Corna D, Zoja C, Longaretti L, Gagliardini E, Perico N, Coffman TM, & Remuzzi G. (2004). Targeted deletion of angiotensin II type 1A receptor does not protect mice from progressive nephropathy of overload proteinuria. *J Am Soc Nephrol,* Vol. 15, No. 10, pp. 2666-74.

Bini EJ, Kinkhabwala A, & Goldfarb DS. (2006). Predictive value of a positive fecal occult blood test increases as the severity of CKD worsens. *Am J Kidney Dis,* Vol. 48, No. 4, pp. 580-6.

Boffa JJ, Lu Y, Placier S, & Stefanski A. (2003). Regression of Renal Vascular and Glomerular Fibrosis: Role of Angiotensin II Receptor Antagonism and Matrix Metalloproteinases. *J Am Soc Nephrol,* Vol. 14, No. 5, pp. 1132-44.

Brandstrom E, Grzegorczyk A, Jacobsson, L, Friberg P, Lindahl A, & Aurell M. (1998). GFR measurement with iohexol and 51Cr-EDTA. A comparison of the two favoured GFR markers in Europe. *Nephrol Dial Transplant,* Vol. 13, No. 5, pp. 1176-82.

Buckalew VM Jr, Berg RL, Wang SR, Porush JG, Rauch S, & Schulman G. (1996). Prevalence of hypertension in 1,795 subjects with chronic renal disease: The Modification of Diet in Renal Disease Study baseline cohort. *Am J Kidney Dis,* Vol. 28, No. pp. 811-21.

Burton C, & Harris KPG. (1996). The role of proteinuria in the progression of chronic renal failure. *Am J Kidney Dis,* Vol. 27, No. 6, pp. 765-75.

Chen J, Muntner P, Hamm LL, & Jones DW. (2004). The metabolic syndrome and chronic kidney disease in U.S. adults. *Ann Intern Med,* Vol. 140, No. 3, pp. 167-74.

Chen J, Chen JK, Neilson EG, & Harris RC. (2006). Role of EGF receptor activation in angiotensin ii-induced renal epithelial cell hypertrophy. *J Am Soc Nephrol,* Vol. 17, No. 6, pp. 1615-23.

Cheung AK, Sarnak MJ, Yan G, Berkoben M, Heyka R, Kaufman A, Lewis J, Rocco M, Toto R, Windus D, Ornt D, & Levey AS. (2004). Cardiac diseases in maintenance hemodialysis patients: Results of the HEMO study. *Kidney Int,* Vol. 65, No.6, pp. 2380-9.

Chitalia VC, Kothari J, Wells EJ, Livesey JH, Robson RA, Searle M, Lynn KL. (2001). Cost-benefit analysis and prediction of 24-hour proteinuria from the spot urine protein-creatinine ratio. *Clin Nephrol,* Vol. 55, No. 6, pp. 436-47.

Chonchol M, Lippi G, Salvagno G, Zoppini G, Muggeo M, & Targher G. (2008). Prevalence of subclinical hypothyroidism in patients with chronic kidney disease. *Clin J Am Soc Nephrol,* Vol. 3, No. 5, pp. 1296-300.

Coresh, J Byrd-Holt D, Astor, BC, Briggs JP, Eggers PW, Lacher DA, & Hostetter TH. (2005). Chronic kidney disease awareness, prevalence, and trends among U.S. adults, 1999 to 2000. *J Am Soc Nephrol,* Vol. 16, No. 1, pp. 180-8.

Centers for Disease Control and Prevention (CDC). (2007). Prevalence of chronic kidney disease and associated risk factors--United States, 1999-2004. *MMWR Morb Mortal Wkly Rep,* Vol. 56, No. 8, pp. 161-5.

Coll E, Botey A, Alvarez L, Poch E, Quintó L, Saurina A, Vera M, Piera C, & Darnell A. (2000). Serum cystatin C as a new marker for noninvasive estimation of glomerular filtration rate and as a marker for early renal impairment. *Am J Kidney Dis,* Vol. 36, No. 1, pp. 29-34.

Constantiner, M, Sehgal, AR, Humbert, L, Constantiner D, Arce L, Sedor JR, & Schelling JR. (2005). A dipstick protein and specific gravity algorithm accurately predicts pathological proteinuria. *Am J Kidney Dis,* Vol. 45, No. 5, pp. 833-41.

Coresh J, Astor BC, Greene T, Eknoyan G, & Levey AS. (2003). Prevalence of chronic kidney disease and decreased kidney function in the adult US population: Third National Health and Nutrition Examination survey. *Am J Kidney Dis,* Vol. 41, No. 1, pp.1-12.

Coresh J, Byrd-Holt D, Astor BC, Briggs JP, Eggers PW, Lacher DA, & Hostetter TH. (2005). Chronic kidney disease awareness, prevalence, and trends among U.S. adults, 1999 to 2000. *J Am Soc Nephrol,* Vol. 16, No. 1, 180-8.

Coresh J, Selvin E, Stevens LA, Manzi J, Kusek JW, Eggers P, Van Lente F, & Levey AS. (2007). Prevalence of chronic kidney disease in the United States. *JAMA,* Vol. 298, No, 17, pp. 2038-47.

Crowley SD, Vasievich MP, Ruiz P, Gould SK, Parsons KK, Pazmino AK, Facemire C, Chen BJ, Kim HS, Tran TT, Pisetsky DS,Barisoni L, Prieto-Carrasquero MC, Jeansson M, Foster MH, & Coffman TM. (2009). Glomerular type 1 angiotensin receptors augment kidney injury and inflammation in murine autoimmune nephritis. *J Clin Invest,* Vol. 119, No. 4, pp. 943-53.

D'Amico G. (1992). Influence of clinical and histological features on actuarial renal survival in adult patients with idiopathic IgA nephropathy, membranous nephropathy, and membranoproliferative glomerulonephritis: Survey of the recent literature. *Am J Kidney Dis,* Vol. 20, No. 4, pp. 315-23.

de Brito-Ashurst I, Varagunam M, Raftery MJ, & Yaqoob MM. (2009). Bicarbonate supplementation slows progression of CKD and improves nutritional status. *J Am Soc Nephrol,* Vol. 20, No. 9, pp. 2075-84.

Dellegrottaglie S, Saran R, Gillespie B, Zhang X, Chung S, Finkelstein F, Kiser M, Sanz J, Eisele G, Hinderliter AL, Kuhlmann M, Levin NW, & Rajagopalan S. (2006). Prevalence and predictors of cardiovascular calcium in chronic kidney disease (from the Prospective Longitudinal RRI-CKD Study). *Am J Cardiol,* Vol. 98, No. 5, pp. 571-6.

De Vriese AS, Endlich K, Elger M, Lameire NH, Atkins RC, Lan HY, Rupin A, Kriz W, & Steinhausen MW. (1999). The role of selectins in glomerular leukocyte recruitment in rat anti-glomerular basement membrane glomerulonephritis. *J Am Soc Nephrol,* Vol. 10, No. 12, pp. 2510-7.

Deinum J, & Derkx FH. (2000). Cystatin for estimation of glomerular filtration rate? *Lancet,* Vol. 356, No. 9242, pp. 1624-5.

Dharnidharka VR, Kwon C, & Stevens G. (2002). Serum cystatin C is superior to serum creatinine as a marker of kidney function: a meta-analysis. *Am J Kidney Dis,* Vol. 40, No. 2, pp. 221-6.

Diamond JR, Karnovsky MJ. (1987). Exacerbation of chronic aminonucleoside nephrosis by dietary cholesterol supplementation. *Kidney Int,* Vol. 32, No. 5, pp. 671-7.

Diemont WL, Vruggink PA, Meuleman EJ, Doesburg WH, Lemmens WA, & Berden JH. (2000). Sexual dysfunction after renal replacement therapy. *Am J Kidney Dis,* Vol. 35, No. 5, pp.845-51.

Eddy AA, McCulloch L, Liu E, & Adams J. (1991). A relationship between proteinuria and active tubulointerstitial disease in rats with experimental nephrotic syndrome. *Am J Pathol,* Vol. 138, No.5, pp. 1111-23.

Eddy AA. (1994). Experimental insights into the tubulointerstitial disease accompanying primary glomerular lesions. *J Am Soc Nephrol,* Vol. 5, No. 6, pp. 1273-87.

Eknoyan G, Hostetter T, Bakris GL, Hebert L, Levey AS, Parving HH, Steffes MW, & Toto R. (2003). Proteinuria and other markers of chronic kidney diseae: A position statement of the National Kidney Foundation (NKF) and the National Institute of Diabetes and Digestive and Kidney Diseases (NIDDK). *Am J Kidney Dis,* Vol. 42, No.4, pp. 617-22.

Eriksen BO, & Ingebretsen OC. (2006). The progression of chronic kidney disease: a 10-year population-based study of the effects of gender and age. *Kidney Int,* Vol. 69, No. 2, pp. 375-82.

Finkelstein, FO, Shirani, S, Wuerth, D, Finkelstein, SH. Therapy Insight: sexual dysfunction in patients with chronic kidney disease. Nat Clin Pract Nephrol 2007; 3, No. 4, pp. 200-7.

Fliser D, & Ritz E. (2001). Serum cystatin C concentration as a marker of renal dysfunction in the elderly. *Am J Kidney Dis,* Vol. 37, No. 1, pp. 79-83.

Fogo AB. (2000). The role of angiotensin II and plasminogen activator inhibitor-1 in progressive glomerulosclerosis. *Am J Kidney Dis,* Vol. 35, No. 2, pp. 179-88.

Fox CS, Larson MG, Leip EP, Culleton B, Wilson PW, & Levy D. (2004). Predictors of new-onset kidney disease in a community-based population. *JAMA,* Vol. 291, No. 7, pp. 844-50.

Freedman BI, Volkova NV, Satko SG, Krisher J, Jurkovitz C, Soucie JM, & McClellan WM. (2005). Population-based screening for family history of end-stage renal disease among incident dialysis patients. *Am J Nephrol,* Vol. 25, No. 6, pp. 529-35.

Fukunishi I, Kitaoka T, Shirai T, Kino K, Kanematsu E, & Sato Y. (2002). Psychiatric disorders among patients undergoing hemodialysis therapy. *Nephron,* Vol. 91, No. 2, pp. 344-7.

Garg AX, Blake PG, Clark WF, Clase CM, Haynes RB, & Moist LM. (2001). Association between renal insufficiency and malnutrition in older adults: Results from the NHANES III. *Kidney Int,* Vol. 60, No. 5, pp. 1867-74.

Gennari FJ, & Segal AS. (2002). Hyperkalemia: An adaptive response in chronic renal insufficiency. *Kidney Int,* Vol. 62, No. 1, pp. 1-9.

Gimenez LF, Solez K, & Walker WG. (1987). Relation between renal calcium content and renal impairment in 246 human renal biopsies. *Kidney Int,* Vol. 31, No. 1, pp. 93-9.

Ginsberg JM, Chang BS, Matarese, RA, & Garella S. (1983). Use of single voided urine samples to estimate quantitative proteinuria. *N Engl J Med,* Vol. 309, No. 25, pp. 1543-6.

Gonick HC, Kleeman CR, Rubini ME, & Maxwell MH. 1971; Functional impairment in chronic renal disease. 3. Studies of potassium excretion. Am J Med Sci 261, No. 5, pp. 281-90.

Groesbeck D, Kottgen A, Parekh R, Selvin E, Schwartz GJ, Coresh J, & Furth S. (2008). Age, gender, and race effects on cystatin C levels in US adolescents. *Clin J Am Soc Nephrol,* Vol. 3, No.6, pp. 1777-85.

Grone EF, & Grone HJ. (2008). Does hyperlipidemia injure the kidney? *Nat Clin Pract Nephrol,* Vol. 4, No. 8, pp. 424-5.

Grubb A, Nyman U, Bjork J, Lindström V, Rippe B, Sterner G, Christensson A. (2005). Simple cystatin C-based prediction equations for glomerular filtration rate compared with the modification of diet in renal disease prediction equation for adults and the Schwartz and the Counahan-Barratt prediction equations for children. *Clin Chem,* Vol. 51, No. 8, pp. 1420-31.

Grubb A, Bjork J, Lindstrom V, Sterner G, Bondesson P, & Nyman U. (2005). A cystatin C-based formula without anthropometric variables estimates glomerular filtration rate better than creatinine clearance using the Cockcroft-Gault formula. *Scand J Clin Lab Invest,* Vol. 65, No. 2, pp. 153-62.

Hallan SI, Coresh J, Astor BC, Asberg A, Powe NR, Romundstad S, Hallan HA, Lydersen S, & Holmen J. (2006). International comparison of the relationship of chronic kidney disease prevalence and ESRD risk. *J Am Soc Nephrol,* Vol. 17, No. 8, pp. 2275-84.

Herzog CA. (2003). How to manage the renal patients with coronary heart disease: The agony and the ecstasy of opinion-based medicine. *J Am Soc Nephrol,* Vol. 14, No. 10, pp. 2556-72.

Hilgers KF, & Mann JF. (2002). ACE inhibitors versus AT(1) receptor antagonists in patients with chronic renal disease. *J Am Soc Nephrol,* Vol. 13. No. 4, pp. 1100-8.

Hirschberg R, & Wang S. (2005). Proteinuria and growth factors in the development of tubulointerstitial injury and scarring in kidney disease. *Curr Opin Nephrol Hypertens,* Vol. 14, No. 1, pp. 43-52.

Hoek FJ, Kemperman FA, & Krediet RT. (2003). A comparison between cystatin C, plasma creatinine and the Cockcroft and Gault formula for the estimation of glomerular filtration rate. *Nephrol Dial Transplant,* Vol. 18, No.10 pp. 2024-31.

Hoffmann S, Podlich D, Hahnel B, Kriz W, & Gretz N. (2004). Angiotensin II type 1 receptor overexpression in podocytes induces glomerulosclerosis in transgenic rats. *J Am Soc Nephrol,* Vol. 15, No. 6, pp. 1475-87.

Holdsworth SR, de Kretser DM, & Atkins RC. (1978). A comparison of hemodialysis and transplantation in reversing the uremic disturbance of male reproductive function. *Clin Nephrol,* Vol. 10, No.4, pp.146-50.

Holley JL, Schmidt RJ, Bender FH, Dumler F, & Schiff M. (1997). Gynecologic and reproductive issues in women on dialysis. *Am J Kidney Dis,* Vol. 29, No. 5, pp. 685-90.

Hooke DH, Gee DC, & Atkins RC. (1987). Leukocyte analysis using monoclonal antibodies in human glomerulonephritis. *Kidney Int,* Vol. 31, No. 4, pp. 964-72.

Hou S. (1999). Pregnancy in chronic renal insufficiency and end-stage renal disease. *Am J Kidney Dis,* Vol. 33, No.2, pp. 235-52.

Hsu CY, & Chertow GM. (2002). Elevations of serum phosphorus and potassium in mild to moderate chronic renal insufficiency. *Nephrol Dial Transplant,* Vol. 17, No. 8, pp. 1419-25.

Hsu CY, Vittinghoff E, Lin F, & Shlipak MG. (2004). The incidence of end-stage renal disease is increasing faster than the prevalence of chronic renal insufficiency. *Ann Intern Med,* Vol. 141, No. 2, pp. 95-101.

Hsu CC, Kao WH, Coresh J, Pankow JS, Marsh-Manzi J, Boerwinkle E, & Bray MS. (2005). Apolipoprotein E and progression of chronic kidney disease. *JAMA,* Vol. 293, No. 23, pp. 2892-9.

Hsu CC, Bray MS, Kao WH, Pankow JS, Boerwinkle E, & Coresh J. (2006). Genetic variation of the renin-angiotensin system and chronic kidney disease progression in black individuals in the atherosclerosis risk in communities study. *J Am Soc Nephrol,* Vol. 17, No. 2, pp. 504-12.

Huang Y, Wongamorntha S, Kasting J, McQuillan D, Owens RT, Yu L, Noble NA, & Border W. (2006). Renin increases mesangial cell transforming growth factor-beta1 and matrix proteins through receptor-mediated, angiotensin II-independent mechanisms. *Kidney Int,* Vol. 69, No. 1, pp. 105-13.

Huugen D, van Esch A, Xiao H, Peutz-Kootstra CJ, Buurman WA, Tervaert JW, Jennette JC, & Heeringa P. (2007). Inhibition of complement factor C5 protects against anti-myeloperoxidase antibody-mediated glomerulonephritis in mice. *Kidney Int,* Vol. 71, No. 7, pp. 646-54.

Ingelfinger JR. (2008). Aliskiren and dual therapy in type 2 diabetes mellitus. *N Engl J Med,* Vol. 358, No. 23, pp. 2503-5.

Iseki K, Ikemiya Y, Inoue T, Iseki C, Kinjo K, & Takishita S. (2004). Significance of hyperuricemia as a risk factor for developing ESRD in a screened cohort. *Am J Kidney Dis,* Vol. 44, No. 4, pp. 642-50.

Ishida-Okawara A, Ito-Ihara T, Muso E, Ono T, Saiga K, Nemoto K, & Suzuki K. (2004). Neutrophil contribution to the crescentic glomerulonephritis in SCG/Kj mice. *Nephrol Dial Transplant,* Vol. 19, No. 7, pp. 1708-15.

Ito I, Yuzawa Y, Mizuno M, Nishikawa K, Tashita A, Jomori T, Hotta N, & Matsuo S. (2001). Effects of a new synthetic selectin blocker in an acute rat thrombotic glomerulonephritis. *Am J Kidney Dis,* Vol. 38, No. 2, pp. 265-73.

Jacobson HR. (1991). Chronic renal failure: pathophysiology. *Lancet,* Vol. 338, No. 8764, pp. 419-23.

Jennette JC, Falk RJ. (2008). New insight into the pathogenesis of vasculitis associated with antineutrophil cytoplasmic autoantibodies. *Curr Opin Rheumatol,* Vol. 20, No. 1, pp. 55-60.

Johnson RJ, Couser WG, Chi EY, Adler S, & Klebanoff SJ. (1987). A new mechanism for glomerular injury: A myeloperoxidase (MPO)-hydrogen peroxide-halide system. *J Clin Invest,* Vol. 79, No. 5, pp.1379-87.

Johnson RJ, Klebanoff SJ, & Couser WG. (2001). Neutrophils (Chapter 25). In: Immunologic Renal Diseases. Neilson, EG, Couser, WG, (Eds), Lippincott-Wilkins, Philadelphia p.579.

Jones CA, McQuillan GM, Kusek JW, Eberhardt MS, Herman WH, Coresh J, Salive M, Jones CP, & Agodoa LY. (1998). Serum creatinine levels in the US population: Third national health and nutrition examination survey. *Am J Kidney Dis,* Vol. 32, No. 6, pp. 992-9.

Jones C, Francis M, Eberhardt M, Chavers B, Coresh J, Engelgau M, Kusek JW, Byrd-Holt D, Narayan KM, Herman WH, Jones CP, Salive M, & Agodoa LY. (2002). Microalbuminuria in the US population: Third national health and nutrition examination survey. *Am J Kidney Dis,* Vol. 39, No. 3, pp. 445-59.

Kazmi WH, Kausz AT, Khan S, Abichandani R, Ruthazer R, Obrador GT & Pereira BJG. (2001). Anemia- an early complication of chronic renal insufficiency. *Am J Kidney Dis,* Vol. 38, No. 4, pp. 803-12.

Kazmi WH, Khan SS, Obrador GT, Pereira BJG, & Kausz AT. (2004). Timing of nephrology referral and mortality among end-stage renal disease patients: A propensity score analysis. *Nephrol Dial Transplant,* Vol. 19, No. 7, pp.1808-14.

Kazmi WH, Shahid K, Yousuf A, Osmani AH, Marmoos TH, Warsi FA, & Khan S. (2007). A higher than expected prevalence of Chronic Kidney Disease in Pakistan. *J Am Soc Nephrol,* Vol. 18, p. 540A.

Kaptein EM, Quion-Verde H, Chooljian CJ, Tang WW, Friedman PE, Rodriquez HJ, & Massry SG. (1988). The thyroid in end-stage renal disease. *Medicine (Baltimore),* Vol. 67, No. 3, pp. 187-97.

KDIGO clinical practice guidelines for the diagnosis, evaluation, prevention, and treatment of chronic kidney disease-mineral and bone disorder (CKD-MBD). (2009). *Kidney Int,* Vol. 76 (Suppl 113), pp. S1-130.

Keane WF. (1994). Lipids and the kidney. *Kidney Int,* Vol. 46, No. 3, pp. 910-20.

Kielstein, JT, Salpeter, SR, Bode-Boeger, SM, Cooke JP, & Fliser D. (2006). Symmetric dimethylarginine (SDMA) as endogenous marker ofrenalfunction--a meta-analysis. *Nephrol Dial Transplant,* Vol. 21, No. 9, pp. 2446-51.

Kimmel PL, Thamer M, Richard CM, & Ray NF. (1998). Psychiatric illness in patients with end-stage renal disease. *Am J Med,* Vol. 105, No. 3, pp. 214-21.

King AJ, & Levey AS. (1993). Dietary protein and renal function. *J Am Soc Nephrol,* Vol. 3, No. 11, pp. 1723-37.

Kitching AR, Ru Huang X, Turner AL, Tipping PG, Dunn AR, & Holdsworth SR. (2002). The requirement for granulocyte-macrophage colony-stimulating factor and granulocyte colony-stimulating factor in leukocyte-mediated immune glomerular injury. *J Am Soc Nephrol,* Vol. 13, No. 2, 350-8.

Knight, EL, Verhave, JC, Spiegelman, D, Hillege HL, de Zeeuw D, Curhan GC, & de Jong PE. (2004). Factors influencing serum cystatin C levels other than renal function and the impact on renal function measurement. *Kidney Int,* Vol. 65, No. 4, pp.1416-21.

Kopple JD, Greene T, Chumlea WC, Hollinger D, Maroni BJ, Merrill D, Scherch LK, Schulman G, Wang SR, & Zimmer GS. (2000). Relationship between nutritional status and the glomerular filtration rate: results from the MDRD study. *Kidney Int,* Vol. 57, No. 4, pp. 1688-703.

Kottgen A, Selvin E, Stevens LA, Levey AS, Van Lente F, Coresh J. (2008). Serum cystatin C in the United States: the Third National Health and Nutrition Examination Survey (NHANES III). *Am J Kidney Dis,* Vol. 51:No. 3, 385-94.

Kurts C, Heymann F, Lukacs-Kornek V, Boor P, & Floege J. (2007). Role of T cells and dendritic cells in glomerular immunopathology. *Semin Immunopathol,* Vol. 29, No. 4, pp. 317-35.

Lan HY, Patterson DJ, & Atkins RC. (1991). Initiation and evolution of interstitial leukocytic infiltration in experimental glomerulonephritis. *Kidney Int,* Vol. 40, No. 3, pp. 425-33.

Lautrette A, Li S, Alili R, Sunnarborg SW, Burtin M, Lee DC, Friedlander G, & Terzi F. (2005). Angiotensin II and EGF receptor cross-talk in chronic kidney diseases: a new therapeutic approach. *Nat Med,* Vol. 11, No. 8, pp. 867-74.

Levey AS. (1990). Measurement of renal function in chronic renal disease. *Kidney Int,* Vol. 38, No.1, pp. 167-84.

Levey AS, Coresh J, Balk E, & Kausz AT. (2003). National Kidney Foundation practice guidelines for chronic kidney disease: evaluation, classification, and stratification. *Ann Intern Med,* Vol. 139, No. 2, pp. 137-47.

Levey AS, Eckardt KU, Tsukamoto Y, Levin A, Coresh J, Rossert J, De Zeeuw D, Hostetter TH, Lameire N, & Eknoyan G. (2005). Definition and classification of chronic kidney disease: A position statement from Kidney Disease: Improving Global Outcomes (KDIGO). *Kidney Int,* Vol. 67, No. 6, :2089-100.

Levin A, Hemmelgarn B, Culleton B, Tobe S, McFarlane P, Ruzicka M, Burns K, Manns B, White C, Madore F, Moist L, Klarenbach S, Barrett B, Foley R, Jindal K, Senior P, Pannu N, Shurraw S, Akbari A, Cohn A, Reslerova M, Deved V,Mendelssohn D, Nesrallah G, Kappel J, & Tonelli M. (2008). Guidelines for the management of chronic kidney disease. *CMAJ,* Vol. 179, No. 11, pp. 1154-62.

Li PK, Leung CB, Chow KM, Cheng YL, Fung SK, Mak SK, Tang AW, Wong TY, Yung CY, Yung JC, Yu AW, & Szeto CC. (2006). Hong Kong study using valsartan in IgA nephropathy (HKVIN): a double-blind, randomized, placebo-controlled study. *Am J Kidney Dis,* Vol. 47, No.5, pp. 751-60.

Ligtenberg G, Blankestijn PJ, Oey L, Klein IH, Dijkhorst-Oei LT, Boomsma F, Wieneke GH, van Huffelen AC, & Koomans HA. (1999). Reduction of sympathetic hyperactivity by enalapril in patients with chronic renal failure. *N Engl J Med,* Vol. 340, No. 17, pp.1321-8.

Lo JC, Chertow GM, Go AS, & Hsu CY. (2005). Increased prevalence of subclinical and clinical hypothyroidism in persons with chronic kidney disease. *Kidney Int,* Vol. 67, No. 3, pp. 1047-52.

Locatelli F, Olivares J, Walker R. (2001). Novel erythropoiesis stimulating protein for treatment of anemia in chronic renal insufficiency. *Kidney Int,* Vol. 60, No. 2, pp.741-7.

Locatelli F, Aljama P, Barany P, Canaud B, Carrera F, Eckardt KU, Hörl WH, Macdougal IC, Macleod A, Wiecek A, & Cameron S. (2004). Revised European best practice guidelines for the management of anaemia in patients with chronic renal failure. *Nephrol Dial Transplant,* Vol. 19 Suppl 2, pp. ii1-47.

Loghman-Adham M. (1993). Role of phosphate retention in the progression of renal failure. *J Lab Clin Med,* Vol. 122, No. 1, pp.16-26.

London G, Guerin A, Pannier B, Marchais S, Benetos A, Safar M. (1992). Increased systolic pressure in chronic uremia. Role of arterial wave reflections. *Hypertension,* Vol. 20, No. 1, pp.10-9.

Macdonald J, Marcora S, Jibani M, Roberts G, Kumwenda M, Glover R, Barron J, & Lemmey A. (2006). GFR estimation using cystatin C is not independent of body composition. *Am J Kidney Dis,* Vol. 48, No. 5, pp. 712-9.

Macdougall IC, Gray SJ, Elston O, Breen C, Jenkins B, Browne J, & Egrie J. (1999). Pharmacokinetics of novel erythropoiesis stimulating protein compared with epoetin alfa in dialysis patients. *J Am Soc Nephrol,* Vol. 10, No. 11, pp. 2392-5.

Mak RH, & DeFronzo RA. (1992). Glucose and insulin metabolism in uremia. *Nephron,* Vol. 61, No. 4, pp. 377-82.

Manetti, L, Pardini, E, Genovesi, M, Campomori A, Grasso L, Morselli LL, Lupi I, Pellegrini G, Bartalena L, Bogazzi F, & Martino E. (2005). Thyroid function differently affects serum cystatin C and creatinine concentrations. *J Endocrinol Invest,* Vol. 28, No. 4, pp. 346-9.

Margolis DM, Saylor JL, Geisse G, DeSchryver-Kecskemeti K, Harter HR, Zuckerman GR. (1978). Upper gastrointestinal disease in chronic renal failure: A prospective evaluation. *Arch Intern Med,* Vol. 138, No. 8, pp. 1214-7.

McCaleb ML, Izzo MS, & Lockwood DH. (1985). Characterization and partial purification of a factor from uremic human serum that induces insulin resistance. *J Clin Invest,* Vol. 75, No. 2, pp. 391-6.

Menon V, Greene T, Wang X, Pereira AA, Marcovina SM, Beck GJ, Kusek JW, Collins AJ, Levey AS, & Sarnak MJ. (2005). C-reactive protein and albumin as predictors of all-cause and cardiovascular mortality in chronic kidney disease. *Kidney Int,* Vol. 68, No. 2, pp. 766-72.

Meyer TW. (2003). Tubular injury in glomerular disease. *Kidney Int,* Vol. 63, No. 2, pp. 774-87.

Michel O, Heudes D, Lamarre I, Masurier C, Lavau M, Bariety J, & Chevalier J. (1997). Reduction of insulin and triglycerides delays glomeruloscerosis in obese Zucker rats. *Kidney Int,* Vol. 52, No. 6, pp. 1532-42.

Moen MF, Zhan M, Hsu VD, Walker LD, Einhorn LM, Seliger SL, & Fink JC. (2009). Frequency of hypoglycemia and its significance in chronic kidney disease. *Clin J Am Soc Nephrol,* Vol. 4, No. 6, pp. 1121-7.

Moran A, Katz R, Jenny NS, Astor B, Bluemke DA, Lima JA, Siscovick D, Bertoni AG, & Shlipak MG. (2008). Left ventricular hypertrophy in mild and moderate reduction in kidney function determined using cardiac magnetic resonance imaging and cystatin C: the multi-ethnic study of atherosclerosis (MESA). *Am J Kidney Dis,* Vol. 52, No. 5, pp. 839-48.

Mussap M, Dalla Vestra M, Fioretto P, Saller A, Varagnolo M, Nosadini R, & Plebani M. (2002). Cystatin C is a more sensitive marker than creatinine for the estimation of GFR in type 2 diabetic patients. *Kidney Int,* Vol. 61, No. 4, pp. 1453-61.

Mussap M, & Plebani M. (2004). Biochemistry and clinical role of human cystatin C. *Crit Rev Clin Lab Sci,* Vol. 41, No. 5-6, pp. 467-550.

Nagata M, & Kriz W. (1992). Glomerular damage after uninephrectomy in young rats. II. Mechanical stress on podocytes as a pathway to sclerosis. *Kidney Int,* Vol. 42, No. 1, pp.148-60.

Nath KA, Hostetter MK, & Hostetter TH. (1985). Pathophysiology of chronic tubulo-interstitial disease in rats. Interactions of dietary acid load, ammonia, and complement component C3. *J Clin Invest,* Vol. 76, No. 2, pp.667-75.

Nath KD. (1992). Tubulointerstitial changes as a major determinant in the progression of renal damage. *Am J Kidney Dis,* Vol. 20, No. 1, pp. 1-17.

Nath KA. (1998). The tubulointerstitium in progressive renal disease (Editorial). *Kidney Int,* Vol. 54, No. 3, pp. 992-4.

National Kidney Foundation. (2002). K/DOQI clinical practice guidelines for chronic kidney disease: evaluation, classification, and stratification. *Am J Kidney Dis,* Vol. 39, No. 2 Suppl 1, pp. S1-266.

Neumann J, Ligtenberg G, Klein II, Koomans HA, & Blankestijn PJ. (2004). Sympathetic hyperactivity in chronic kidney disease: Pathogenesis, clinical relevance, and treatment. *Kidney Int,* Vol. 65, No. 5, pp. 1568-76.

Newman DJ, Thakkar H, Edwards RG, Wilkie M, White T, Grubb AO, & Price CP. (1995). Serum cystatin C measured by automated immunoassay: A more sensitive marker of changes in GFR than serum creatinine. *Kidney Int,* Vol. 47, No. 1, pp. 312-8.

NKF-DOQI Clinical Practice Guidelines for Anemia of Chronic Renal Failure. (2001). IV. Administration of epoetin. Am J Kidney Dis, Vol. 37 (Suppl 1), pp. S207.

Nissenson AR, Pereira BJ, Collins AJ, & Steinberg EP. (2001). Prevalence and characteristics of individuals with chronic kidney disease in a large health maintenance organization. *Am J Kidney Dis,* Vol. 37, No. 6, pp. 1177-83.

Nordfors L, Lindholm B, Stenvinkel P. (2005). End-stage renal disease--not an equal opportunity disease: the role of genetic polymorphisms. *J Intern Med,* Vol. 258, No. 1:1-12.

Oddoze C, Morange S, Portugal H, Berland Y, & Dussol B. (2001). Cystatin C is not more sensitive than creatinine for detecting early renal impairment in patients with diabetes. *Am J Kidney Dis,* Vol. 38, No. 2, pp. 310-6.

Ohno I, Hosoya T, Gomi H, Ichida K, Okabe H, & Hikita M. (2001). Serum uric acid and renal prognosis in patients with IgA nephropathy. *Nephron,* Vol. 87, No.4, pp. 333-9.

Ohtake T, Kobayashi S, Moriya H, Negishi K, Okamoto K, Maesato K, Saito S. (2005). High prevalence of occult coronary artery stenosis in patients with chronic kidney disease at the initiation of renal replacement therapy: An angiographic examination. *J Am Soc Nephrol,* Vol. 16, No. 4, pp. 1141-8.

Okada H, Moriwaki K, Konishi K, Kobayashi T, Sugahara S, Nakamoto H, Saruta T, & Suzuki H. (2000). Tubular osteopontin expression in human glomerulonephritis and renal vasculitis. *Am J Kidney Dis,* Vol. 36, No. 3, pp. 498-506.

Ong AC, & Fine LG. (1994). Loss of glomerular function and tubulointerstitial fibrosis: Cause or effect. *Kidney Int,* Vol. 45, No. 2, pp. 345-51.

Palmer BF. (2003). Sexual dysfunction in men and women with chronic kidney disease and end-stage kidney disease. *Adv Renal Rep Therapy,* Vol. 10, No. 1, pp. 48-60.

Parfrey PS, & Foley RN. (1999). The clinical epidemiology of cardiac disease in chronic renal failure. *J Am Soc Nephrol,* Vol. 10, No. 7, pp. 1606-15.

Parving HH, Persson F, Lewis JB, Lewis EJ, & Hollenberg NK. (2008). Aliskiren combined with losartan in type 2 diabetes and nephropathy. *N Engl J Med,* Vol. 358, No. 23, pp. 2433-46.

Passauer J, Pistrosch F, & Bussemaker E. (2005). Nitric oxide in chronic renal failure. *Kidney Int,* Vol. 67, No. 5, pp.1665-7.

Passauer J, Pistrosch F, Bussemaker E, Lässig G, Herbrig K, & Gross P. (2005). Reduced agonist-induced endothelium-dependent vasodilation in uremia is attributable to an impairment of vascular nitric oxide. *J Am Soc Nephrol,* Vol. 16, No. 4, 959-65.

Peng YS, Chiang CK, Kao TW, Hung KY, Lu CS, Chiang SS, Yang CS, Huang YC, Wu KD, Wu MS, Lien YR, Yang CC, Tsai DM, Chen PY, Liao CS, Tsai TJ, & Chen WY. (2005). Sexual dysfunction in female hemodialysis patients: A multicenter study. *Kidney Int,* Vol. 68, No. 2, pp. 760-5.

Perkins BA, Nelson RG, Ostrander BE, Blouch KL, Krolewski AS, Myers BD, & Warram JH. (2005). Detection of Renal Function Decline in Patients with Diabetes and Normal or Elevated GFR by Serial Measurements of Serum Cystatin C Concentration: Results of a 4-Year Follow-Up Study. *J Am Soc Nephrol,* Vol. 16, No. 5, pp. 1404-12.

Poge U, Gerhardt T, Stoffel-Wagner B, Klehr HU, Sauerbruch T, Woitas RP. (2006). Calculation of glomerular filtration rate based on cystatin C in cirrhotic patients. *Nephrol Dial Transplant,* Vol. 21, No.3, pp. 660-4.

Poge U, Gerhardt T, Stoffel-Wagner B, Palmedo H, Klehr HU, Sauerbruch T, Woitas RP. (2006). Cystatin C-based calculation of glomerular filtration rate in kidney transplant recipients. *Kidney Int,* Vol. 70, No. 1, pp. 204-10.

Rahman SN, Heifner KJ, Fadem SZ, et al. (2002). HRQOL improvements in anemic CKD patients treated with darbepoetin alfa (Aranesp™). National Kidney Foundation Clinical Nephrology Meeting, Chicago (IL), USA, April 17–21,

Rahn KH, Heidenreich S, & Bruckner D. (1999). How to assess glomerular function and damage in humans. *J Hypertens,* Vol. 17, No. 3, pp. 309-17.

Raine AE, Bedford L, Simpson AW, Ashley CC, Brown R, Woodhead JS, & Ledingham JG. (1993). Hyperparathyroidism, platelet intracellular free calcium and hypertension in chronic renal failure. *Kidney Int,* Vol. 43, No. 3, pp. 700-5.

Rastaldi MP, Ferrario F, Crippa A, Dell'Antonio G, Casartelli D, Grillo C, & D'Amico G. (2000). Glomerular monocyte-macrophage features in ANCA-positive renal vasculitis and cryoglobulinemic nephritis. *J Am Soc Nephrol,* Vol. 11, No. 11, pp. 2036-43.

Remuzzi A, Puntorieri S, Battaglia C, Bertani T, & Remuzzi G. (1990). Angiotensin converting enzyme inhibition ameliorates glomerular filtration of macromolecules and water and lessens glomerular injury in the rat. *J Clin Invest,* Vol. 85, No. 2, pp. 541-9.

Remuzzi A, Gagliardini E, Donadoni C, Fassi A, Sangalli F, Lepre MS, Remuzzi G, & Benigni A. (2002). Effect of angiotensin II antagonism on the regression of kidney disease in the rat. Kidney Int, Vol. 62, No. 3, pp. 885-94.

Rennke HG, Anderson S, & Brenner BM. (1989). Structural and functional correlations in the progression of renal disease. In: Renal Pathology, Tisher, CC, Brenner, BM (Eds), Lippincott, Philadelphia, pp. 43-66.

Rennke HG, Klein PS, Sandstrom DJ, & Mendrick DL. (1994). Cell-mediated immune injury in the kidney: Acute nephritis induced in the rat by azobenzenearsonate. *Kidney Int,* Vol. 45, No. 4, pp. 1044-56.

Rops AL, van der Vlag J, Lensen JF, Wijnhoven TJ, van den Heuvel LP, van Kuppevelt TH, & Berden JH. (2004). Heparan sulfate proteoglycans in glomerular inflammation. *Kidney Int,* Vol. 65, No. 3, pp. 768-85.

Rosas SE, Joffe M, Franklin E, Strom BL, Kotzker W, Brensinger C, Grossman E, Glasser DB, & Feldman HI. (2003). Association of decreased quality of life and erectile dysfunction in hemodialysis patients. *Kidney Int,* Vol. 64, No. 1, pp. 232-8.

Rose BD. (1987). Pathophysiology of Renal Disease, 2nd ed, McGraw-Hill, New York p.11.

Rubin R, Silbiger S, Sablay L, & Neugarten J. (1994). Combined antihypertensive and lipid-lowering therapy in experimental glomerulonephritis. *Hypertension,* Vol. 23, No. 1, pp. 92-5.

Ruiz-Ortega M, Ruperez M, Esteban V, Rodríguez-Vita J, Sánchez-López E, Carvajal G, & Egido J. (2006). Angiotensin II: a key factor in the inflammatory and fibrotic response in kidney diseases. *Nephrol Dial Transplant,* Vol. 21, No. 1, pp. 16-20.

Russo LM, Sandoval RM, McKee M, Osicka TM, Collins AB, Brown D, Molitoris BA, & Comper WD. (2007). The normal kidney filters nephrotic levels of albumin retrieved by proximal tubule cells: retrieval is disrupted in nephrotic states. *Kidney Int,* Vol. 71, No. 6, pp. 504-13.

Sanchez-Lozada LG, Tapia E, Santamaria J, Avila-Casado C, Soto V, Nepomuceno T, Rodríguez-Iturbe B, Johnson RJ, & Herrera-Acosta J. (2005). Mild hyperuricemia induces vasoconstriction and maintains glomerular hypertension in normal and remnant kidney rats. *Kidney Int,* Vol. 67, No. 1, pp. 237-47.

Sarnak, MJ, Greene, T, Wang, X, Beck G, Kusek JW, Collins AJ, & Levey AS. (2005). The effect of a lower target blood pressure on the progression of kidney disease: Long-term follow-up of the Modification of Diet in Renal Disease Study. *Ann Intern Med,* Vol. 142, No.5, pp. 342-51.

Schanstra JP, Neau E, Drogoz P, Arevalo Gomez MA, Lopez Novoa JM, Calise D, Pecher C, Bader M, Girolami JP, & Bascands JL. (2002). In vivo bradykinin B2 receptor activation reduces renal fibrosis. *J Clin Invest,* Vol. 110, No. 3, pp. 371-9.

Schwab SJ, Christensen RL, Dougherty K, & Klahr S. (1987). Quantitation of proteinuria by the use of protein-to-creatinine ratios in single urine samples. *Arch Intern Med,* Vol. 147, No. 5, pp. 943-4.

Schwarz S, Trivedi BK, Kalantar-Zadeh K, & Kovesdy CP. (2006). Association of disorders in mineral metabolism with progression of chronic kidney disease. *Clin J Am Soc Nephrol,* Vol. 1, No. 4, pp.825-31.

Segerer S, Nelson PJ, & Schlondorff D. (2000). Chemokines, chemokine receptors, and renal disease: from basic science to pathophysiologic and therapeutic studies. *J Am Soc Nephrol,* Vol. 11, No. 1, pp. 152-76.

Segerer, S, & Schlondorff, D. (2007). Role of chemokines for the localization of leukocyte subsets in the kidney. *Semin Nephrol,* Vol. 27, No. 3, pp. 260-74.

Sjostrom P, Tidman M, & Jones I. (2005). Determination of the production rate and non-renal clearance of cystatin C and estimation of the glomerular filtration rate from the serum concentration of cystatin C in humans. *Scand J Clin Lab Invest,* Vol. 65, No. 2, pp. 111-24.

Shlipak MG, Sarnak MJ, Katz R, Fried LF, Seliger SL, Newman AB, Siscovick DS, & Stehman-Breen C. (2005). Cystatin C and the risk of death and cardiovascular events among elderly persons. *N Engl J Med,* Vol. 352, No.20, pp. 2049-60.

Shimizu, H, Maruyama, S, Yuzawa, Y, Kato T, Miki Y, Suzuki S, Sato W, Morita Y, Maruyama H, Egashira K, Matsuo S. Anti-monocyte chemoattractant protein-1 gene therapy attenuates renal injury induced by protein-overload proteinuria. J Am Soc Nephrol 2003; 14, No. 6, pp. 1496-505.

Smith D, & DeFronzo RA. (1982). Insulin resistance in uremia mediated by postbinding defects. *Kidney Int,* Vol. 22, No. 1, pp. 54-62.

Stevens LA, Coresh J, Schmid CH, Feldman HI, Froissart M, Kusek J, Rossert J, Van Lente F, Bruce RD 3rd, Zhang YL,Greene T, & Levey AS. (2008). Estimating GFR using serum cystatin C alone and in combination with serum creatinine: a pooled analysis of 3,418 individuals with CKD. *Am J Kidney Dis,* Vol. 51, No.3, pp. 395-406.

Stevens LA, Schmid CH, Greene T, Li L, Beck GJ, Joffe MM, Froissart M, Kusek JW, Zhang YL, Coresh J, & Levey AS. (2009). Factors other than glomerular filtration rate affect serum cystatin C levels. *Kidney Int,* Vol. 75, No. 6, pp.652-60.

Steinhauslin F, & Wauters JP. (1995). Quantification of proteinuria in kidney transplant recipients: Accuracy of the urine protein/creatinine ratio. *Clin Nephrol,* Vol. 43, No. 2, pp.110-5.

Timoshanko JR, Kitching AR, Semple TJ, Holdsworth SR, & Tipping PG. (2005). Granulocyte macrophage colony-stimulating factor expression by both renal parenchymal and immune cells mediates murine crescentic glomerulonephritis. *J Am Soc Nephrol,* Vol. 16, No. 9, pp. 2646-56.

Tipping PG, & Holdsworth SR. (2003). T Cells in glomurulonephritis. *Springer Semin Immunopathol,* Vol. 24, No. 4, pp. 377-93.

Trespalacios FC, Taylor AJ, Agodoa LY, & Abbott KC. (2002). Incident acute coronary syndromes in chronic dialysis patients in the United States. *Kidney Int,* Vol. 62, No. 5, pp. 1799-805.

Uhlig K, Macleod A, Craig J, Lau J, Levey AS, Levin A, Moist L, Steinberg E, Walker R, Wanner C, Lameire N, & Eknoyan G. (2006). Grading evidence and recommendations for clinical practice guidelines in nephrology. A position statement from Kidney Disease: Improving Global Outcomes (KDIGO). *Kidney Int,* Vol. 70, No. 12, pp. 2058-65.

Uribarri J, Douton H, & Oh MS. (1995). A re-evaluation of the urinary parameters of acid production and excretion in patients with chronic renal acidosis. *Kidney Int,* Vol. 47, No. 2, pp. 624-7.

US Renal Data System. (2010). USRDS 2009 Annual Data report: Atlas of end-stage renal disease in the United States. Am J Kidney Dis, Vol. 55 (Suppl 1): S1.

Vadas O, Hartl, O, & Rose K. (2008). Characterization of new multimeric erythropoietin receptor agonists. *Biopolymers,* Vol. 90, No. 4, pp. 496-502.

Wallia R, Greenberg AS, Piraino B, Mitro R, Puschett JB. (1986). Serum electrolyte patterns in end-stage renal disease. *Am J Kidney Dis,* Vol. 8, No. 2, pp. 98-104.

Wang Y, Chen J, Chen L, Tay YC, Rangan GK, & Harris DC. (1997). Induction of monocyte chemoattractant protein-1 in proximal tubule cells by urinary protein. *J Am Soc Nephrol,* Vol. 8, No. 10, pp. 1537-45.

Warnock, DG. Uremic acidosis. Kidney Int 1988; 34, No. 2, pp. 278-87.

White C, Akbari A, Hussain N, Dinh L, Filler G, Lepage N, & Knoll GA. (2005). Estimating glomerular filtration rate in kidney transplantation: A comparison between serum creatinine and cystatin c-based methods. *J Am Soc Nephrol,* Vol. 16, No, 12, pp. 3763-70.

Widmer B, Gerhardt RE, Harrington JT, & Cohen JJ. (1979). Serum electrolyte and acid-base composition: The influence of graded degrees of chronic renal failure. *Arch Intern Med,* Vol. 139, No. 10, pp.1099-102.

Witte EC, Lambers Heerspink HJ, de Zeeuw D, Bakker SJ, de Jong PE, & Gansevoort R. (2009). First morning voids are more reliable than spot urine samples to assess microalbuminuria. *J Am Soc Nephrol,* Vol. 20, No. 2, pp. 436-43.

Woods LL. (1993). Mechanisms of renal hemodynamic regulation in response to protein feeding. *Kidney Int,* Vol. 44, No. 4, pp. 659-75.

Xiao H, Heeringa P, Liu Z, Huugen D, Hu P, Maeda N, Falk RJ, & Jennette JC. (2005). The role of neutrophils in the induction of glomerulonephritis by anti-myeloperoxidase antibodies. *Am J Pathol,* Vol. 167, No. 1, pp. 39-45.

Young JM, Terrin N, Wang X, Greene T, Beck GJ, Kusek JW, Collins AJ, Sarnak MJ, & Menon V. (2009). Asymmetric dimethylarginine and mortality in stages 3 to 4 chronic kidney disease. *Clin J Am Soc Nephrol,* Vol. 4, No. 6, pp. 1115-20.

Yu HT. (2003). Progression of chronic renal failure. *Arch Intern Med,* Vol. 163, No. 12, pp. 1417-29.

Zelmanovitz T, Gross JL, Oliveira J, & de Azevedo MJ. (1998). Proteinuria is still useful for the screening and diagnosis of overt diabetic nephropathy. *Diabetes Care,* Vol. 21, No. 7,1076-9.

Zelmanovitz T, Gross JL, Oliveira JR, Paggi A, Tatsch M, & Azevedo MJ. (1997). The receiver operating characteristics curve in the evaluation of a random urine specimen as a screening test for diabetic nephropathy. *Diabetes Care,* Vol. 20, No. 4, pp. 516-9.

# 13

# Acute Renal Cortical Necrosis

Manohar Lal
*Jinnah Postgraduate Medical Center, Karachi*
*Pakistan*

## 1. Introduction

Acute renal cortical necrosis is a rare cause of acute renal failure secondary to ischemic necrosis of the renal cortex. It accounts for only 2% of all causes of acute renal failure in developed countries (Grünfeld et al., 1981), but occurs more frequently in developing world (Chugh et al., 1976; Chugh et al., 1983; Hassan et al., 2009; Parkash et al., 1995). The obstetric complications are the commonest (50 - 70%) cause of renal cortical necrosis (Hassan et al., 2009), non-obstetric causes account for 20-30% of all cases of cortical necrosis and in these circumstances the incidence is higher in men than in women (Duff & More, 1941). Majority of the patients become dialysis dependent and occasional patients may recover partial kidney function and are dialysis-independent.

Acute cortical necrosis is usually a bilateral condition, rarely being unilateral (Blau et al., 1971). The lesions are usually caused by significant prolonged diminished renal arterial perfusion secondary to vascular spasm, micro-vascular injury, or intravascular coagulation.

Renal cortical necrosis is usually extensive although local or localized forms occur.

Most of the patients present as acute renal failure and suspicion of the condition arises following prolonged oliguria and/or anuria. The kidney biopsy is the gold standard for the diagnosis.

## 2. Etiology

### 2.1 Pregnancy related

- Abruptio placentae
- Severe pre-eclampsia / eclampsia
- Criminal / Septic Abortion (Gram negative septicemia)
- Hyperemesis gravidarum
- Prolonged intrauterine death

### 2.2 Infections

#### 2.2.1 Children

- Diarrhea, vomiting (Dehydration)
- Peritonitis
- Septicemia
- Congenital heart disease
- Fetal maternal transfusion

- Dehydration.
- Perinatal asphyxia
- Placental hemorrhage
- Hemolytic uremic syndrome (HUS).

#### 2.2.2 Adults & adolescents

- Scarlet fever
- Streptococcal Infections
- Peritonitis
- Cholera

### 2.3 Hemodynamic causes

Acute tubular necrosis progressing to acute cortical necrosis with shock and crush injury.

### 2.4 Trauma

- Head injuries
- Burns
- Gastrointestinal hemorrhage
- Thrombotic thrombocytopenic purpura
- Pancreatitis
- Dissecting aneurysm

### 2.5 Snake bite

Due to direct toxic effect or shock, hemorrhage, haemoptysis

### 2.6 Drugs

Nonsteroidal anti-inflammatory drugs and contrast media.

### 2.7 Hyper acute kidney transplant rejection

### 2.8 Poisonous plants

- Fava Beans
- Exposure to Sap of Marking-nut tree
- Almond Extract (? Cyanide)

### 2.9 Glycol poisoning

- Dioxane
- Di ethylene Glycol (anti freeze)

### 2.10 Metallic & other poisoning

- Arsenic
- Cadmium
- Lithium Carmine
- Pyrazolene
- Camphor
- Phosphorus

### 2.11 Idiopathic

In a small number of cases, no cause is apparent even after extensive search. These cases are labeled as idiopathic in origin.

## 3. Pathology

The classic description of this condition by Sheehan & Moore (1952) still holds true to this day. They described the lesion at different stages in evolution as seen in autopsy material. They divided the fully developed form into various types, depending on the extent of the lesion.

### 3.1 Focal form

In this small scattered foci of necrosis are seen that vary from lesion of individual glomeruli to areas of cortical necrosis 0.5 mm in diameter. On gross examination kidneys usually are slightly enlarged and have punctuate red areas on cut section and on the sub capsular surface. Histologically, only few glomeruli in any one focus are affected, showing necrosis often with thrombosis at the vascular pole (Figure 1). Proximal convoluted tubules are always necrotic, and the distal tubules are affected similarly in the centre of larger lesions. In the remainder of the cortex, many proximal convoluted tubules appear necrotic, but glomeruli and distal convoluted tubules show no changes of consequence. There may be an over lap between acute tubular necrosis and cortical necrosis (Sheehan & Moore, 1952).

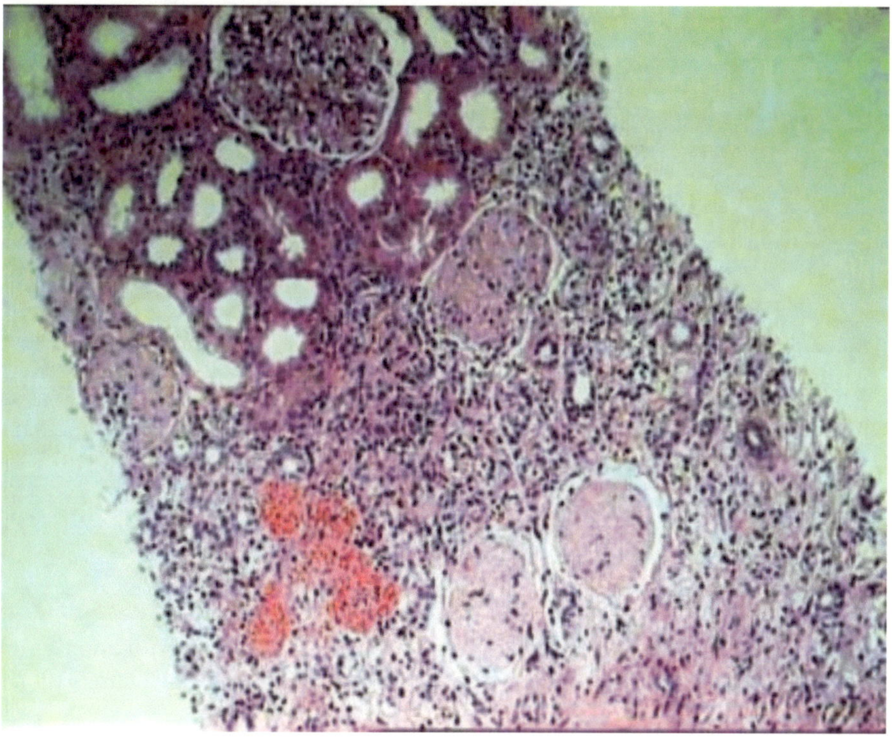

Fig. 1. Low-power view showing part of renal cortex. Three glomeruli in the lower part of the field are infarcted, while one glomerulus along with surrounding tubules, is still viable, in a case of focal cortical necrosis. (H&E stain, ×100).

### 3.2 Minor form

The changes are similar to those described previously on gross description, except that lesions upto 3 mm in diameter are found.

Grossly, the affected foci have white centers with a red congested rim.

Histologically, in the affected foci there is necrosis of all elements including afferent arteriole, and interlobular artery. These and the glomeruli often contain thrombus material. Polymorphonuclear leucocytes are found sometime in portions of the necrotic lesion analogous to the peripheral dead zone of small infarct. Extensive proximal tubular necrosis is found in the remainder of the cortex.

### 3.3 Patchy form

Numerous larger polar areas of necrosis are found, sometimes occupying most of the width of the cortex, with a zone of congestion and hemorrhage around the periphery. The congestion is particularly pronounced in the inner cortex. The patches of cortical necrosis occupy about one third to two thirds of the cortex, but the columns of Bertini are usually spared. The kidneys are moderately enlarged.

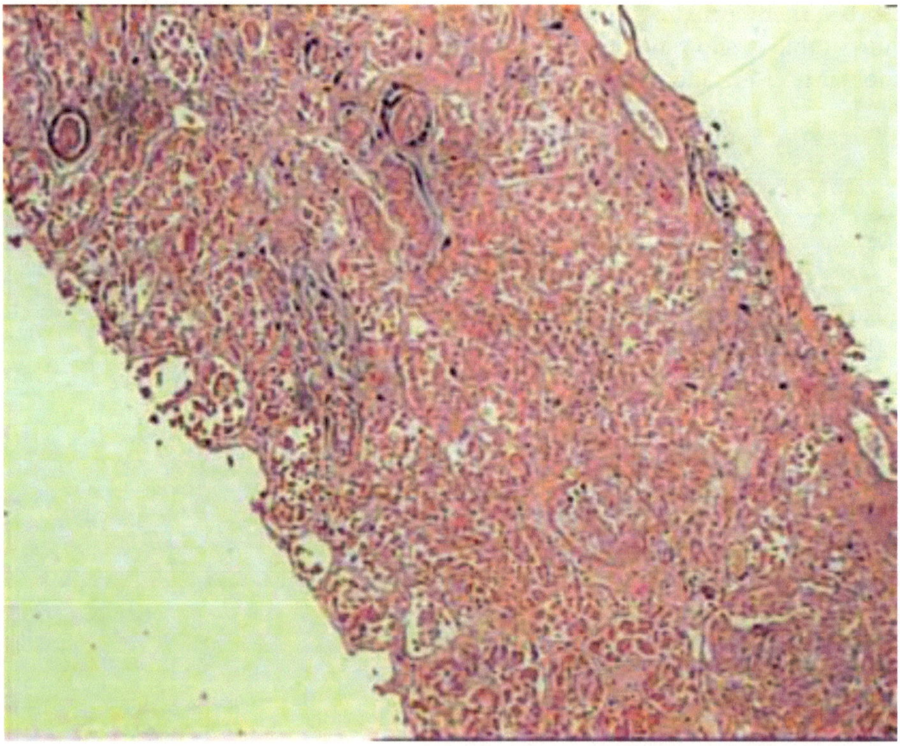

Fig. 2. Low-power view showing complete infarction of both the glomeruli and the surrounding renal parenchyma in a case of acute cortical necrosis. (H&E stain, ×100).

Histologically the foci of cortical necrosis are large enough to show a central dead zone. All the structures within the necrotic areas usually are necrotic although occasionally collecting ducts appear undamaged. The arteries and arterioles are necrotic and dilated, and contain thrombus material in cases seen more than 2 days after onset.

### 3.4 Gross renal cortical necrosis

The cortex is almost entirely necrotic with the exception of thin surviving areas immediately under the capsule & at the cortico-medullary junctions. The kidneys are usually enlarged when the condition is well developed. Almost the entire cortex is yellowish white except from the spared zones in the sub capsular and juxtamedullay cortex. If seen earlier, the affected cortex is somewhat hemorrhagic or congested with whitish yellow streaks. The columns of Bertini are necrotic.

Histologically, changes similar to those seen in the patchy form are seen, but with arteries showing necrosis and thrombosis over a greater length than in the patchy form (Figure 2).

### 3.5 Confluent focal cortical necrosis

This condition is very common in those not associated with abruptio placentae (Sheehan & Moore, 1952). In this type there are widespread lesions of glomeruli and tubules, but there is no involvement of arteries. The lesions vary greatly from nephron to nephron both in severity and in apparent age. The glomeruli either appear normal or show various changes such as congestion, thrombosis of capillaries or of the vascular pole, or frank necrosis. Many proximal convoluted tubules appear normal but others are necrotic. Distal convoluted tubules appear normal. On gross inspection in the early stages the kidney has a red congested cortex with punctuate hemorrhages or pale mottling, but no white infracted areas.

### 3.6 Calcification in cortical necrosis

In some cases, in which partial recovery occurs & patient survives for several weeks/months calcification of necrotic cortex may occur which can be seen on radiology (Alwall et al., 1958; Effersoe et al., 1962; Oram et al., 1964; Phillips, 1962).

### 3.7 Necrosis in other organs

Other organs may show necrosis in cases of renal cortical necrosis e.g., anterior lobe of pituitary, adrenals, spleen, lungs, gastro intestinal tract, liver, pancreas etc. (Sheldon & Hertig, 1942).

## 4. Pathogenesis

The pathogenesis of cortical necrosis is far from clear, and probably many factors are involved.

### 4.1 Vasospasm

Following abruptio placentae, there is an initial vaso spasm that reduces blood flow for periods varying from several minutes to six hours. The spasm then abates and recirculation of blood occurs. If the spasm is of short duration and good flow is re-established, acute tubular necrosis occurs. However in patients who develop cortical necrosis, a new spasm is thought to occur, this time more proximally in the vascular tree & lasting for upto 30 hours, causing necrosis of the arteries beyond the obstruction. Then thrombosis occurs, with permanent blockage to the circulation (Matlin & Gary, 1974; Schrieiner, 1979).

It has long been suggested that vasculature in pregnancy is more prone than usual to vaso-constriction which may partly account for the greater frequency of cortical necrosis in this state.

### 4.2 Generalized Schwartzman reaction

Similarity has been shown between cortical necrosis & the generalized Schwartzman reaction in rabbits. In this reaction, two small doses of bacterial endotoxin given 24 hours apart, cause microscopic thrombosis that involves the glomerular capillaries and leads to development of renal cortical necrosis (Moss et al., 1977; Sporn, 1978). This mechanism may be active during septic abortions.

The sequence of events starts with sudden widespread dilation of glomerular capillaries, follows by an escape of plasma by filtration. Increased viscosity of the blood follows, with stasis and formation of thrombi, which extend backward to arteries of increasing size, which become necrotic.

### 4.3 Vascular thrombosis

The importance of fibrin and fibrinogen deposition in the glomeruli and small vessels has been demonstrated. This may result from mechanical obstruction with blood flow through the glomeruli.

However, there is disagreement about the chain of events; whether coagulation or vasomotor dependence phenomena occur earlier. Endotoxaemia and/or bacterial sepsis is by far the most common factor responsible for intravascular coagulation.

Immunologic mechanisms also may play a role in the pathogenesis of acute cortical necrosis. Gelfand et al. (1970) found lymphocytotoxic antibody in 27% of patients with acute cortical necrosis and anti-platelet antibody in 79%.

## 5. Clinical features

In those cases of acute cortical necrosis associated with abruptio placentae patient may present with:

- Severe lower abdominal pain
- Per vaginal bleeding
- Hypotension / Shock
- Oliguria / anuria.

Without abruptio placentae:

- Oliguria / anuria
- Infection / diarrhea / symptoms of predisposing disease.

Acute renal failure as a result of acute cortical necrosis cannot be distinguished readily from other forms of acute renal failure such as acute tubular necrosis and renal biopsy is the only sure way of making the diagnosis during life (Lauler & Schreiner, 1958).

## 6. Diagnosis

### 6.1 Ultrasonography

Initially shows enlarged, swollen kidneys with reduced blood flow. Cortical tissue becomes shrunken later in the course of disease (Sefczek et al., 1984).

### 6.2 KUB X-ray

Plain X ray of the kidney shows calcification weeks or months later (Moell, 1973).

### 6.3 Contrast enhanced CT scanning

Contrast enhanced CT scanning is the most sensitive modality. Diagnostic features include absent opacification of the renal cortex and enhancement of sub-capsular and juxtamedullary areas and of the medulla without excretion of contrast medium (Kleinknecht et al., 1973).

### 6.4 DTPA renal scan

It reveals markedly diminished perfusion with delayed or no function. It is more helpful in transplant kidneys.

### 6.5 Kidney biopsy

Kidney biopsy provides the definitive diagnosis and prognostic information.

## 7. Unilateral cortical necrosis

Unilateral cortical necrosis may occur rarely with ureteric obstruction on the uninvolved side (Blau et al., 1971). The mechanism is not clear, but experimentally, ureteric occlusion has a similar effect on the cortical necrosis found in the generalized Schwartzman reaction.

## 8. Recovery from cortical necrosis

Partial recovery of renal function has been reported and it is likely that recovery is governed by the extent of the lesion (Walls et al., 1968). Schrieiner (1979) emphasized that there is high evidence of hypertension in patients who recover from cortical necrosis and Kleinknecht et al. (1973) found that patients who recover, may exhibit a slower decline in renal functions associated with a progressive reduction in renal mass.

## 9. References

Alwall N, Erlanson P, Tornberg A, Moell H, & Fajers CM. (1958). Two cases of gross renal cortical necrosis in pregnancy with severe oliguria and anuria for 116 and 79 days respectively; clinical course, roentgenological studies of the kidneys (size, outlines and calcifications), and post-mortem findings. *Acta Med Scand,* Vol. 161, No. 2, pp. 93-8.

Blau EB, Dysart N, Fish A, Michael A, & Vernier R. (1971). Unilateral renal cortical necrosis. Case report and experimental observations. *Am J Dis Child,* Vol. 122, No. 1, pp. 31-3.

Chugh KS, Singhal PC, Kher VK, Gupta VK, Malik GH, Narayan G, & Datta BN. (1983). Spectrum of acute cortical necrosis in Indian patients. *Am J Med Sci,* Vol. 286, No. 1, pp. 10-20.

Chugh KS, Singhal PC, Sharma BK, Pal Y, Mathew MT, Dhall K, & Datta BN. (1976). Acute renal failure of obstetric origin. Obstet Gynecol, Vol. 48, No.6, pp.642-6.

Duff GL, & More RH. (1941). Bilateral cortical necrosis of the kidney. *Am J Med Sci,* Vol. 201, pp. 429.

Effersoe P, Raaschou F, Thomsen AC. (1962). Bilateral renal cortical necrosis. A patient followed up over eight years. *Am J Med,* Vol. 33, pp. 455-8.

Gelfand MC, & Friedman EA. (1970). Prognosis of renal allotransplants in patients with bilateral renal cortical necrosis. *Transplantation,* Vol. 10, No. 5, pp. 442-6.

Grünfeld JP, Ganeval D, & Bournérias F. (1980). Acute renal failure in pregnancy. *Kidney Int,* Vol. 18, No. 2, pp. 179-91.

Hassan I, Junejo AM, & Dawani ML. (2009). Etiology and outcome of acute renal failure in pregnancy. *J Coll Physicians Surg Pak,* Vol. 19, No. 11, pp. 714-7.

Kleinknecht D, Grünfeld JP, Gomez PC, Moreau JF, & Garcia-Torres R. (1973). Diagnostic procedures and long-term prognosis in bilateral renal cortical necrosis. Kidney Int, Vol. 4, No. 6, pp. 390–400.

Lauler DP, Schreiner GE. (1958). Bilateral renal cortical necrosis. Am J Med, Vol. 24, No. 4, pp. 519–29.

Matlin RA, & Gary NE. (1974). Acute cortical necrosis. Case report and review of the literature. Am J Med, Vol. 56, No. 1, pp. 110-8.

Moell H. (1957). Gross bilateral renal cortical necrosis during long periods of oliguria-anuria; roentgenologic observations in two cases. Acta radiol, Vol. 48, No. 5, pp.355-60.

Oram S, Ross G, Pell L, Winterler J. (1964). Renal cortical calcification after snake bite. *Am Heart J,* Vol. 67, pp. 714-5.

Phillips MJ. (1962). Bilateral renal corticol necrosis associated with calcification: report of a case and a review of etiology. *J Clin Pathol,* Vol. 15, No. 1, pp. 31-5.

Prakash J, Tripathi K, Pandey LK, Sahai S, Usha, & Srivastava PK. (1995). Spectrum of renal cortical necrosis in acute renal failure in eastern India. *Postgrad Med J,* Vol. 71, No. 834, pp. 208-10.

Schreiner GE. (1979) Bilateral cortical necrosis. In: Hamburger J, Crosnier J, Grunfeld JP (Eds): *Nephrology.* New York, Wiley, pp. 411-30.

Sefczek RJ, Beckman I, Lupetin AR, & Dash N. (1984). Sonography of acute renal cortical necrosis. AJR Am J Roentgenol, Vol. 142, No. 3, pp. 553-4.

Sheehan HL, & Moore HC. (1952). *Renal cortical necrosis and the kidney of concealed accidental haemorrhage.* Blackwell, Oxford.

Sheldon WH, & Hertig A. (1942). Bilateral cortical necrosis of the kidney. A report of 2 cases. *Arch Pathol,* Vol. 34, pp. 866.

Sporn IN. (1978). Renal cortical necrosis. Arch Intern Med, Vol. 138, No.12, pp. 1866.

Moss SW, Gary NE, & Eisinger RP. (1977). Renal cortical necrosis following streptococcal infection. Arch Intern Med, Vol. 137, No. 9, pp. 1196-7.

Walls J, Schorr WJ, Kerr DN. (1968). Prolonged oliguria with survival in acute bilateral cortical necrosis. *Br Med J,* Vol. 26, No. 4, pp. 220-2.

# 14

# Pathophysiological Approach to Acid Base Disorders

Absar Ali
*Aga Khan University*
*Karachi*
*Pakistan*

## 1. Introduction

In this chapter, we are presenting the review of the acid base disorders. The emphasis is on the pathophysiology and the underlying concepts.
The complicated formulas and graphs are avoided and things are explained in the simple language. The basic acid base disorders namely metabolic acidosis, metabolic alkalosis, respiratory acidosis and respiratory alkalosis are discussed in detail. When appropriate the information is presented in the table forms to make it clear. Important references are also given for the interested readers.

## 2. Basic concepts

### 2.1 Acid and base

According to the standard definitions, acid is a substance which can donate $H^+$ ion and base is a substance which can accept $H^+$ ion (Ali, 1994; Boron, 2006; Kellum, 2007).
Acids are of two types.

1. Volatile acids for example carbon dioxide ($CO_2$) which is regulated by the alveolar ventilation in the lungs.
2. Non-volatile acids for example lactic acid, sulfuric acid, phosphoric acid, uric acid and, keto acid. These acids may not be converted to $CO_2$ and hence must be removed from the body by the kidneys to keep the acid base in balance.

Acids and bases are also categorized according to their chemical behavior in the blood. They are called strong and weak. The strong acids and bases are completely ionized at the pH of 7.4. The weak acids and bases are ionized only partially at the pH of 7.4, depending upon their dissociation constant (pKa). Hydrochloric Acid (HCl) is a strong acid and Sodium Hydroxide (NaOH) is a strong base. Sodium Bicarbonate (Na $HCO^-_3$) is a weak acid (Boron, 2006; DuBose & Hamm, 1999; Kellum, 2007).

#### 2.1.1 Acidemia

Acidemia is defined as an increase in $H^+$ concentration of the blood. Acidemia may also be defined as a decrease in arterial pH.

### 2.1.2 Alkalemia

Alkalemia is defined as a decrease in the $H^+$ concentration of the blood. Alkalemia may also be defined as an increase in arterial pH.

## 2.2 Normal concentrations

The normal concentration of $H^+$ in plasma or serum is 40 nmol/liter and it varies inversely with the $HCO^-_3$ concentration.
The pH (Plasma concentration of $H^+$) is the negative log of H concentration. Thus,

$$pH = - \log ( H^+ ).$$

The normal arterial pH is 7.40, normal partial pressure of carbon dioxide ($PCO_2$) is 40 mmHg. Normal serum bicarbonate ($HCO^-_3$) concentration is 24 mEq/L.
Concentration of ions in a solution should be written in brackets. For example, for hydrogen ions as ($H^+$). However for the convenience it is often written with out brackets.

When coagulation factors are removed from the plasma, it is called serum. For practical purposes, plasma and serum are the same as far as the clinical medicine is concerned (DuBose & Hamm, 1999).

## 2.3 Buffers

Buffers are weak acids, i.e. they do not dissociate completely at the pH of 7.4. They accept or donate $H^+$ ions to prevent large changes in the free $H^+$ ion concentration.
The body buffers are divided into 3 groups:
(1) Extracellular (2) intracellular, and (3) bone

### 2.3.1 Extracellular buffers

Bicarbonate is the most important extracellular buffer due to its high concentration and also due to its ability to control the $PCO_2$ by alveolar ventilation. This system plays a central role in the maintenance of acid-base balance. $HCO^-_3$ is regulated by renal $H^+$ excretion and $PCO_2$ by the ventilation of lungs. Clinically, the acid base status of a person is expressed in terms of the principal extracellular buffer, the bicarbonate/$CO_2$ system.
Relationship between acid and base is expressed by the following equation:

$$(H^+) = 24 \times CO_2 \div (HCO^-_3)$$

Henderson-Hasselbalch equation is the modified form of the above simpler equation:
Henderson-Hasselbalch equation:

$$pH = 6.10 + \log ( HCO_3^- ) \div (0.03 \times PCO_2)$$

pH is (-log $H^+$ ), 6.10 is the pKa, 0.03 is solubility constant for $CO_2$ in the extracellular fluid, and $PCO_2$ is the partial pressure of carbon dioxide in the extracellular fluid.
Other, less important buffers in the extracellular fluid are phosphates and the plasma proteins.

### 2.3.2 Intracellular buffers

The intracellular buffers are phosphates, hemoglobin (Hgb), and proteins.

$$H^+ + HPO4^{-2} \quad <-> \quad H2PO4^-$$

$$H^+ + Hgb^- \quad <-> \quad HHgb$$

$$H^+ + Protein^- \quad <-> \quad HProtein$$

#### 2.3.3 Bone

It is an important buffer for acid and base loads with as much as 40 percent contribution in buffering (Halperin & Goldstein, 2002; Kellum, 2005).

## 3. Types of acid base disorers

There are four types of acid base disorders. A patient may present with one (simple) or more than one (mixed) disorder.
Metabolic Acidosis
Metabolic Alkalosis
Respiratory Acidosis
Respiratory Alkalosis

### 3.1 Acidosis

Acidosis is a process which tends to raise the hydrogen ion (H+) concentration.

#### 3.1.1 Metabolic acidosis

When the process of acidosis is primarily due to retention of non volatile acid or due to bicarbonate loss, it is called metabolic acidosis. The arterial pH is low as well as serum bicarbonate concentration (Kraut & Madias, 2010).

#### 3.1.2 Respiratory acidosis

When the process of acidosis is primarily due to CO2 retention, it is called respiratory acidosis. The arterial pH is low and $PCO_2$ is high (Corey, 2005).

### 3.2 Alkalosis

Alkalosis is a process which tends to lower the hydrogen ($H^+$) concentration.

#### 3.2.1 Metabolic alkalosis

When the process of alkalosis is primarily due to loss of non volatile acid or due to retention of bicarbonate, it is called metabolic alkalosis. The arterial pH is high as well as serum bicarbonate concentration (Corey, 2005).

#### 3.2.2 Respiratory alkalosis

When the process of alkalosis is primarily due to $CO_2$ loss, it is called respiratory alkalosis. The arterial pH is high and $PCO_2$ is low.
Acidosis and alkalosis are the processes. Acidemia and alkalemia are the end result of these processes. Acidosis induces acidemia and alkalosis induces alkalemia.
In the body, these processes of acidosis and alkalosis never stop and one should use the terms acidosis and alkalosis rather than acidemia and alkalemia.

### 3.3 Compensations

The body responds to acid and base disorder by changes to bring the pH towards normal value. In respiratory disorders, bicarbonate (HCO3) changes to compensate. In metabolic disorders, partial pressure of carbon dioxide (P $CO_2$) changes to compensate. It is worthy of note that compensation always occurs in the same direction as the primary disorder (Adrogue & Madias, 1998; Corey, 2005).

## 4. Acute and chronic

Respiratory acidosis and respiratory alkalosis are divided into two groups, acute and chronic, on the basis of their compensation. There are no plasma buffers for respiratory acidosis or alkalosis. The role of intracellular buffers and bone buffers is minor. The renal compensation takes about 3 to 5 days to complete.

Hence the acute phase continues for 3 to 5 days. Once full renal compensation is in place, the respiratory acidosis and respiratory alkalosis are called chronic.

On the other hand, metabolic acidosis and metabolic alkalosis are not divided into acute and chronic groups. However, sometimes the terms acute metabolic acidosis or alkalosis, and chronic metabolic acidosis or alkalosis are used. They indicate the time period, and not the compensatory response. In the metabolic disorders, the plasma buffers act immediately and respiratory compensation occurs quickly with in minutes to hours, so the acute phase, if any, is very brief (Schrier, 2003).

## 5. Diagnosis of acid base disorders

Evaluation of any acid-base disorder requires measurement of arterial blood gases (ABGs) and serum bicarbonate ($HCO^-_3$) concentration. The Henderson-Hasselbalch equation shows that the pH is determined by the ratio of $HCO^-_3$ concentration to $PCO_2$.

In metabolic acidosis, the primary event is a drop in the serum $HCO^-_3$ and P $CO_2$ drops as a secondary response. In respiratory alkalosis, the primary event is a drop in $PCO_2$ and bicarbonate drops as a secondary event. $PCO_2$ and $HCO^-_3$ both will be low in metabolic acidosis as well as in respiratory alkalosis. The pH will be low in metabolic acidosis and high in respiratory alkalosis (Boron, 2006; Corey, 2005; DuBose & Hamm, 1999; Kellum, 2007; Lowenstein, 1993).

Similarly, $PCO_2$ and $HCO^-_3$ will be high in metabolic alkalosis as well as in respiratory acidosis. The pH will be high in metabolic alkalosis and low in respiratory acidosis.

| Disorder | Primary Event | Secondary Event | pH |
|---|---|---|---|
| Metabolic Acidosis | $HCO^-_3$ Low | $PCO_2$ Low | Low |
| Metabolic Alkalosis | $HCO^-_3$ High | $PCO_2$ High | High |
| Respiratory Acidosis | $PCO_2$ High | $HCO^-_3$ High | Low |
| Respiratory Alkalosis | $PCO_2$ Low | $HCO^-_3$ Low | High |

Table 1. Compensation in Simple Acid Base Disorders (Direction of primary and secondary event is always same)

The second step in the diagnosis of acid base disorders is to evaluate the degree of compensation. Once the disorder is diagnosed, the degree of compensation should be assessed. The expected degree of compensation is predefined on the basis of studies and experiments done by the scientists (Table 2).

| Type of Disorder | Primary Change | Compensation Response | Expected pH |
|---|---|---|---|
| Metabolic Acidosis | Low $HCO^-_3$ | 1.2 mm Hg drop in $PCO_2$ for every 1 mEq/L drop in $HCO^-_3$ (1.2 : 1) OR $PCO_2 = 1.5\ HCO^-_3 + 8 \pm .2$ | Last 2 digits of $PCO_2$ |
| Metabolic Alkalosis | High $HCO^-_3$ | 0.7 mm Hg rise in $PCO_2$ for every 1 mEq/L rise in $HCO^-_3$ (0.7 : 1) | From Henderson-Hasselbalch equation |
| Acute Respiratory Acidosis | High $PCO_2$ | 1 mEq/L rise in $HCO^-_3$ for every 10 mm Hg rise in $PCO_2$ (1 : 10) | 0.08 drop in pH for every 10 mm Hg rise in $PCO_2$ |
| Chronic Respiratory Acidosis | High $PCO_2$ | 3.5 mEq/L rise in $HCO^-_3$ for every 10 mm Hg rise in $PCO_2$ (3.5 : 10) | 0.03 drop in pH for every 10 mm Hg rise in $PCO_2$ |
| Acute Respiratory Alkalosis | Low $PCO_2$ | 2 mEq/L drop in $HCO^-_3$ for every 10 mm Hg drop in $PCO_2$ (2 : 10) | 0.08 rise in pH for every 10 mm Hg drop in $PCO_2$ |
| Chronic Respiratory Alkalosis | Low $PCO_2$ | 4 mEq/L drop in $HCO_3$ for every 10-mm Hg drop in $PCO_2$ ( 4 : 10) | 0.03 rise in pH for every 10 mm Hg drop in $PCO_2$ |

Table 2. Expected Degree of Compensatory Responses

### 5.1 Metabolic acidosis

The diagnosis of a simple metabolic acidosis requires low serum bicarbonate and a low extracellular pH.

#### 5.1.1 Mechanism of acid production

The pathophsiology is better understood if we classify the metabolic acidosis on the basis of the mechanisms of acid production (Table 3).

**(1) Increased Acid (H+) Generation**

In these disorders, there is either an increased $H^+$ generation due to deranged metabolism in the body or by the increased administration of chemicals which are the source of $H^+$ ions. Examples of the first are lactic acidosis, keto acidosis and examples of the later are methanol poisoning, ethylene glycol poisoning, and salicylate poisoning.

**(2) Increased Loss of HCO-3**

In these disorders, the primary event is loss of $HCO^-_3$, which in turn leaves behind $H^+$ ions. Examples are diarrhea, ureteral diversion, and proximal renal tubular acidosis (RTA type 2).

**(3) Diminished Renal Acid (H+) Excretion**

In these disorders, there is decreased excretion of acid ($H^+$) from the kidneys. The kidneys are responsible for removing the daily non volatile acid load and to increase the $H^+$ excretion in case of metabolic acidosis. Obviously, when kidneys themselves are not competent, metabolic acidosis will occur. Examples of decreased acid ($H^+$) excretion are renal failure, distal renal tubular acidosis (RTA type 1), and RTA type 4.

| Increased Acid ( $H^+$) Generation |
| --- |
| Lactic acidosis<br>Ketoacidosis<br>Methanol Poisoning<br>Ehylene Glycol Poisoning<br>Salicylate Poisoning |
| **Increased Loss Of $HCO^-_3$** |
| Diarrhea<br>Ureteral diversion<br>Proximal renal tubular acidosis(Type 2) |
| **Diminished Renal Acid (H+) Excretion** |
| Renal failure<br>Distal renal tubular acidosis (type 1)<br>Renal tubular acidosis type 4 |

Table 3. Important Causes of Metabolic Acidosis (According to the Mechanism )

### 5.1.2 High and normal anion gap

Metabolic Acidosis may also be divided in two groups according to the serum anion gap.

1. High Serum Anion Gap Metabolic Acidosis
2. Normal Serum Anion Gap Metabolic Acidosis (Table 4)

The terms gap and non gap metabolic acidosis are used sometimes. There is always an anion gap, normal, high, low, or negative. The gap/no gap terminologies should be abandoned.

| Increased Anion Gap |
| --- |
| Advaned Renal Failure<br>Lactic acidosis<br>Ketoacidosis<br>Methanol Poisoning<br>Ehylene Glycol Poisoning<br>Salicylate Poisoning |
| **Normal Anion Gap** |
| Early Stages of Renal Failure<br>Renal Tubular Acidosis (all types)<br>Diarrhea<br>Ureteral diversion |

Table 4. Important Causes of Metabolic Acidosis (According to the Serum Anion Gap)

Serum Anion Gap (Serum AG) is the difference between the routinely measured cations i.e. sodium (Na) and sum of routinely measured anions i.e. chloride (Cl) and bicarbonate ($HCO^-_3$). It can be calculated from the following formula:

Serum AG = Routinely Measured Cations – Routinely Measured Anions

$$\text{Serum AG} = Na - (Cl + HCO^-_3)$$

Although, serum potassium (K) is also routinely measured but it is omitted from calculations. The reasons for omission of K from calculation are twofold. First, its serum concentration range is small, and second, if it is changed drastically, patient will succumb to its consequences before the change in the anion gap is considered.
The serum anion gap may also be written as following.

Serum AG = Unmeasured anions - Unmeasured cations

Unmeasured anions are albumin, lactate, sulfate, urate, phosphate, and other anions. Unmeasured cations are potassium, magnesium, calcium, and other cations. Serum AG will increase when there is a rise in the unmeasured anions or fall in the unmeasured cations.
The serum anion gap (AG) will not increase if the $H^+$ ion is accompanied by chloride. Serum AG will increase if acid $H^+$ accompanies an anion other than chloride.
The normal range of the serum AG is 10± 3 meq/L. Negatively charged serum albumin contributes most of the serum AG. One g/dL of serum albumin is equal to 2.5 meq/L of anion gap.
Examples of normal AG metabolic acidosis are diarrhea and RTA.
Examples of high AG metabolic acidosis are lactic acidosis, keto acidosis, renal failure, methanol poisoning, and ethylene glycol poisoning (Corey, 2005; Emmett & Narins, 1997; Fidkowski & Helstrom, 2009).

### 5.1.3 Delta anion gap/delta bicarbonate

The ratio of increase in serum Anion Gap to decrease in plasma bicarbonate is called Delta AG ($\Delta$ AG)/Delta $HCO^-_3$($\Delta$ $HCO^-_3$)) ratio, or just $\Delta/\Delta$ ratio. It is a useful tool in sorting out the cause of metabolic acidosis.
In case of high anion gap metabolic acidosis, the drop in $HCO^-_3$ should match the rise in the AG. In other words, the $\Delta/\Delta$ ratio should be 1:1. In lactic acidosis, AG increases more than the drop in serum $HCO^-_3$ and $\Delta/\Delta$ ratio may be as high as 1.6:1.
The reason for this discrepancy is buffering of the part of the $H^+$ by the intracellular and bone buffers. The part of the $H^+$ which is taken care by the intracellular and bone buffers does not lower the serum $HCO^-_3$ concentration. The accompanied anion (lactate) remains in the extracellular fluid and raises the AG.
In ketoacidosis, the $\Delta$ AG/$\Delta$ $HCO^-_3$ ratio is usually 1:1 due to partial excretion of ketones from the kidneys which balance out the intracellular and bone buffering. In mixed high anion gap and normal anion gap metabolic acidosis, the $\Delta$ AG/$\Delta$ $HCO^-_3$ ratio will be less than one (Fidkowski & Helstrom, 2009; Kellum, 2007; Rastegar, 2007).
In mixed metabolic alkadosis and metabolic acidosis, the $\Delta$ AG/$\Delta$ $HCO^-_3$ ratio will be more than 2. It this case, the drop in $HCO^-_3$ is much less than the rise in AG due to concomitant metabolic alkalosis.

In the following paragraphs urinary anion gap, urinary osmolar gap, and serum osmolar gap are explained. These are the commonly used investigations in solving the complicated acid base disorders.

### 5.1.4 Urinary anion gap

The urinary anion gap is the difference between major urinary cations (sodium and potassium) and major urinary anions (chloride). It is calculated as follows:

$$\text{Urinary Anion Gap} = (Na + K) - (Cl)$$

Urinary AG is an indirect measurement of urinary ammonium ($NH^+_4$) excretion. Negative value means chloride concentration of urine is higher than the sum of sodium and potassium. Negative urine AG is an appropriate response to metabolic acidosis. An increased $NH^+_4$ excretion results in enhanced acid removal from the kidney, for example, in diarrhea (DuBose TD Jr, et al. 1991; Oh & Carrol, 2002; Rose et al., 2001; Schoolwerth, 1991). Positive value means chloride concentration of urine is less than the sum of sodium and potassium. Positive urine anion gap indicates decreased $NH^+_4$ excretion, and decreased acid removal from the kidney, for example in renal tubular acidosis (Batlle et al., 1988).

### 5.1.5 Urinary osmolar gap

Just like urinary AG the urine osmolar gap (UAG) is a measure of urinary $NH^+_4$ excretion. An advantage of urine osmolar gap is that, it is not dependent on urinary chloride. It takes account of all the urinary anions accompanied with ammonium. It is calculated as follows:

$$\text{Urinary Osmolar Gap} = \text{Measured urine osmolality} - \text{Calculated urine osmolality}$$

$$\text{Calculated urine osmolality} = 2 \times (Na + K) + \frac{\text{Urine Urea Nitrogen}}{2.8} + \frac{\text{Urine Glucose}}{18}$$

In the above formula, 2 indicates the anions accompanying sodium and potassium. Na and K are in meq/L , Urea Nitrogen and glucose are in mg / dl. (Kamel et al., 1990).

### 5.1.6 Serum osmolar gap

It is the difference between measured serum osmolality and calculated serum osmolality. Measured serum osmolality includes all the serum osmoles. Calculted osmolality includes only some selected ones (Kamel et al., 1990).

Calculated Serum Osmolality=

$$2 \times Na + \frac{\text{Blood Urea Nitrogen mg/dl}}{2.8} + \frac{\text{Blood Glucose mg/dl}}{18}$$

In the above formulas, 2 indicates the anions accompanying sodium.

Normal serum osmolar gap is about 5 to 10. Examlpes of high osmolar gap metabolic acidosis are methanol and ethlylene glycol intoxication. There are conditions when serum osmolar gap is high with out acidosis, eg. mannitol infusion and ethanol ingestion (Lynd et al., 2008).

## 6. Stewart approach

Traditionally, the hydrogen ion concentration (pH) of blood is expressed as a function of the ratio of $PCO_2$ and serum $HCO^-_3$ based upon Henderson-Hasselbalch equation.
An alternative approach was proposed by Stewart, which is called Stewart's approach or strong ion difference (SID) approach.
The SID is the difference between the concentration of strong cations and concentration of strong anions in the plasma. Major strong cations are $Na^+$, $K^+$, $Ca^{++}$, $Mg^{++}$, and the major strong anions are $Cl^-$ and lactate$^-$.
According to SID approach, there are six primary acid-base disturbances. These are respiratory acidosis, respiratory alkalosis, strong ion acidosis, strong ion alkalosis, nonvolatile buffer ion acidosis, and nonvolatile buffer ion alkalosis.
Stewart proposed that the serum bicarbonate concentration is not independent and does not play an active role in the determination of the $H^+$ concentration. According to Stewart's theory of SID, the plasma concentrations of nonvolatile weak acids and PCO2 are independent variables. Nonvolatile total weak acids are phosphate and charges of albumin. The pH depends upon these three variables and not on HCO3/ $PCO_2$ ratio.
The SID method was presented by Stewart as an alternative to serum AG method for solving the acid-base problems. However, it did not get the popularity. Many physiologists believe that Stewart's method does not give any additional information if serum AG is corrected for serum albumin concentration (Fidkowski & Helstrom, 2009; Kellum et al., 1995).

## 7. Modified base excess method

Base excess is the amount of acid or base that must be added to the solution to bring the pH to 7.4 at $PCO_2$ of 40 mmHg and temperature of 37$^\circ$ C. Negative base excess means there is acidemia and positive base excess means there is alkalemia. The modified or sometimes called "standardized base excess method" is based upon Stewart's theory. It may be defined as the amount of strong acid or strong base required to bring the pH to 7.4 and $PCO_2$ to 40 mmHg (Fidkowski & Helstrom, 2009; Kraut & Madias, 2007; Rastegar, 2009).
Arterial Blood Gas machine gives a calculated base excess value. Any therapeutic decision can not be taken on this calculated value because of two reasons. First, it may give a false value of zero when metabolic acidosis and metabolic alkalosis coexist. Second, it is impossible to predict the PCO2 level and pH after correcting the base excess or deficit.
This standardized base excess method does not give any advantage over traditional Henderson-Hasselbalch equation based methods.
*In the following paragraphs important causes of metabolic acidosis are discussed.*

## 8. Chronic and acute renal failure

The new name for chronic renal failure is chronic kidney disease and the new name for acute renal failure is acute kidney injury. Metabolic acidosis in renal failure results from reduced number of functioning nephrons. The single nephron function is intact.
The initial stages of renal dysfunction give rise to normal anion gap and later stages give rise to high anion gap metabolic acidosis. The anions accompanying the acid are sulfate, phosphate and urates. In early stages of renal failure, these anions are excreted without problem; thus the anion gap remains normal.

In latter stages of renal failure, there is retention of these unmeasured anions and high anion gap metabolic acidosis develops (Kraut & Kurtz, 2005; Narins & Emmett, 1980).

## 9. Methanol and ethylene glycol intoxication

Methanol and ethylene glycol are ingested for pleasure as a substitute for ethanol , and also in the suicidal attempts, or taken accidently. Moonshine is a nick name of methanol when it is made illegally or locally using the radiators of the motor vehicles. Antifreeze solution contains high concentration of ethylene glycol (Lynd et al., 2008).

### 9.1 Methanol

Methanol is oxidized to formate by alcohol dehydrogenase and aldehyde dehydrogenase. Formate causes retinal injury with optic disc edema, blindness which may be permanent and basal ganglia injury.

High anion gap metabolic acidosis develops, due to accumulation of formate (formic acid). Serum AG is increased. (Kraut & Kurtz, 2008). Serum osmolar gap is increased.

### 9.2 Ethylene Glycol

Ethylene Glycol is metabolized to glycolate (glycolic acid), oxalate (oxalic acid), and glyoxylate by alcohol dehydrogenase and aldehyde dehydrogenase. Renal failure occurs due to renal tabular damage by glycolic acid and precipitation of oxalate crystals in the kidneys. High anion gap metabolic acidosis develops due to accumulation of glycolic acid and oxalic acid . Serum AG is increased. (Kraut & Kurtz, 2008). Serum osmolar gap is increased.

## 10. Lactic acidosis

Lactic acidosis is one of the most common causes of metabolic acidosis. Lactic acid is derived from the metabolism of pyruvic acid, which is generated from glucose and amino acids. Increased anaerobic metabolism lead to increased lactate production. The lactate produced in lactic acidosis is L-Lactate type, the accumulation of which gives rise to high anion gap.

The causes of lactic acidosis can be divided into type A, and type B. Type A lactic acidosis is associated with obviously impaired tissue oxygenation, for example, in shock, sepsis, hypovolemia, and cardiac failure.

In type B lactic acidosis, the impairment in oxygenation is not apparent. There is mitochondrial dysfunction due to toxins and drugs like metformin and nucleoside reverse transcriptase inhibitors (NRTIs).

### 10.1 D-lactic acidosis

D-lactate is produced in the colon from metabolism of starch and glucose by the gram-positive anaerobes. In the setting of short bowel syndrome and malignancy, over production of D-lactate with severe metabolic acidosis may occur. Diagnosis may be difficult because the usual assays used in laboratories detect only L-lactate.

## 11. Ketoacidosis

Ketoacids are derived from metabolism of fatty acids in the liver. Normal metabolism of fatty acids give rise to formation of triglycerides, $CO_2$, water, and ketoacids. However in the absence of insulin, ketoacids are produced out of proportion and cause acidosis.

Ketoacids are; (1) β-Hydroxy butyric acid, and (2) Acetoacetic acid. Acetone is often grouped with Ketoacids but it is not an acid.
Uncontrolled Diabetes Mellitus is the most common cause of Ketoacidosis. Starvation and excessive alcohol intake may also give rise to mild to moderate ketoacidosis. Diagnosis of Ketoacidosis requires documentation of Ketones in the blood or urine (Arieff & Carroll, 1972).

## 12. Dilutional metabolic acidosis

It is due to a fall in the serum bicarbonate concentration secondary to extracellular volume expansion by non bicarbonate fluid. Massive amounts of normal saline infusion may produce dilutional acidosis. It is not a clinically significant entity and only of academic interest

## 13. Salicylate poisoning

Aspirin (acetyl salicylic acid) poisoning results in mixed respiratory alkalosis and metabolic acidosis. Metabolic acidosis is due to accumulation of salicylic acid as well as lactic acid and ketoacids. Liver plays an important role in the detoxification of salicylate. In case of overdose, this system of detoxification saturates and results in deposition of salicylates in the tissues including brain.

## 14. Renal Tubular Acidosis (RTA)

There are 3 types of RTA:
Distal RTA (type 1)
Proximal RTA (type 2)
Hyporenin hypoaldosteronism (RTA type 4)
There is a Type 3 RTA also which is a rare autosomal recessive disorder due to carbonic anhydrase II deficiency and has features of both distal and proximal RTA (Table 5).

| | **Type I Distal RTA** | **Type II Proximal RTA** | **Type IV RTA** |
|---|---|---|---|
| Primary defect | Decreased distal acidification | Decreased proximal $HCO_3^-$ reabsorption | Aldosterone deficiency Rennin deficiency |
| Urine pH | > 5.3 | Variable | Usually < 5.3 |
| Plasma $HCO_3^-$ meq/L | Usually < 10 | Usually 15-20 | Usually > 15 |
| Fractional excretion of $HCO_3^-$ | < 3% | 15 to 20 % | < 3 % |
| Other abnormalities | Nephrocalcinosis, nephrolithiasis | Osteomalacia | Common in diabetics |
| Plasma Potassium | Usually low | Usually low | High |

Table 5. Comparison of Renal Tubular Acidosis

### 14.1 Distal RTA (type 1)

In distal RTA, the main problem is impaired secretion of acid ($H^+$) from the intercalated cells of the collecting tubules. Collecting tubules has two types of cells (1) principal cells, which are responsible for sodium and potassium balance, and (2) intercalated cells which are responsible for ($H^+$) secretion and maintenance of acid base balance.
As a result of decreased $H^+$ secretion, there is decreased ammonium ($NH^+_4$) and decreased titratable acid excretion. Titratable acid means the acid removed by phosphate buffer system of urine. Anion Gap is normal because of retention of chloride along with $H^+$ ions.
Nephrocalcinosis and nephrolithiasis are known complication of RTA type 1. High urine pH facilitates calcium phosphate precipitation and stone formation in the renal tubules and urinary collecting system (Batlle et al., 2006; Karet, 2009; Rodríguez, 2002).

### 14.2 Proximal RTA (type 2)

In RTA type 2, the proximal bicarbonate ($HCO^-_3$) reabsorption threshold is reduced and this results in the loss of filtered $HCO^-_3$. Once a new steady state is achieved with low serum $HCO^-_3$ the loss of bicarbonates ceases. Urine pH is initially high due to bicarbnonaturia and later may drop to less than 5.3 in untreated persons.

### 14.3 Type 4 RTA

In type 4 RTA, the primary defect is decreased potassium (K) secretion from the distal nephron, mainly collecting tubules due to aldosterone deficiency or resistance. The decreased $H^+$ secretion and subsequent metabolic acidosis is secondary to defective K secretion. Most common cause of Type 4 RTA is hyporenin hypoaldosteronism syndrome. A decreased K secretion results in hyperkalemia and its treatment improves metabolic acidosis (Rodríguez, 2002).

## 15. Metabolic alkalosis

There are two stages of metabolic alkalosis:
(1) Generation of alkalosis, and (2) Maintenance of alkalosis
The kidneys are very efficient in correcting the metabolic alkalosis by excreting out the extra bicarbonate. Only generation of alkalosis is not sufficient to produce alkalemia. There must be some other factors present to maintain the alkalosis. Hypovolemia and hypochloremia are the most important etiologies responsible for maintenance of alkalosis (Table 6 and 7) (Khanna & Kurtzman, 2006).

### 15.1 Urine chloride

Measurement of urine chloride concentration is a key test used in solving the differential diagnosis of metabolic alkalosis. It differentiates between hypovolemic and euvolemic states. In metabolic alkalosis, urine chloride is more reliable indicator of volume status as compared to urine sodium. Urine sodium may be high in spite of hypovolemia in metabolic alkalosis. It is due to the obligatory loss of sodium along with bicarbonate spill over.
Based upon urine chloride concentration, the causes of metabolic alkalosis may be divided in two groups (Table 8).

### 15.2 Saline responsiveness

Metabolic alkalosis may also be classified according to the response to saline administration. Urine chloride will be low in saline responsive alkalosis. Urine chloride may be high or low in saline resistant alkalosis.

| |
|---|
| **Renal Loss of Acid ( $H^+$)** |
| Diuretics |
| Hypermineralcoricoidosis |
| Post Hypercapnia |
| **Gastriointestinal Loss of Acid ($H^+$ )** |
| Vomiting |
| Nasogastric Suction |
| Chloride Loosing Diarrhea |
| **Addition of Bicarbonate** |
| Administration of Sodium Bicarbonate |
| Blood transfusion |
| Milk Alkali Syndrome |
| **Trans cellular Shift** |
| Hypokalemia |
| **Excessive Hypotonic Fluid Loss** |
| Contraction Alkalosis |

Table 6. Important Causes of Metabolic Alkalosis (According to the mechanism)

| **Factors Responsible for Maintenance of Metabolic Alkalosis** |
|---|
| Volume Depletion |
| Effective Circulatory Volume Depletion |
| Chloride Depletion |
| Hyperaldosteronism |
| Hypokalemia |

Table 7. Factors Responsible for Maintenance of Metabolic Alkalosis.

| **Causes of Metabolic Alkalosis** (According to Urine Chloride Concentration) | |
|---|---|
| Urine Chloride Concentration | |
| **Less Than 20 meq/L** | **More than 40 meq/L** |
| Hypovolumia | Diuretics |
| Vomiting | Hyperaldosteronism |
| Nasogastric Suction | Bicarbonate Administration |
| Posthypercapnia | Bartter's Syndrome |
| | Gitelman's Syndrome |

Table 8. Causes of Metabolic Alkalosis

### 15.3 Saline responsive

In these conditions, correction of hypovolemia will result in increased delivery of chloride and sodium to the distal nephron which will result in increased sodium bicarbonate excretion. Examples: Vomiting, Nasogastric Suction, Diuretics, Posthypercapnia.

### 15.4 Saline resistant

In these conditions, the specific treatment of underlying cause is required to correct the alkalosis. Edematous states may respond to saline but may develop pulmonary edema and worsening of peripheral edema.
Examples: Congestive heart failure, Cirrhosis, Mineralocorticoid excess, Hypokalemia and Renal Failure.
*Pathophysiology of the important causes of metabolic alkalosis is discussed below.*

### 15.5 Gastrointestinal losses

The secretion of bicarbonate from the pancreas depends upon stimuli by the acid coming from stomach to the duodenum. Vomiting or nasogastric tube drainage prevents the acid from reaching the duodenum resulting in the decreased secretion of bicarbonate. The hdrochloric acid (HCl) loss and retention of bicarbonate results in metabolic alkalosis.

### 15.6 Diuretics

The loop diuretics are the common cause of metabolic alkalosis. They produce alkalosis by volume contraction, increased urinary $H^+$ loss and hypokalemia.

### 15.7 Hyperaldosteronism

Primary and secondary mineralocorticoid excess results in metabolic alkalosis. It is primarily due to increased acid secretion from the distal nephron.

### 15.8 Post hypercapnic alkalosis

Rapid lowering of the blood carbon dioxide ($CO_2$) in chronic $CO_2$ retainers will cause post hypercapnic metabolic alkalosis. Chronic retention of $CO_2$ stimulates renal HCO3 retention to compensate for respiratory acidosis. Once $CO_2$ content of the blood is reduced quickly, for example, by ventilator, the compensated $HCO_3$ component is unmasked resulting in metabolic alkalosis.

### 15.9 Milk alkali syndrome

Excessive intake of calcium salts, for example calcium carbonate, may result in metabolic alkalosis, especially in renal failure. Carbonate is converted to $HCO_3$ in the body and calcium decreases $HCO_3$ excretion from the kidneys. It is called milk alkali syndrome because of its association with milk intake which contains large amounts of calcium.

### 15.10 Hypokalemia

Decreased plasma potassium ($K^+$) level causes shift of $K^+$ from intracellular to extra cellular fluid, in an attempt to correct hypokalemia. To keep the electrical neutrality, $H^+$ shifts from outside to the inside of the cells. This loss of $H^+$ from extracellular fluid results in metabolic alkalosis.
It is interesting to note that metabolic alkalosis itself perpetuates hypokalemia. In metabolic alkalosis of any cause, transcellular shift of $H^+$ and $K^+$ takes place. $H^+$ ions move out of the cells to correct alkalosis and $K^+$ moves inside the cells producing hypokalemia.

### 15.11 Bicarbonate administration

As mentioned above, in euvolemic persons with normal renal function, it is impossible to produce alkalosis due to rapid renal excretion of any administered $HCO_3$. However, in hypovolemia or in renal failure, administration of bicarbonates results in metabolic alkalosis simply due to inability of the kidneys to excrete the extra bicarbonates.

### 15.12 Multiple blood transfusions

Massive blood transfusion occasionally results in metabolic alkalosis. Citrate which is used as an anticoagulant in blood is converted to bicarbonate in the liver resulting in metabolic alkalosis.

### 15.13 Contraction alkalosis

Loss of water around a fixed amount of $HCO^-_3$ results in increased concentration of $HCO^-_3$ and metabolic alkalosis. The increased pure water loss and hypotonic fluid loss by loop diuretics, excessive sweating and congenital chloride diarrhea are examples of conditions associated with contraction alkalosis.

### 15.14 Bartter's syndrome and Gitelman's syndrome

These are the autosomal recessive disorders characterized by hypokalemia and metabolic alkalosis.

In Bartter's syndrome, there is a defect in the sodium chloride transport in the thick ascending limb of the loop of Henle at the site of action of loop diuretics. The characteristic abnormalities include hypokalemia, metabolic alkalosis and increased urinary calcium excretion.

In Gitelman's syndrome, there is a defect in the sodium chloride transport in the distal tubule which is the site of action of thiazide diuretics. The characteristic abnormalities include hypokalemia, metabolic alkalosis, decreased urinary calcium excretion, and hypomagnesaemia.

## 16. Respiratory acidosis and alkalosis

### 16.1 Respiratory acidosis

The primary event in respiratory acidosis is retention of $CO_2$. Metabolism of carbohydrates and fats results in the production of $CO_2$ which combines with H2O to form $H_2\ HCO^-_3$. It then dissociate into acid ( $H^+$) and bicarbonate ($HCO^-_3$).

$$CO_2 x\ 0.03 + H2O \ <-> \ H_2\ HCO^-_3 \ <-> HCO^-_3 + H^+$$

Kidneys compensate to respiratory acidosis by increasing acid ($H^+$) excretion.

Lungs through alveolar ventilation remove $CO_2$. In the absence of ventilation, $CO_2$ will accumulate in the body and will result in severe acidosis (rise of free $H^+$ ions and drop of pH). This type of acidosis is called respiratory acidosis (Arieff & Carroll, 1972).

According to the Henderson-Hasselbalch equation, pH depends upon the ratio of bicarbonate and $PCO_2$.

$$\left(H^+\right) = 24 x\ \frac{PCO_2}{HCO^-_3}$$

$$pH = 6.10 + \log \frac{HCO^-_3}{0.03\ P\ CO_2}$$

The partial pressure of $CO_2$ ($PCO_2$) in the arterial blood is in equilibrium with that in the alveolar air. Normal arterial PCO2 is approximately 40 mmHg. CO2 is not an acid. It increases the acidity of the solution through the formation of $H_2CO_3$. Increased $PCO_2$ will increases the $H_2CO3$ concentration. It then dissociates into the acid ($H^+$) and bicarbonate ($HCO^-_3$).
In contrast to metabolic acidosis, bicarbonate ($HCO^-_3$) does not act as a buffer in respiratory acidosis. It is part of the problem, not part of the solution. Sodium bicarbonate administration in respiratory acidosis is not beneficial, rather may be harmful. Administration of bicarbonate will result in an initial transient rise in pH due to the left shift. Then, $H_2CO_3$ will immediately dissociate and the net result will be higher $PCO_2$, higher $HCO^-_3$, higher $H^+$, and lower pH.
Intracellular buffers mostly hemoglobin (Hgb) bind free $H^+$ and form $H^+$-Hgb which is carried to lungs by the blood circulation. In the lungs, $H^+$ is released form Hgb and combines with available $HCO^-_3$ to form $CO_2$, which is exhaled by lungs to the atmosphere.
Increasing ventilation is the only treatment of respiratory acidosis. Renal response to increased $H^+$ excretion takes about 3 to 5 days to complete. At this stage, the respiratory acidosis is termed chronic. The $PCO_2/HCO^-_3$ ratio improves to settle pH at a higher level than it was in acute phase. This renal compensation is always suboptimal. If the pH is 7.4 or above, it means that there is a concomitant component of metabolic alkalosis.
The degree of compensation and expected pH after compensation are predefined (Table 2).

### 16.1.1 Causes of respiratory acidosis

The cause of respiratory acidosis is only one, that is, decreased ventilation. Several conditions can lead to decreased ventilation and respiratory acidosis. Causes of decreased ventilation may be divided into three groups. Important ones are listed here:
Central: Norcotics, Sedatives, Anaesthesia,
Peripheral: Neuropathies, Muscle weakness, Myopathies
Pulmonary and Airway Pathology: Pneumnia, Pneumothorax,Sleep apnea, and Emphysema.

### 16.2 Respiratory alkalosis

The primary event in respiratory alkalosis is decreased $PCO_2$. According to the Henderson-Hasselbalch equation, pH depends upon the ratio of bicarbonate and $PCO_2$ as mentioned above. Lower the $PCO_2$, the higher the pH and vice versa.
Extracellular buffers are not efficient in respiratory alkalosis. Intracellular buffers e.g. protein, phosphate and Hgb act to release intracellular $H^+$ in an attempt to correct the alkalosis. This response also is not very efficient. Renal response of decreasing $H^+$ secretion takes 3 to 5 days to complete. At this stage, it is called chronic respiratory alkalosis.

### 16.2.1 Causes of respiratory alkalosis

Like respiratory acidosis, the cause of respiratory alkalosis is only one, that is, increased ventilation. Important causes of increased ventilation are listed here:
Hypoxemia, Sepsis, Salicylate intoxication, Pregnancy, stroke, Liver Failure, Psychological Causes, Artificial by ventilator (Kaplan & Frangos, 2005).

## 17. Conclusion

Primary acid base disorders are metabolic acidosis, metabolic alkalosis, respiratory acidosis, and respiratory alkalosis. In practice, patients often present with mixed and complex acid